KAPLAN & STUDY GUIDE AND SELF-EXAMINATION REVIEW IN PSYCHIATRY

TENTH EDITION

KAPLAN & SADOCK'S
STUDY GUIDE AND SELF-EXAMINATION
REVIEW IN PSYCHIATRY

TENTH EDITION

ERIC R. WILLIAMS, M.D.
Associate Dean for Student Affairs
Clinical Associate Professor
Neuropsychiatry & Behavioral Science
University of South Carolina
School of Medicine Columbia
Columbia, South Carolina

LINDSAY MOSKOWITZ, M.D., L.L.C.
Private Practice
Tarrytown, New York
Psychiatric Director of Residential Program
  at Backcountry Wellness
Greenwich, Connecticut
Staff Psychiatrist Clementine, Monte Nido
Briarcliff Manor, New York

SERIES EDITORS

ROBERT BOLAND, M.D.
Senior Vice President and Chief of Staff,
  The Menninger Clinic
Professor and Vice Chair, Menninger
  Department of Psychiatry and
  Behavioral Sciences
The Brown Foundation Endowed Chair in
  Psychiatry
Baylor College of Medicine
Houston, Texas

MARCIA L. VERDUIN, M.D.
Associate Dean for Students
Professor of Psychiatry
Departments of Medical Education and
  Clinical Sciences
University of Central Florida College of
  Medicine
Orlando, Florida

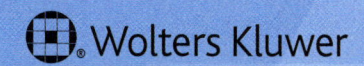

Wolters Kluwer

Philadelphia · Baltimore · New York · London
Buenos Aires · Hong Kong · Sydney · Tokyo

Acquisitions Editor: Chris Teja
Development Editor: Ariel S. Winter
Editorial Coordinator: Sean Hanrahan
Editorial Assistant: Kristen Kardoley
Marketing Manager: Kirsten Watrud
Production Project Manager: Matt West
Manager, Graphic Arts & Design: Stephen Druding
Manufacturing Coordinator: Beth Welsh
Prepress Vendor: Aptara, Inc.

10th edition

Copyright © 2024 Wolters Kluwer.

© 2011 by LIPPINCOTT WILLIAMS & WILKINS, a WOLTERS KLUWER business
© 2007, 2003 by LIPPINCOTT WILLIAMS & WILKINS
Two Commerce Square
2001 Market Street
Philadelphia, PA 19103 USA
LWW.com

All rights reserved. This book is protected by copyright. No part of this book may be reproduced or transmitted in any form or by any means, including as photocopies or scanned-in or other electronic copies, or utilized by any information storage and retrieval system without written permission from the copyright owner, except for brief quotations embodied in critical articles and reviews. Materials appearing in this book prepared by individuals as part of their official duties as U.S. government employees are not covered by the above-mentioned copyright. To request permission, please contact Wolters Kluwer at Two Commerce Square, 2001 Market Street, Philadelphia, PA 19103, via email at permissions@lww.com, or via our website at shop.lww.com (products and services).

9 8 7 6 5 4 3 2 1

Printed in Singapore

Library of Congress Cataloging-in-Publication Data available upon request.

978-1-9751-9911-1

This work is provided "as is," and the publisher disclaims any and all warranties, express or implied, including any warranties as to accuracy, comprehensiveness, or currency of the content of this work.

This work is no substitute for individual patient assessment based upon healthcare professionals' examination of each patient and consideration of, among other things, age, weight, gender, current or prior medical conditions, medication history, laboratory data and other factors unique to the patient. The publisher does not provide medical advice or guidance and this work is merely a reference tool. Healthcare professionals, and not the publisher, are solely responsible for the use of this work including all medical judgments and for any resulting diagnosis and treatments.

Given continuous, rapid advances in medical science and health information, independent professional verification of medical diagnoses, indications, appropriate pharmaceutical selections and dosages, and treatment options should be made and healthcare professionals should consult a variety of sources. When prescribing medication, healthcare professionals are advised to consult the product information sheet (the manufacturer's package insert) accompanying each drug to verify, among other things, conditions of use, warnings and side effects and identify any changes in dosage schedule or contraindications, particularly if the medication to be administered is new, infrequently used or has a narrow therapeutic range. To the maximum extent permitted under applicable law, no responsibility is assumed by the publisher for any injury and/or damage to persons or property, as a matter of products liability, negligence law or otherwise, or from any reference to or use by any person of this work.

shop.lww.com

Preface

Now in its 10th edition, *Kaplan and Sadock's Study Guide and Self-Examination Review in Psychiatry* again stands alone as a separate book from the *Synopsis* and *Comprehensive* in the Kaplan series. However, this book is best used in conjunction with the 12th edition of the *Synopsis of Psychiatry*, as the chapters align and the source material for the questions is the *Synopsis*. Answer explanations cover the rationale of the correct and incorrect choices and also provide a corresponding page number in the *Synopsis* where the test-taker can read more about the subject matter.

The questions are all written in a multiple-choice, one-best-answer format, and cover etiology, diagnosis, and treatment of psychiatric disorders across the DSM-5-TR. In addition, topics such as history taking, ethics, forensics issues, community psychiatry, normal development and aging, neurosciences and behavioral sciences are also included.

This book was written to meet the needs of medical students, residents, practicing physicians, and mental health professionals from all fields. It is designed to help those preparing for the United States Medical Licensing Examination (USMLE), Psychiatry Resident In-Training Examination (PRITE), and the American Board of Psychiatry and Neurology (ABPN) licensing and maintenance-of-certification exams. The authors have experience in writing for each of those examinations, as well as for the Focus Self-Assessment exam and *Journal of the American Academy of Child and Adolescent Psychiatry* CME articles. Completing the questions in this book serves as a valuable way to test knowledge in psychiatry as part of the continuing medical education process.

All 600 questions in this edition are completely new. Question stems are a mixture of USMLE-style vignettes and more direct ABPN and PRITE formats. New to the *Study Guide* are twenty video interviews with five additional corresponding questions per video.

COMPREHENSIVE TEACHING SYSTEM

Study Guide forms one part of a comprehensive system developed by the founding editors of the Kaplan and Sadock series to facilitate the teaching of psychiatry and the behavioral sciences. At the head of the system is the *Comprehensive Textbook of Psychiatry*, which is global in depth and scope; it is designed for and used by psychiatrists, behavioral scientists, and all other workers in the mental health field. *Kaplan & Sadock's Synopsis of Psychiatry* is a relatively brief, highly modified, original, and current version useful for medical students, psychiatric residents, practicing psychiatrists, and other mental health professionals. A special edition of *Synopsis*, the *Concise Textbook of Clinical Psychiatry* covers just the diagnosis and treatment of all psychiatric disorders. Other parts of the system are the pocket handbooks: *Pocket Handbook of Clinical Psychiatry* and *Pocket Handbook of Psychiatric Drug Treatment*. These books cover the diagnosis and the treatment of mental disorders, and psychopharmacology, respectively, and are compactly designed and concisely written to be carried in the pocket by clinical clerks and practicing physicians of all specialties to provide a quick reference. Together, these books create a multi-pronged approach to teaching, studying, and learning psychiatry.

HOW TO USE THIS BOOK

To use this book most effectively in preparation for a standardized exam, the test-taker should allot between 60 and 90 seconds per question. A test-taker who knows the material well should be able to cover up the answer choices and generate the correct response to the question themselves. The answers should be verified by referring to the corresponding answer section in each chapter, paying particular attention to the discussion of the wrong answers. If further information is needed, the reader is referred to the relevant pages of the 12th edition of the *Synopsis of Psychiatry*. For those new to the material, it may be most helpful to start with the *Synopsis*, then do the questions in the *Study Guide* for that chapter. After all questions in the book have been completed, watch the videos and complete those questions, as they are not linked to a specific chapter.

ACKNOWLEDGMENTS

The authors wish to thank Drs. Bob Boland and Marcy Verduin for trusting us to write this companion guide to the *Synopsis*, which they edited. They have served as friends and mentors dating back to when we were all on the PRITE Editorial Board, and later the Focus Editorial Board.

We also thank the Wolters Kluwer editorial team, who did not give us too much of a side eye when we asked for an extension of the deliverables: Chris Teja (Acquisitions Editor), Ariel S. Winter (Development Editor), and Sean Hanrahan (Editorial Coordinator). We also thank Matt Rubin of Symptom Media for production of the video content.

Thank you to my partner Ara for proofreading and making suggestions to my questions, and for putting up with 3 years of talk about "The Book."—Eric

Many thanks to my family for their love and support, and especially my three little ones—Belle, Ryder, and Chance—who are looking forward to hearing their new favorite bedtime story. A special thank you to Eric for getting me involved in question writing and this book!—Lindsay

Contents

A. CLINICAL PSYCHIATRY

1. Examination and Diagnosis of the Psychiatric Patient............. 3
2. Neurodevelopmental Disorders and Other Childhood Disorders.......... 14
3. Neurocognitive Disorders........... 27
4. Substance Use and Addictive Disorders...................... 35
5. Schizophrenia Spectrum and Other Psychotic Disorders........... 44
6. Bipolar Disorders 51
7. Depressive Disorder 54
8. Anxiety Disorders................. 59
9. Obsessive-Compulsive and Related Disorders 62
10. Trauma- and Stressor-Related Disorders...................... 65
11. Dissociative Disorders.............. 68
12. Somatic Symptom and Related Disorders...................... 72
13. Feeding and Eating Disorders........ 77
14. Elimination Disorders.............. 83
15. Sleep–Wake Disorders 87

16. Human Sexuality and Sexual Dysfunctions..................... 92
17. Gender Dysphoria, Gender Identity, and Related Conditions............. 97
18. Disruptive, Impulse Control, and Conduct Disorders................. 99
19. Personality Disorders 102
20. Other Conditions that May Be a Focus of Clinical Attention........ 108

B. TREATMENT ACROSS THE LIFESPAN

21. Psychopharmacology 115
22. Other Somatic Therapies........... 139
23. Psychotherapy................... 144
24. Psychiatric Rehabilitation and Other Interventions 151
25. Consult to Other Disciplines........ 154
26. Level of Care.................... 161

C. OTHER ISSUES RELEVANT TO PSYCHIATRY

27. Ethics and Professionalism 165
28. Forensic and Legal Issues 170
29. End-of-Life Issues and Palliative Care................... 176

30. Community Psychiatry 180

31. Global and Cultural Issues
    in Psychiatry 183

D. CONTRIBUTIONS FROM THE SCIENCES AND SOCIAL SCIENCES TO PSYCHIATRY

32. Normal Development and Aging..... 187

33. Contributions from the
    Neurosciences 193

34. Contributions from the Behavioral
    and Social Sciences............... 203

Index   215

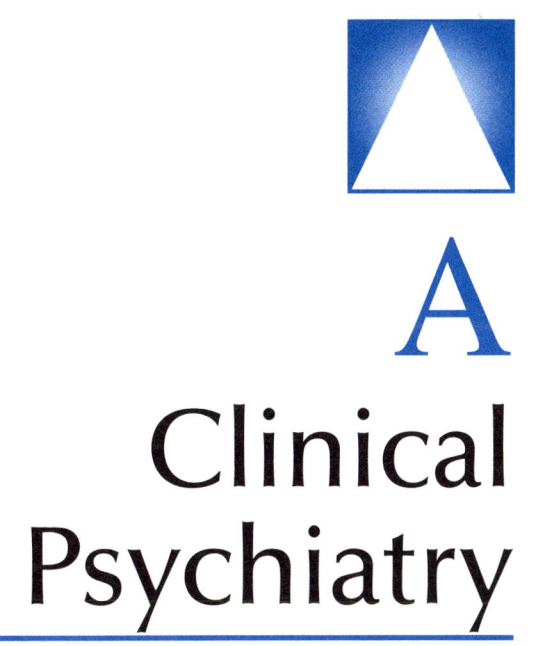

A
Clinical Psychiatry

1

Examination and Diagnosis of the Psychiatric Patient

1.1. Which of the following first steps is most appropriate in conducting a psychiatric interview of a patient?

A. Obtain consent from the patient
B. Offer to meet with family and patient together
C. Identify elements of the process the patient wishes to alter
D. Perform a safety assessment
E. Review HIPAA laws and limits of confidentiality

1.2. Which of the following elements differentiates empathy from identification?

A. Ability to maintain objectivity
B. Association with poor boundaries
C. Being able to experience the emotion
D. High association with physician burnout
E. True understanding of the situation

1.3. A person-centered approach, as opposed to a traditional medial one, focuses on which of the following aspects during an interview?

A. Deficits
B. Illness
C. Safety
D. Strengths
E. Transference

1.4. Which question is a part of the the Rapid Alcohol Problem Screen 4 (RAPS4) screening tool for substance use?

A. Have you ever been arrested for your drinking?
B. Have people annoyed you by criticizing your drinking?
C. Have you ever cut down on your drinking?
D. Have you ever driven drunk?
E. Have you ever failed to remember things after drinking?

1.5. Which of the following medical conditions can resemble an anxiety disorder?

A. Arthritis
B. Hyperthyroidism
C. Lupus
D. Malnutrition
E. Transient ischemic attacks

1.6. A family history of which illness might affect the choice of an antipsychotic medication?

A. Diabetes
B. Cancer
C. Hyperkalemia
D. Hypothyroidism
E. Kidney stones

1.7. An increase in amount of speech noted on mental status examination can be a sign of which of the following psychiatric symptoms?

A. Depression
B. Disinterest
C. Mania
D. Paranoia
E. Thought blocking

1.8. A patient with manic symptoms replies in this manner when asked what he did yesterday- "I hiked and biked with Mike and Mat and ate rat that sat cat." This is an example of which of the following types of thought processes?

A. Clang association
B. Neologism
C. Perseveration
D. Tangentiality
E. Thought blocking

1.9. Asking a patient a hypothetical example of what they would do upon finding a stamped envelope on the street can help test for which of the following cognitive functions?

A. Abstract reasoning
B. Impulse control
C. Fund of knowledge
D. Insight
E. Judgment

1.10. Using empathy to convey understanding and noting the patient's strengths, along with exploring their ambivalence and conflicts about change is a part of which of the following techniques?

A. Acknowledgment of emotions
B. Minimizing patients' concerns
C. Motivational interviewing
D. Premature interpretation
E. Summarizing

1.11. Which of the following elements would constitute a passive suicidal statement?

A. Being able to state many reasons to live
B. Denial of intent to act on the thoughts
C. Lack of having a plan
D. Not possessing the means to do it
E. Not taking preparatory steps toward the plan

1.12. A patient presenting with anxiety has a mental status examination notable for a tremor and pallor. Vital signs are significant for an elevated heart rate. Which of the following medical conditions should be ruled out?

A. Hypothyroidism
B. Normal pressure hydrocephalus
C. Pheochromocytoma
D. Temporal arteritis
E. Ulcerative colitis

1.13. What is an element that is included in a psychotherapy note, but not a progress note?

A. A detailed assessment and plan
B. Comments on countertransference and dreams
C. Data that can be disclosed to the patient
D. Inclusion with the rest of the medical record
E. Information about third-party payer access

1.14. Reliability data on the Structured Clinical Interview for the DSM (SCID) suggests that it performs better on more severe disorders for which of the following diagnoses?

A. Alcohol abuse
B. Bipolar disorder
C. Dysthymia
D. Social phobia
E. Unspecified eating disorder

1.15. What rating scale was designed to assess change in psychotic inpatients with significant impairment, and cover a broad range of symptoms of depression and anxiety, with flaws including needing a large amount of clinical training to achieve good reliability?

A. Brief Psychiatric Rating Scale (BPRS)
B. Hamilton Anxiety Rating Scale (HAM-A)
C. Positive and Negative Syndrome Scale (PANSS)
D. Scale for the Assessment of Positive Symptoms (SAPS)
E. Structured Clinical Interview for DSM (SCID)

1.16. The Child Behavior Checklist (CBCL) is unable to assess which of the following elements?

A. A clinical diagnosis
B. Cutoff scores for problems
C. Parent ratings
D. Symptoms within a clinical range
E. Teacher ratings

1.17. The Connors Rating Scale is most commonly used in the assessment of which psychiatric disorder?

A. Attention deficit hyperactivity
B. Bipolar
C. Major depressive
D. Obsessive compulsive
E. Substance use

1.18. Finger agnosia, dyscalculia, dysgraphia, and right–left disorientation are components of which of the following syndromes?

A. Dressing apraxia
B. Gerstmann
C. Hurler
D. Neglect
E. Pickwickian

1.19. Impairment in which of the following features is unique to Broca aphasia as opposed to other types of aphasias?

A. Awareness of deficit
B. Breakdown of syntactic structure
C. Comprehension
D. Fluency
E. Repetition

1.20. A patient is unable to bisect a line placed midline. This is most commonly indicative of a lesion in which of the following areas of the brain?

A. Cerebellum
B. Medulla
C. Parietal
D. Pons
E. Temporal

1.21. For older individuals, the technique of having them draw a clock is a sensitive measure of which of the following neuropsychological functions?

A. Attention and concentration
B. Planning and organization
C. Remote and recent memory
D. Sensory and motor
E. Speech and language

1.22. A high level of which of the following types of validity would be shown if a test measuring hypochondria demonstrates the patient with high scores had more doctor's visits due to symptoms of physical complaints?

A. Criterion validity
B. Discriminant
C. Face validity
D. Factor
E. Predictive validity

1.23. Which type of neuroimaging measures blood flow by using heme molecules as an endogenous contrast agent?

A. fMRI (functional magnetic resonance imaging)
B. MRA (magnetic resonance angiography)
C. MRS (magnetic resonance spectroscopy)
D. PET (positron emission tomography)
E. SPECT (single-photon emission computed tomography)

1.24. A young adult with chronic substance use has an MRI of the brain which is significant for loss of gray-white matter and atrophy. Mental status examination demonstrates abnormalities in short-term memory, "scanning" speech, and a notable tremor. Which of the following substances is most likely being abused?

A. Alcohol
B. Amphetamines
C. Cannabis
D. MDMA (ecstasy)
E. Toluene

1.25. A patient recently started on valproate seems confused and lethargic. Which of the following blood levels should be checked urgently?

A. Ammonia
B. BUN
C. Platelets
D. Sodium
E. WBC

1.26. Which of the following blood tests should be obtained at the initiation of treatment with an MAOI (monoamine oxidase inhibitor) and periodically after?

A. Basal metabolic panel
B. Complete blood count
C. Lipid panel
D. Liver function tests (LFTs)
E. Renal function panel

1.27. Which vitamin or mineral level should be tested as part of a standard workup for dementia?

A. Magnesium
B. Vitamin B12
C. Vitamin C
D. Vitamin D
E. Zinc

1.28. Which of the following lab or vital sign abnormalities might also contribute to prolongation of the QTc interval in a patient on antipsychotic medications?

A. Hyperkalemia
B. Hypertension
C. Hypomagnesemia
D. Hyponatremia
E. Tachycardia

1.29. Oral ziprasidone is contraindicated in patients with a history of which of the following medical conditions?

A. A recent myocardial infarction
B. Hypoglycemia
C. Hyperprolactinemia
D. Leukocytosis
E. Renal failure

1.30. Which is the only abnormality of the brain that is better seen on CT scans as compared to MRIs?

A. Atrophy
B. Calcifications
C. Inflammation
D. Strokes
E. Tumors

1.31. When using developmental tests on older infants and preschoolers, which of the following areas should be the main focus?

A. Language
B. Motor
C. Perceptual
D. Sensory
E. Social

1.32. Which test measures communication, daily living skills, socialization, and motor domains for typical children and adolescents as well as those who are visual or hearing, emotionally, or intellectually impaired?

A. Behavior Assessment System for Children (BASC)
B. Home Situations Questionnaire-Revised (HSQ-R)
C. Luria-Nebraska Neuropsychological Battery (LNNB:C)
D. Thematic Apperception Test (TAT)
E. Vineland Adaptive Behavior Scale

1.33. An obese child with hypotonia and small hands and feet along with hoarding, excessive daytime sleepiness, compulsive behavior, and skin picking likely has a deletion in which of the following chromosomes?

A. Elastin focus on 7q11-23
B. Microdeletion at 16q13.3
C. Paternal origin of 15q12
D. Paternal on 5p
E. Pregnancy-associated plasma protein-A (PAPPA)

1.34. A child is being evaluated for ADHD. Mental status examination is noted for a long face with large ears. Medical history is significant for mitral valve prolapse and intellectual disability. Which of the following genetic mutations is most likely present in this child?

A. Deletion on 7q11-23
B. Deletion on 15q12 of maternal origin
C. Inactivation of the FMR-1 gene
D. Partial deletion chromosome 5
E. Trisomy 21

1.35. What is the most common reason cited by elderly adults who consider suicide?

A. Anxiety
B. Financial difficulties
C. Loneliness
D. Pain
E. Sickness

1.36. A pill-rolling tremor is most commonly associated with which of the following classes of psychiatric medications?

A. Benzodiazepines
B. Phenothiazine
C. Selective serotonin reuptake inhibitors
D. Stimulants
E. Tricyclics

1.37. Which type of agnosia involves inability to recognize faces?

A. Anosognosia
B. Anosmia
C. Atopognosia
D. Prosopagnosia
E. Visual agnosia

1.38. A fair skin, blue-eyed, blond-hair child presents with language delays, hyperactivity, self-injury, and new-onset seizures. She most likely has a genetic condition caused by the buildup of which of the following substances?

A. Galactose
B. Iduronate 2-sulfatase
C. L-iduronidase
D. Phenylalanine
E. Uric acid

1.39. A child presents with dysmorphic facial features consisting of a broad forehead, a depressed nasal bridge, and widely spaced teeth and is described as having elfin-like facies. The patient has a medical history significant for cardiac and thyroid abnormalities and a psychiatric history significant for hyperactivity and anxiety though is very social and makes friends easily. The child most likely has which of the following genetic syndromes?

A. Cri-du-chat
B. Fragile X
C. Prader–Willi
D. Smith–Magenis
E. Williams

1.40. Which neuropsychological test measures sensory-motor, perceptual, and cognitive functioning?

A. Luria-Nebraska
B. Millon Adolescent
C. Mullen
D. Rotter
E. Thematic Apperception

1.41. Suicidality falls under what category on the mental status examination?

A. Judgment
B. Mood
C. Perception
D. Thought content
E. Thought process

1.42. Which of the following respiratory symptoms is more indicative of depression rather than an underlying pulmonary disorder?

A. Breathlessness while active
B. Breathlessness with little changes with exertion
C. Difficulty with expiration
D. Fluctuation in breathlessness over hours
E. Insidious onset of breathlessness

ANSWERS

1.1. A. Obtain consent from the patient
After introductions, consent to proceed with the interview should be obtained. The nature of the interview and length of time should be discussed and then the patient should be encouraged to give feedback regarding altering elements in the process. While discussion of limits of confidentiality and performing a safety assessment should be included in all interviews, these are not the initial steps that need to be done. If a family member wants to be involved, it is typically best to have the patient present, though this is often best suited for the end of the interview. (1)

1.2. A. Ability to maintain objectivity
The ability to maintain objectivity is crucial in a therapeutic relationship and can differentiate empathy from identification. With identification, psychiatrists experience as well as understand the emotion, which can lead to boundary problems along with physician burnout. (2)

1.3. D. Strengths
A psychiatric interview should be person centered to best help understand the patient and their goals. A person-centered approach focuses on strengths and assets, as well as deficits, compared to a traditional medical approach focusing only on illness and deficits. (4)

1.4. E. Have you ever failed to remember things after drinking?
The RAPS4 and CAGE are brief standardized questionnaires that psychiatrists can use to assess substance abuse or dependence. There is some overlap between the two. The RAPS4 includes the following four questions: Have you ever felt guilty after drinking (Remorse), could not remember things did or said (Amnesia), failed to do what was normally expected after drinking (Perform), or had a morning drink (Starter)? The CAGE also includes four questions: Have you ever cut down on your drinking (Cut)? Have people annoyed you by criticizing your drinking (Annoyed)? Have you ever felt bad about your drinking (Guilty)? Have you ever needed a drink first thing in the morning (Eye-opener)? Though driving drunk or getting arrested for drinking can be a sign of abuse or dependence, it is not part of these screening tools. (7)

1.5. B. Hyperthyroidism
Obtaining a past medical history is a key part of all psychiatric interviews. Some medical illness can contribute to or mimic psychiatric disorders, or they might be caused by treatment of a psychiatric disorder. A classic psychiatric disorder that can resemble an anxiety disorder is hyperthyroidism. The other disorders listed are more likely to mimic or cause depressive symptoms. (7)

1.6. A. Diabetes
Obtaining a family history is essential in helping to define the patient's risk factors for psychiatric illness and can also be useful in guiding medication choices. A family history of diabetes or hyperlipidemia might make one utilize an atypical antipsychotic with caution due to risk of worsening both conditions, along with causing other metabolic side effects. (8)

1.7. C. Mania
An increase in the amount of speech on mental status examinations could be a sign of mania or hypomania. A decrease in the amount of speech can be from depression, anxiety, or disinterest. Decreased speech could also be a sign of thought blocking or psychosis. (9)

1.8. A. Clang associations
Thought process is the way in which thoughts are organized, formed, or expressed. Clang associations are when words are put together by the sound of the words rather than for the meaning (i.e., rhyming is prominent). Neologisms are new words or combinations of a few words that are not actually understandable or true words. Perseveration is the repetition of words out of context. Tangential thought process means never returning to the previous statement. Thought blocking appears when a patient stops and the thought is unable to come out, often leading to a stop midsentence. (10)

1.9. E. Judgment
Judgment refers to a person's ability to make good decisions and act on them. A classic example of a question to test judgment is, "What would you do if you found a stamped envelope on the street?" Abstract reasoning is the ability to shift between concepts and examples, identifying similarities between like objects, for example. Fund of knowledge can be tested by fact-based questions (i.e., "Who is the president of the United States?").

Insight refers to the patient's understanding of how they are functioning and potential contributing factors to their illness. (11)

1.10. C. Motivational interviewing
Motivational interviewing is a technique used to motivate the patient to change maladaptive behaviors. Relaying empathy and highlighting ambivalence and conflicting feelings are key to motivating change. Nonverbal actions, such as moving a tissue box, can sometimes be used to help acknowledge emotions. Minimizing the patient's concerns might happen when attempting to reassure patients; thus, concerns should be explored. Premature interpretations, even if accurate, should be avoided as they can lead to the patient becoming defensive and feeling misunderstood. Summarizing is a useful technique that should be done periodically to help clarify understanding. (16)

1.11. B. Denial of intent to act on the thoughts
A suicide assessment should be performed for all patients during the initial interview. The patient should be asked about any current thoughts of suicide and if present, what the intent is. If a patient has thoughts of suicide but denies intent to act on these thoughts or denies a wish to be dead, that is referred to as passive suicidal ideation. Higher-risk patients include those who have specific plans to end their life and access to the means to complete the plan, along with those who have taken preparatory steps to move forward with the plan. (17)

1.12. C. Pheochromocytoma
Pheochromocytomas produce symptoms that mimic anxiety including rapid heartbeat, tremors, and pallor. Increased urinary catecholamines are diagnostic for a pheochromocytoma. Hyper, not hypothyroidism can lead to anxiety. Normal pressure hydrocephalus can be present with dementia, shuffling gait, and incontinence. Temporal arteritis can cause unilateral throbbing headaches and can lead to blindness. Ulcerative colitis can present as weight loss and depressive symptoms. (19)

1.13. C. Data that can be disclosed to the patient
Psychotherapy notes include details of transference, countertransference, fantasies, dreams, and personal information about name of contacts of the patient, etc., which would not be included in the actual progress notes in the medical record. Unlike progress notes, psychotherapy notes should be kept separate from the rest of the medical record and the data in them should not be disclosed to any person, including the patient. Detailed assessments and plans should be included in progress notes, not the psychotherapy note. (27)

1.14. B. Bipolar disorder
The SCID, Structured Clinical Interview for DSM, is designed to be administered by an experienced clinician, requires training and is primarily focused on research and is used to verify diagnoses in clinical trials. Reliability data suggests that it performs better on more severe disorders and alcohol dependence compared to milder disorders, such as dysthymia. (31)

1.15. A. Brief Psychiatric Rating Scale (BPRS)
The BPRS was developed in the late 1960s as a short scale to measure the severity of psychiatric symptomatology and is primarily designed to assess changes in psychotic inpatients. However, good reliability is difficult to achieve without extensive training and this scale is often only suitable for patients with a fairly significant level of clinical impairment. The HAM-A is often used to monitor treatment response in clinical trials and in some clinical settings for generalized anxiety disorders. The PANSS was designed to remedy the deficits in the BPRS in the assessment of positive and negative symptoms in schizophrenia and other psychotic disorders by adding additional items and providing anchors for each. It is a highly reliable tool which has become the standard for assessing clinical outcomes in treatment studies for schizophrenia and other psychotic disorders. The SAPS and the Scale for the Assessment of Negative Symptoms (SANS) provide a detailed assessment of positive and negative symptoms in schizophrenia, with the SAPS assessing for hallucinations, delusions, thought disorders, etc., and the SANS assessing for poverty of speech, apathy, anhedonia, etc. The SCID, Structured Clinical Interview for DSM, is primarily used in research and to verify a variety of diagnoses in clinical trials. (38)

1.16. A. A clinical diagnosis
The CBCL includes different self-rated versions for parents, teachers, and children to help assess preschoolers through adolescents. It does not generate diagnoses, rather it suggests cut-off scores for problems in the clinical range and provides a good overall view of symptomatology and can be used to track changes over time. (45, 46)

1.17. A. Attention deficit hyperactivity
The Connors Rating Scale includes teacher-, parent-, and self-reported measures and assesses a range of childhood and adolescent psychopathology. The Connors Scale is most commonly used in screening for ADHD in schools and in clinical populations, and can be used to follow changes in symptom severity over time. (47)

1.18. B. Gerstmann
Aside from language, the left hemisphere is responsible for limb apraxia. Lesions in the left hemisphere can result in finger agnosia, dyscalculia, dysgraphia, and right–left disorientation, referred to as Gerstmann syndrome. Dressing apraxia is associated with special deficits from right hemisphere damage and include right–left confusion and difficulty putting limbs into clothing. Hurler syndrome, an autosomal recessive condition, includes symptoms such as hirsutism, corneal clouding, coarse facial features, and moderate-to-severe intellectual disability. Neglect syndromes are most commonly associated with right hemisphere damage in the parietal region and include failure to detect visual or tactile stimuli, or to move the limb in the contralateral hemispace. Pickwickian syndrome is recognized by a puffy appearance, as seen in hypothyroidism, obesity, and periodic respirations. (21, 47, 49, 87)

1.19. D. Fluency
Broca aphasia, or nonfluent or expressive aphasia, caused by a left inferior frontal convolution lesion, is characterized by nonfluent speech (i.e., telegraphic or agrammatism) with intact auditory comprehension. This is in contrast to Wernicke aphasia, caused by a superior temporal gyrus lesion, which has fluent speech but impaired comprehension. Repetition can be somewhat impaired in both aphasias. Unlike those with Broca aphasia, those with Wernicke are not typically aware of their communication deficits. (48)

1.20. C. Parietal lobe
Failure to bisect a line placed midline is an example of a neglect syndrome. It is characterized by failure to detect visual or tactile stimuli or move the limb in the contralateral hemisphere. It is most commonly associated with right hemisphere damage in the parietal region, though other areas in the cortex and subcortical areas can also cause it. (49)

1.21. B. Planning and organization
The clock-drawing technique is widely used in elderly individuals at risk for dementia as a test that is a sensitive measure of planning and organization. More subtle difficulties can also be detected when comparing performance to premorbid expectations such as perseveration and neglect. Double simultaneous stimulation of visual and auditory modalities can test for sensory and motor functions and can also test for neglect. The WMS-III can measure attention, memory, and new learning. Expressive language is often measured by testing verbal fluency, via generating words within semantic and phonetic categories. Conducting a digit span is a measure of attention. (54)

1.22. A. Criterion validity
Face validity refers to the content of the test items and if they measure what they intend to measure. While it refers to the degree the items on the surface measure what the instrument is supposed to, criterion validity uses data outside the test to measure validity. Discriminant validity tells whether the test can discriminate between groups of patients at times (i.e., discriminate between mild, moderate, vs. severe major depressive disorder). Factor validity utilizes a multivariate statistical technique, factor analysis, to determine if a group of items on a test empirically cluster together. (56/57)

1.23. A. fMRI (functional magnetic resonance imaging)
fMRIs measure regional cerebral blood flow by measuring heme molecules as an endogenous contrast agent. MRA creates a 3-D map of brain blood flow and is typically used by neurologists and neurosurgeons. MRS is a research method used to measure brain metabolism and is done in an MRI machine with additional software to allow signals from protons to be suppressed and signals from other compounds to be measured. PET scans involve the detection of emitted positron radiation, typically by using FDG (fluorodeoxyglucose) to measure regional brain glucose metabolism. SPECT scans are not typically used to study the brain. They are more commonly used to study other organs. (61)

1.24. E. Toluene
Inhalants, such as toluene, as found in paints, glues, and cleaning solutions, can cause significant brain damage, as well as damage to other organs, such as the liver, kidneys, lung, bone marrow, etc. It can

lead to hypoxia and can cause a loss of gray-white matter and brain atrophy on MRIs. Chronic use can also be associated with panic attacks and personality changes. (63)

1.25. A. Ammonia
While valproate (valproic acid, Depakene; divalproex, Depakote) can cause hematologic abnormalities including leukopenia and thrombocytopenia, if a patient is presenting as lethargic or has a change in mental status, ammonia levels should be checked urgently, as valproate can increase ammonia levels. Elevated liver function tests (LFTs) and acute pancreatitis are also risks of valproate treatment. (64)

1.26. D. Liver function tests (LFTs)
Treatment with MAOIs can occasionally be associated with hepatotoxicity. Thus, LFTs are usually obtained at the initiation of treatment and periodically after. Blood pressure should also be obtained before initiating treatment and monitored afterward. (64)

1.27. B. Vitamin B12
Vitamin B12 and folate deficiencies are associated with dementia, delirium, psychosis, and paranoia and should be checked as part of a workup. These deficiencies are especially common in patients who abuse alcohol. (66)

1.28. C. Hypomagnesemia
A QTc measurement on an EKG greater than 500 milliseconds is considered prolonged and can increase the risk of a severe arrhythmia. Factors that can prolong QTc include certain drugs, in addition to bradycardia, hypokalemia, or hypomagnesemia. (67)

1.29. A. A recent myocardial infarction
Ziprasidone (Geodon) is associated with a dose-related prolongation of the QTc interval and can lead to fatal arrhythmias. An EKG should be checked before initiation. Ziprasidone is contraindicated in patients with a history of known QTc prolongation, recent myocardial infarctions, and uncompensated heart failure. It should also be used with caution in those with bradycardia, hypokalemia, hypomagnesemia, or those on other QTc prolonging drugs. (67)

1.30. B. Calcifications
MRIs are typically preferred over CTs for most purposes due to a lack of radiation exposure. CTs are primarily used in emergent situations. The only component of the brain seen better on CT scans are calcifications, which can be invisible on MRIs. (70)

1.31. A. Language
When using instruments such as the Gesell Infact Scale, the Bayley Cales of Infant and Toddler Development, and the Denver Developmental Screening Test with very young infants the tests focus on sensorimotor and social responses to objects and interactions. When used for older infants and preschoolers, the emphasis is on language acquisition. (81)

1.32. E. Vineland adaptive behavior scale
The Vineland Adaptive Behavior Scale is used for those 0 to 19 years old to provide a standard score measuring adaptive behavior and communication, skills of daily living, and socialization. There are separate standardization groups for normal, visually handicapped, hearing impaired, emotionally disturbed, and those with intellectual disability. The BASC has teacher and parent rating scales as well as a child self-report of personality across various domains at home, school, and the community in those ages 4 to 18 years. The HSQ-R is a test of attentional capacity in which parents rate the child's specific problems with attention and concentration. The LNNB:C tests sensory-motor, perceptual and cognitive functioning. The TAT is a type of projective test that can assess interpersonal functioning. (82, 83)

1.33. C. Paternal origin of 15q12
Prader–Willi syndrome involves a deletion in 15q2 of paternal origin and presents with hypotonia, failure to thrive in infancy, then obesity, small hands and feet, and microorchidism. Compulsive behavior, hyperphagia, hoarding, and anxiety/aggression, and skin picking are also features of Prader–Willi syndrome. Rubinstein–Taybi syndrome is sporadic or likely autosomal dominated, though there have been microdeletions documented in some cases at 16q13.3. It presents with short stature, microcephaly, broad thumb, big toes, etc., feeding difficulties, seizures, distractibility and expressive language difficulties. Often these kids are loving and responsive to music. Cri-du-chat syndrome is from a partial deletion on 5p including the elastin locus on 7q11-23 and presents with a round face, hypertelorism, epicanthal folds, slanting palpebral fissures, a broad flat nose, etc. along with congenital heart disease, severe intellectual disability, self-injury, and an infant-like cry. Cornelia de Lange

syndrome is due to a lack of PAPPA linked to chromosome 9q33 and presents with a continuous eyebrow, thin downturning of the upper lip, microcephaly and short stature, etc. along with failure to thrive, self-injury, language delays, profound intellectual disability, etc. (86)

1.34. C. Inactivation of the FMR-1 gene

The child depicted has fragile X syndrome, which is caused by an inactivation of the FMR-1 gene at X q27.3. Features consist of a long face, large ears, midface hypoplasia, a high-arched palate, short stature, and macroorchidism. Mitral valve prolapse, joint laxity, and strabismus are other features. ADHD symptoms of hyperactivity and inattention are often noted along with anxiety, speech and language delays, and learning disorders. Deletion of 15q12 of maternal origin causes Angelman syndrome. Fair hair and blue eyes are common along with dysmorphic facial features of wide-smiling mouth, thin upper lip, and pointed chin. The syndrome is notable for a happy disposition and paroxysmal laughter and hand flapping. Deletions that include the elastin locus on chromones 7q11-23 include features such as short stature, broad forehead, depressed nasal bridge, and elf-like features. It presents with anxiety and hyperactivity. Cri-du chat involves a partial deletion on 5p and signs include an infantile cry, severe intellectual disability, and a round face with hypertelorism and epicanthal folds. Down syndrome features include upward-slanted palpebral fissures, midface depression, and a flat, wide nausea bridge, along with short stature. Hyperactivity and increased depression and Alzheimer are notable in down syndrome which is caused by trisomy 21. (86)

1.35. C. Loneliness

Suicide is a leading cause of death in the elderly, and loneliness is the most common reason cited by older adults who consider suicide. Feelings of loneliness, worthlessness, hopelessness, and helplessness are all symptoms of depression, which is highly linked to suicide. Approximately 75% of those who complete suicide suffer from depression and/or alcohol abuse. (88)

1.36. B. Phenothiazine

Mental status examination symptoms of adverse effects of phenothiazine medication include a pill-rolling tremor, shuffling gait, stooped posture, and body asymmetry, along with abnormal movements of the mouth and tongue. (88)

1.37. D. Prosopagnosia

Prosopagnosia is the inability to recognize faces. A denial of illness is called anosognosia. A denial of a body part is atopognosia and an inability to recognize objects is called visual agnosia. Anosmia is the loss of smell. (88)

1.38. D. Phenylalanine

Phenylketonuria involves a defect in phenylalanine hydroxylase or biopterin, resulting in accumulation of phenylalanine. It typically presents in those with fair skin, blue eyes, blond hair, and rashes and if untreated can lead to intellectual disability, language delays, self-injury, and hyperactivity. Generalized seizures can occur later in development. Galactosemia is caused by a defect in galactose-1-phosphate uridyltransferase or galactokinase and presents as vomiting, jaundice, hepatosplenomegaly, cataracts, food refusal, increased intracranial pressure, langue disorders, behavioral problems, and anxiety. Hurler syndrome is caused by a deficiency in alpha-L-iduronidase activity resulting in short stature, hepatosplenomegaly, hirsutism, corneal clouding, dwarfism, coarse facial features, and typically death before 10 years old. Hunter syndrome is caused by a deficiency in iduronate sulfatase resulting in a coarse face with flat nasal bridge, hearing loss, ataxia, enlarged liver and spleen, recurrent infections, hyperactivity, sleep abnormalities and intellectual disability. Uric acid builds up in Lesch–Nyhan syndrome due to a defect in hypoxanthine guanine phosphoribosyl-transferase, resulting in ataxia, chorea, kidney failure, gout, along with aggression and self-biting. (87)

1.39. E. Williams

The symptoms are consistent with a diagnosis of Williams syndrome, caused by a deletion that includes the elastin locus on chromosome 7q11-23 and is inherited in an autosomal dominant fashion. Cri-du-chat syndrome, caused by a partial deletion in 5p presents with a round face with hypertelorism, epicanthal folds and slanting palpebral fissures along with heart disease, GI abnormalities, severe intellectual disability, self-injury, and cat-like cries. Fragile X is due to inactivation of FMR-1 gene at Xq27.3 de ot CGG base repeats, accounts for 10% to 12% of intellectual disability in males and presents with a long face, large ears, midface hypoplasia, a high-arched palate, etc. Prader–Willi syndrome presents with a 15q12 deletion of paternal origin and symptoms include hypotonia, obesity, small hands and feet, microorchidism, short stature, almond-shaped eyes, hyperphagia, hoarding, aggression and skin picking. Smith–Magenis syndrome is caused by a complete or partial deletion of 17p11.2 and presents with a broad face and hands, small toes, a deep voice, severe intellectual disability, hyperactivity, severe self-injury including hand biting and head banging. (86)

1.40. A. Luria-Nebraska

The Luria-Nebraska Neuropsychological Battery: Children's Revision (LNNB:C) provides standard measure for sensory–motor, perceptual, and cognitive tests. The Millon Adolescent Personality Inventory (MAPI) provides standard scores for personality styles, expressed concerns, and behavioral correlates. The Mullen Scales of Early Learning is a test of language and visual scales for receptive and expressive ability in newborns to 5 year olds. The Rotter Incomplete Sentences Blank Test is a qualitative projective test for children and adolescents, with an adult version as well. The Thematic Apperception Test (TAT) is also a projective test involving generating stories for 6 year olds and up and can give data regarding interpersonal functioning. (83)

1.41. D. Thought content

Both suicidality and homicidality fall under the category of thought content. Obsessional thoughts and compulsions also go under thought content, along with delusions. Mood is what the patient reports as their internal emotional state. Thought process does not describe what the patient is thinking, rather how the thoughts are formulated, organized, or expressed. Perceptual disturbances include hallucinations, illusions, depersonalization, and derealization. Judgment refers to the patient's capacity to make good decision and act on them. (10)

1.42. B. Breathlessness with little changes in exertion

In conducting a medical review of systems during a psychiatric interview it is important to tease apart obstructive airway and other organic pulmonary diseases from breathing problems due to psychiatric conditions. In depression, breathlessness is experienced at rest and shows little change with exertion and can fluctuate in minutes. Often, a history can show the breathing problems coincided with the depressive episode and is accompanied by panic attacks including symptoms such as dizziness, sweating, palpitations, and paresthesias. Often with depression, the emphasis is placed on struggles with inspiration, whereas in true pulmonary disease the difficulty is with expiration. In pulmonary obstructive airway disease, the onset is typically insidious. Of course, when in doubt of the origin of respiratory symptoms, a referral should be made to the primary care doctor or pulmonologist. (19)

Neurodevelopmental Disorders and Other Childhood Disorders

2.1. The parents of an 8-year-old girl meet with their daughter's teacher due to concerns that the child is not keeping up with her peers in school. Her teacher says that the child is reading below the kindergarten level, and cannot perform basic addition. The parents add that their daughter did not start talking until age 2. All are concerned that the child may be intellectually disabled. Cognitive testing by the school psychologist reveals an IQ of 64. The child's hearing and vision are normal, and there are no known medical illnesses. What further history must be elicited before the diagnosis is made?

A. Her exposure to language prior to starting school
B. The extent of her social functioning
C. The progression of her motor milestones
D. The source of the family's drinking water
E. The age of the parents' home

2.2. The majority of individuals with a diagnosis of intellectual disability have an IQ in what range?

A. <20
B. 20 to 34
C. 35 to 49
D. 50 to 69
E. 70 to 80

2.3. A 7-year-old child with autism spectrum disorder and intellectual disability presents to the outpatient clinic with his parents, who report that their son has become increasingly aggressive over the last 6 months. They state that when an unexpected change in routine occurs, such as having to take a different route home due to traffic, he starts to bite himself and sometimes attacks them. The mother reports that he once tried to grab the wheel of the car while they were driving. Behavioral interventions have been minimally effective. What medication has the most evidence for short-term management of the child's behaviors?

A. Gabapentin
B. Risperidone
C. Melatonin
D. Haloperidol
E. Olanzapine

2.4. Which of the following cerebral abnormalities would most likely be found following the death of a 50-year-old individual with Down syndrome?

A. Arteriovenous malformations
B. Senile plaques
C. Enlarged ventricles
D. Decreased pigmentation in the substantia nigra
E. Optic gliomas

2.5. The parents of an 18-month-old boy present to an outpatient clinic with concerns for their child's repeated seizures. They state that he usually comes out of them after a few seconds, but they are becoming more frequent. They report that he is often irritable, which they attribute to him not being able to communicate, as he has no language skills. The child was born at home, and there was no prenatal or follow-up care. Physical examination is challenging because he has difficulty remaining still, but reveals a fair-skinned child with eczema and a prominent musty odor on his breath. Motor development is at the level of a 6 month old. What is the most likely diagnosis?

A. Fragile X syndrome
B. Rett syndrome
C. Childhood disintegrative disorder
D. Phenylketonuria (PKU)
E. Adrenoleukodystrophy

2.6. The most common inherited cause of intellectual disability involves what genetic abnormality?

A. A mutation of the FMR1 gene
B. A deletion in chromosome 5
C. A deletion in chromosome 15
D. The presence of the NF2 gene
E. A nondisjunction of chromosome 21

2.7. An 18-month-old boy is brought to the primary care clinic because he is not yet able to say "mama" or "dada" clearly and communicates mostly through grunts and whines. He is responsive to the presence of his parents and others and will cry if they leave the room. He cannot follow simple commands. When his name is called, he sometimes turns his head toward the caller. He has met his motor milestones. The mother received adequate prenatal care, and the child had no known illnesses. What should be the first step in the workup of this child?

A. Chromosome analysis
B. Neuropsychological testing
C. Head imaging
D. Hearing test
E. Speech evaluation

2.8. A 6-year-old boy has difficulty pronouncing certain sounds, most notably the letter *r*. He says "meah-wuh" instead of "mirror," and "bwake" instead of "break." His pronunciations are not common in the cultural dialect. He has no difficulty with other phonemes, and shows no motor, social, or intellectual delays. He makes As and Bs in his first-grade class. What is the most appropriate intervention for this child?

A. Observation only
B. Initiate speech therapy
C. Obtain hearing testing
D. Obtain IQ testing
E. Obtain neurologic testing

2.9. A child with autism spectrum disorder would most likely have difficulty with what domain of language?

A. Phonology
B. Grammar
C. Semantics
D. Pragmatics

2.10. Parents bring their 6-year-old son to the primary care clinic due to concerns that "he doesn't show any affection towards us. He barely even looks at us when we talk to him, and sometimes will not speak back when spoken to." They state that he does not play cooperatively with children his age, and though he may be physically next to other children, he will play by himself with the same toy truck. "He doesn't use it as a truck, he just holds it up and spins the wheels over and over. He would do that all day if you let him." They add that he often suddenly flaps his hands with no provocation. They report that he was evaluated by the school psychologist and found to have an IQ of 85. Though his verbal abilities were tested as normal, they lagged behind other cognitive domains. The child has no known medical illnesses and is on no medications. What is the most likely diagnosis?

A. Mild intellectual disability
B. Social communication disorder
C. Hearing difficulty
D. Autism spectrum disorder (ASD)
E. Stereotypic movement disorder

2.11. A 9-year-old girl is brought to the outpatient clinic by her father, who reports that her grades in school consist of Cs and Ds because she forgets to turn in her homework and makes careless mistakes on her class assignments. Notes from her teacher say that she is disorganized, as evidenced by her messy desk and bookbag, and that she often loses or forgets to bring her notebook and writing utensils. The teacher has moved her to the front of the classroom in an effort to keep her from being distracted by the other children, but this has not been successful. Her father reports that the symptoms were present during the last school year, but that they have gotten worse. There is no history of medical illness and she takes no medications. What is the first-line treatment for this child's condition?

A. Behavioral modification
B. Parent management training
C. Stimulant medication
D. Anticonvulsant medication
E. Alpha-agonist medication

2.12. What treatment is considered first-line therapy for attention-deficit hyperactivity disorder (ADHD) in adults?

A. Stimulant medication
B. Atomoxetine
C. Alpha-agonist medication
D. Bupropion
E. Modafinil

2.13. A 10-year-old boy is referred by his teacher to the school psychologist due to poor reading and spelling abilities. The child says that the letters in words appear "jumbled up" on paper, and that he has difficulty distinguishing between some letters such as *b* and *d*. He has started to become frustrated when asked to read out loud in class, and once yelled at the teacher when she called on him to read. His latest report card consists of an "A" in math, art, and music, and a "B" in geography. What evaluation is necessary to make the diagnosis?

A. IQ testing
B. Standardized reading testing
C. Observation of the child in the classroom
D. Adaptive functioning testing
E. Continuous performance testing

2.14. An 8-year-old girl is brought to the outpatient clinic for an evaluation of tics. Her parents state the tics began 3 years ago, and that they were hoping that she would just "grow out of them." They report that the tics began with eye blinking and winking and have since progressed to fist clenching. One year ago, she started clearing her throat. The child states that she has gotten used to the eye movements and that they no longer bother her. She adds that she used to bother the other kids in her class with the throat clearing, but that she can now "hold it in until I get home," at which time she clears her throat for several minutes. She makes grades of As and Bs, and has several friends who sometimes sleep over on the weekends. What is the treatment for this child?

A. Risperidone therapy
B. Habit reversal training
C. Aripiprazole therapy
D. Parental psychoeducation
E. Cognitive behavioral therapy

2.15. Parents bring their 3-month-old daughter to the pediatrician because of poor weight gain since birth. This is their first child. They state that she does not seem to be interested in feeding, despite attempting both breast milk and bottle formula. The mother reports that the child is irritable when they try to feed her, and that the child often pushes away, but will sometimes take formula. The mother adds that she feels guilty because her daughter's lack of engagement is starting to make her feel like she wants to be less engaged in her daughter's care. There were no complications during the pregnancy or delivery, and the child came home from the hospital the day after birth. At 1 month old, she was 40th percentile for length and weight. She is currently 35th percentile for weight and 40th percentile for length. Physical examination reveals a healthy infant in no acute distress. She responds appropriately to both parents. What is the most appropriate next step in management?

A. Contact child protective services
B. Admit the child to the hospital
C. Order a swallowing study
D. Refer the family to a psychiatrist
E. Arrange for a home health nurse to help with feeding

2.16. A 3-year-old girl is found by child protective services locked alone in the dark basement of a house after a neighbor called to report suspected abuse and neglect. When questioned by police, the parents state that they keep her there for many hours at a time, and sometimes overnight, as punishment because "she often misbehaves." A social worker leads the child out of the basement, and the child leaps into the social worker's arms and gives her a kiss. She appears thin. She does not cry when separated from her parents. The child is then taken to a foster home, where she immediately runs up to the foster father, sits on his lap, and gives him a kiss. What is the most likely explanation for the child's behavior?

A. Normal development
B. Expected behavior given the child's recent circumstances
C. Posttraumatic stress disorder (PTSD)
D. Disinhibited social engagement disorder
E. Reactive attachment disorder

2.17. What is the first-line treatment for posttraumatic stress disorder (PTSD) of infancy, childhood, and adolescence?

A. Risperidone therapy
B. Cognitive behavioral therapy (CBT)
C. Sertraline therapy
D. Eye movement desensitization and reprocessing (EMDR)
E. Prazosin therapy

2.18. According to the DSM-5, what symptom can replace depressed mood in a diagnosis of major disorder in a child as opposed to in an adult?

A. Aggression
B. Behavioral regression
C. Crying
D. Oppositional behavior
E. Irritability

2.19. A 15-year-old girl is brought to the outpatient clinic by her parents due to concern that she has been "in a funk" for several months, which they attribute to her not making the cheerleading team at school. They note that she has not been eating as much in order to lose weight before next year's tryouts. When the parents leave the room, the girl says that she did not make the cheerleading team because she did not have the energy to "give it my all, and I'm not trying to lose weight, I just don't feel hungry. I actually love to eat." She is worried that she will never feel better, and worries about her grades, which have dropped from As and Bs last school year to mostly Cs this year. "I can't concentrate. I'll get to the end of the page in a book and have no idea what I read. My parents think this has been going on for a few months, but it's been over a year." She denies suicidal ideation. She states that she has been taking an SSRI as prescribed by her previous doctor for the last 3 months, "and I feel the same, despite increasing the dose twice." What is the next step in treatment?

A. Electroconvulsive therapy
B. Change to serotonin norepinephrine reuptake inhibitor (SNRI)
C. Change to another selective serotonin reuptake inhibitor (SSRI)
D. Augment with cognitive behavioral therapy
E. Augment with interpersonal therapy

2.20. A 16-year-old boy is brought to the urgent care center by his parents after he told them that he wanted to kill himself. He says that he has been depressed for the last 3 months, "and I don't see the point of living any longer if this is going to continue." His parents state that they offered to buy him a car "in the hopes that it would make him snap out of it." He missed the last week of school 2 months ago and has stayed to himself in his room, even though friends have tried to engage him in playing video games, his favorite hobby. He has lost about 5 pounds and rarely eats. Though he sleeps much of the day, he still has little energy. When asked about his mood, he starts crying and says, "I can't stand this anymore. I want to die," and voices a plan to shoot himself. His parents confirm that they have a gun in the house, but they have hidden it. What is the most appropriate disposition?

A. Discharge to home with a psychiatry appointment in the morning
B. Emergently admit the child to a hospital
C. Begin an SSRI and have him follow-up in 2 to 3 weeks with a psychiatrist
D. Refer to a therapist for cognitive behavioral or interpersonal psychotherapy
E. Send the family to a local emergency room (ER) for further evaluation

2.21. The school resource officer (SRO) is called to the classroom of a 9-year-old boy who is throwing books, pushing over desks, and yelling. The teacher tells the SRO that, "one minute he was fine, then the next he's doing this. All I told him to do was use a pencil instead of a pen on his writing assignment. I feel like I'm always walking on eggshells with him!" The parents are called to the school once the acute situation has resolved, and confirm what the teacher says about his temperament. They report to the principal that he has these tantrums several times a week at home that begin "over nothing," and that he is always irritable. They once called the police because he was so out of control after an argument with his younger sister that he broke windows in the house. What is the most likely diagnosis?

A. Bipolar disorder
B. Oppositional defiant disorder (ODD)
C. Intermittent explosive disorder
D. Disruptive mood dysregulation disorder (DMDD)
E. Conduct disorder

2.22. Normal separation anxiety, as opposed to separation anxiety disorder, typically diminishes around what age?

A. 9 months
B. 1.5 years
C. 2.5 years
D. 4 years
E. 5 years

2.23. The Food and Drug Administration (FDA) placed a "black-box" warning on antidepressants for use in children out of concern for what adverse effect?

A. Serotonin syndrome
B. Suicidality
C. Aggression
D. Cognitive dulling
E. Cardiac arrhythmias

2.24. A 14-year-old girl presents with her parents to the school counselor because she refuses to give a required speech in her language arts class. She says that everyone will laugh at her and think she is stupid because she will "mess up and say something wrong." The teacher, her parents, and peers have tried to convince her that this will not be the case, but she is undeterred. Her parents note that she will not attend a group sleepover or let herself become romantically interested in anyone for the same reason. When told that not giving the speech will severely impact her grade, she says that she would rather fail. In addition to an SSRI, what is the most evidence-based treatment for this child?

A. Administration of a beta-blocker 30 minutes prior to giving the speech
B. Cognitive behavioral therapy (CBT)
C. Administration of buspirone
D. Exposure and response prevention therapy
E. Interpersonal therapy

2.25. The teacher of a 5-year-old boy contacts the boy's parents after the first week of kindergarten due to concern about the child's hearing. The teacher notes that the child does not say anything in class, but will shake his head and nod when addressed. His parents are shocked, and say that he talks at home all the time. The child is called into the meeting during which he says nothing. On the way home, when asked why he isn't talking, he starts to cry. What is the first-line treatment for this child?

A. Cognitive behavioral therapy
B. Speech therapy
C. SSRI therapy
D. Family therapy
E. Beta-blocker therapy

2.26. OCD is comorbid with attention-deficit hyperactivity disorder (ADHD), anxiety disorders, and what other disorder?

A. Major depression
B. Tourette
C. Oppositional defiant
D. Bipolar
E. Substance use

2.27. A 12-year-old boy is brought from school to the emergency department by emergency medical services (EMS) due to a sudden behavioral outburst that could not be controlled. Thirty minutes before EMS arrived, the child suddenly jumped up from his desk and screamed, "Get away from me monster!" He then jumped on a classmate and started biting him. Staff managed to free the other child and get everyone out of the room while the patient threw chairs, desks, and other items at a fixed point in the room as he screamed, "I'll kill you!" The teacher told the emergency medical technician (EMT) that the boy has scared her for months with the way he looked blankly at her and others, and that the other children had largely avoided him. On arrival, the child is sedated with haloperidol and lorazepam. Vital signs are then within normal limits. Complete blood count (CBC), comprehensive metabolic panel (CMP), heavy metals, urine drug screen (UDS), lumbar puncture, and head CT are all negative. His parents are contacted and confirm the symptoms seen by the teacher, and add that he was "fine until about 8 months ago, when he started withdrawing from everyone and his grades started falling." What is the most likely course of the child's illness?

A. Spontaneous remission
B. Gradual remission
C. Waxing and waning
D. Maintenance of current symptoms
E. Chronic deterioration

2.28. What recreational drug has been found to correlate with an increased risk of psychiatric disorders, notably schizophrenia?

A. Alcohol
B. Cocaine
C. Marijuana
D. Heroin
E. Lysergic acid diethylamide (LSD)

2.29. A 30-year-old man stocks shelves and carries bags out to the cars of patrons of a local grocery store. He lives with his parents, who drive him to and from work, cook for him, remind him to bathe, and help him manage his money. He is able to stay at the house by himself while they are at work. Though he received a certificate of completion for high school, he last tested at the second-grade level for reading, third-grade level for math, and first-grade level for writing. He is able to speak clearly and makes his needs known, but with a limited vocabulary. What is the most likely level of the man's intellectual disability?

A. Borderline
B. Mild
C. Moderate
D. Severe
E. Profound

2.30. An individual with intellectual disability suffers from what neurologic problem more frequently than that found in the general population?

A. Hypotonia
B. Ataxia
C. Alzheimer disease
D. Parkinson disease
E. Seizures

2.31. A 26-year-old G1 P1 A0 woman who received no prenatal care gives birth to a child with microcephaly. APGAR scores are 6 and 8 at 1 and 5 minutes, respectively. The infant's respirations are labored, and a patent ductus arteriosus is revealed in the workup. The infant also has cataracts. The mother recalls having a low-grade fever and sore throat for about 3 days during the first month of the pregnancy. What is the most likely acquired cause of the infant's symptoms?

A. Syphilis
B. Herpes simplex
C. Toxoplasmosis
D. HIV
E. Rubella

2.32. The level of intellectual disability in children with autism spectrum disorder is usually in what range?

A. 70 to 85
B. 50 to 69
C. 35 to 49
D. <34

2.33. Parents are concerned about their 15-month-old daughter who has not yet developed meaningful verbal communication. She says a few words, but mostly repeats the last word or two that her parents say when they address her. She does not initiate engagement with them unless she needs something. She is content rocking on a rocking horse toy almost continuously for hours on end. When told she has to stop and go to bed or eat, she screams until she either tires herself out or is allowed back onto the toy. She also screams if they try to feed her something other than strained peas and soggy cereal flakes. A hearing test is normal, and a nonverbal cognitive test for young children reveals an IQ of 70 and average adaptive skills. Chromosome testing is negative for abnormalities. What type of therapy is necessary for the best possible prognosis for this child?

A. Speech therapy
B. Social skills training
C. Cognitive behavioral therapy (CBT)
D. Neurofeedback
E. Risperidone therapy

2.34. Atomoxetine treats ADHD by what mechanism?

A. Alpha-2 agonism
B. Norepinephrine and dopamine reuptake inhibition
C. Norepinephrine reuptake inhibition
D. Dopamine reuptake inhibition
E. Facilitation of dopamine release

2.35. A 17-year-old boy is taken to the ER by his parents after they found him shivering in the bathroom and vomiting. When they tried to lift him up, he winced in pain and vomited. His parents state that they are sure he has been using drugs again because "he went to a party 2 days ago and did not come home until yesterday." He refuses to answer questions. Temperature is 98.8F, BP 140/90, pulse 105, respirations 20. On examination, the patient is diaphoretic and tremulous, with piloerection. He guards during the abdominal examination. Pupils are dilated. What is the most likely diagnosis?

A. LSD overdose
B. Alcohol withdrawal
C. 3,4-methylenedioxymethamphetamine (MDMA) overdose
D. Heroin withdrawal
E. Cocaine overdose

2.36. What is the most commonly tried substance by high school seniors?

A. Marijuana
B. Cigarettes
C. Alcohol
D. Inhalants
E. Vaping

ANSWERS

2.1. B. The extent of her social functioning
In addition to cognitive testing, which provides an IQ score, a diagnosis of intellectual disability requires an assessment of adaptive functioning, which includes social functioning and performance of everyday tasks. The psychological testing should include a standardized measure of adaptive functioning. As the concern is whether or not the child has an intellectual disability, the etiology, such as from chronic exposure to leaded paint in an old home, or low exposure to language, would not alter the diagnosis, though it could alter the prognosis. A child can have an intellectual disability with or without difficulty with physical milestones. (93, 96)

2.2. D. 50 to 69
Approximately 85% of individuals with intellectual disability are in the mild range, with an IQ between 50 and 69, and mild deficits in social and communication skills. About 10% are in the moderate range, with an IQ between 35 and 49. About 4% are in the severe range, with an IQ between 20 and 34, and about 1% fall in the profound range, with an IQ less than 20. An IQ between 70 and 80 was called borderline intellectual functioning in the DSM-IV. This is now no longer a diagnosis in the DSM-V-TR. (95)

2.3. B. Risperidone
Antipsychotics, particularly risperidone and aripiprazole, have shown effectiveness in the reduction of aggressive and self-injurious behaviors and explosive rage. Though the antipsychotics haloperidol and olanzapine could theoretically be effective, they have not been as studied for this indication in children as risperidone and aripiprazole. Melatonin is often used in children with autism spectrum disorder to help regulate sleep, but has no evidence for helping with aggression. Anticonvulsants do not have conclusive data for aggression. (99)

2.4. B. Senile plaques
Individuals with Down syndrome who are over age 40 have a high incidence of neurofibrillary tangles and senile plaques, which correlates with a decline in memory, self-care skills, and language, similar to that seen in individuals with Alzheimer dementia. There are anecdotal reports of arteriovenous malformations in individuals with Down syndrome, but this is not common. Decreased pigmentation of the substantia nigra is associated with Rett syndrome. Ventriculomegaly has been shown in some Down syndrome mice, but is not common in humans. Optic gliomas are seen in neurofibromatosis. (102)

2.5. D. Phenylketonuria (PKU)
This child's presentation is classic for PKU, which presents with severe intellectual disability if not diagnosed in the first few months of life. The musty breath is caused by a buildup of phenylketones in the body. Eczema is often present. Pale skin is due to phenylalanine not being converted into melanin. Neurologic problems can include seizures. Treatment consists of a low-phenylalanine diet. Though fragile X, Rett, autism spectrum disorder, and adrenoleukodystrophy all are causes of intellectual disability, their presentations are markedly different from PKU. Persons with fragile X have relatively strong communication skills. Rett overwhelmingly affects females, and presents with a decrease in communication skills around 12 months, as opposed to failure to develop those skills. Adrenoleukodystrophy symptoms begin around 5 to 8 years old, and intellectual disability is mild. The intellectual deficits of childhood disintegrative disorder begin around 3 to 4 years of age after normal intellectual development. (102)

2.6. A. A mutation of the FMR1 gene
A mutation of the FMR1 gene is the cause of fragile X syndrome, which is inherited from the mother, as opposed to Down syndrome, which is not inherited and usually caused by a nondisjunction during meiosis. A deletion in chromosome 5 is the cause of Cri-du-chat syndrome, and a deletion in chromosome 15 is the cause of Prader–Willi syndrome. The presence of the NF2 gene on chromosome 22 leads to neurofibromatosis type 2. A nondisjunction of chromosome 21 leads to one of the chromosomal aberrations in Down syndrome. (100–103)

2.7. D. Hearing test
Though the child appears to have a mixed receptive and expressive language disorder, an audiogram must be done first to rule out a hearing impairment, as deafness or hard of hearing can account for the child's presentation. Once that step has been completed, further laboratory and imaging procedures may be warranted based on history and observation of the child. (112)

2.8. A. Observation only
The child has speech sound disorder, which he will likely naturally outgrow in a year or two. If the

phonologic difficulty continues past that time, he should start speech therapy. Given that he is showing no other speech difficulties, an audiogram or neurologic testing is not needed at this time. He is showing no signs of intellectual delay, so an IQ test is not needed. (116)

2.9. D. Pragmatics
Autism spectrum disorder, by definition, includes social communication deficits. Pragmatics involves the skill of using language, including discerning intent behind words and understanding the context of what is being expressed. Phonology is the ability to produce sounds to make words. Deficits in this domain are seen in language disorders such as expressive (such as speech sound disorder) or mixed expressive–receptive language disorders. Grammar refers to the organization and rules of word placement to form language. Semantics involves the acquisition of words and the meaning of words or sentences. (107, 120)

2.10. D. Autism spectrum disorder (ASD)
The confluence of symptoms is most consistent with ASD. About 30% of children with ASD are intellectually disabled, so this is not a necessary feature of the diagnosis. An IQ of 85 is not in the range of mild intellectual disability. Though he has difficulty with social communication, it is in the context of other symptoms of ASD such as repetitive movements and restricted interests. Given that his verbal abilities are normal, it is unlikely that he has a hearing deficit. He demonstrates stereotypic movements, but similar to the social communication deficits, this is in the context of ASD, so that is the most likely diagnosis. (125–127)

2.11. C. Stimulant medication
The child is exhibiting symptoms of attention-deficit hyperactivity disorder (ADHD), inattentive type, for which stimulant medication is the first-line treatment. Nonstimulant medications, such as atomoxetine or alpha-agonists, are considered second or third line. If she were to show features of absence seizures, then a neurologic referral, and possibly an anticonvulsant, would be warranted. Behavior modification and parent management training can be helpful psychosocial treatment adjuncts to medication. (135–138)

2.12. A. Stimulant medication
Similar to pharmacological treatment of ADHD in children, stimulant medications, particularly long-acting preparations, are first line. Modafinil has scant evidence for treatment efficacy in adults and no FDA approval for ADHD. (141)

2.13. B. Standardized reading testing
IQ testing is helpful in that it allows for comparison of the child's specific deficits to their overall cognitive performance. However, for all specific learning disorders, standardized testing in that cognitive domain (also known as achievement testing) must be obtained. For specific learning disorder with impairment in reading, that would include spelling, writing, language, and design copying assessments. Observation of the child could be helpful to assist with student and teacher strategies to help him become less frustrated with reading. Adaptive function testing is used to assess social and life-skills functioning, and is necessary for the diagnosis of intellectual disability. Continuous performance testing is used to track progress with treatment for attention-deficit hyperactivity disorder (ADHD). (142–143)

2.14. D. Parental psychoeducation
This child's presentation and time course of tics are consistent with a diagnosis of Tourette syndrome. Because the child does not appear bothered by the motor and vocal tics, and social and school functioning do not appear to be impaired, treatment is not necessary. Instead, the parents should be given information about Tourette, including the most likely course of the disorder and when treatment should begin. If the tics were of moderate severity, behavioral interventions such as habit reversal training would be indicated. If they were severe and causing disruptions in school and social functioning, medication, such as risperidone, which is considered first-line pharmacologic treatment due to evidence and efficacy, may be warranted. Cognitive behavioral therapy has not been shown to reduce tics without some other concurrent intervention. (159–160)

2.15. C. Order a swallowing study
The child is displaying signs of avoidant/restrictive food intake disorder (ARFID), which consists of a lack of interest in and/or avoidance of food. Signs include failure to gain weight as expected, food refusal, and eating too little. Because infants with ARFID become irritable or withdrawn when feeding, mothers may subsequently not engage as much during feeding as they would otherwise. This child is starting to fall off of her growth curve, but not drastically, so hospitalization is not warranted at

this time. There are no signs of abuse or neglect, so child protective services does not need to be involved. One of the first steps in the workup is to rule out medical causes, so a swallowing study should be ordered to make sure there is not a structural etiology. Though referral to a psychiatrist or a home health nurse may eventually become part of the treatment plan, a medical cause should still first be ruled out. (166–167)

2.16. D. Disinhibited social engagement disorder
The child is displaying signs of disinhibited social engagement disorder, in which she has little hesitation around adult strangers, willingness to go off with an adult stranger, increased familiarity with adult strangers, and lack of checking back with her parents in this unfamiliar situation. She also has been subject to neglect and likely deprivation. A normally developing child would protest being taken away from her parents by a stranger, even from abusive parents, and would not be overly familiar with adult strangers. These same circumstances could have resulted in reactive attachment disorder and caused her to behave in the opposite manner toward adults, that of not responding to comfort and showing little affect and social responsiveness. Not enough is known about her history or current functioning to diagnose PTSD, and given that she was just rescued, it would be difficult to argue that the traumatic event is truly over. (167–168)

2.17. B. Cognitive behavioral therapy (CBT)
Though sertraline is FDA approved for PTSD in adults, there is little evidence to support its use in children and adolescents. There is also little to no evidence for alpha-agonists and antipsychotics for the core symptoms of PTSD in children. CBT, specifically trauma-focused CBT, has demonstrated efficacy in the treatment of childhood PTSD. Though EMDR shows efficacy in some studies, it is not considered first line, and is somewhat controversial. (172)

2.18. E. Irritability
The criteria for major depressive disorder in children are the same for that in adults with the exception that irritability can be used as a symptom instead of depressed mood. Though depressed children may demonstrate aggression, regression, crying, and oppositional behavior, those behaviors are not sufficient to make the diagnosis. (174)

2.19. C. Change to another SSRI
The child displays symptoms consistent with a diagnosis of persistent depressive disorder that is resistant to treatment. According to both the Treatment of SSRI-Resistant Depression in Adolescents (TORDIA) study and a consensus group from the Texas Children's Medication Algorithm Project (TMAP), the next step is a change to another SSRI. If this is unsuccessful, the next step would be to consider augmenting with psychotherapy and/or changing from an SSRI to a different class of medication, though the argument could be made that she should have been started on a combination of an SSRI and psychotherapy. (175, 177–179)

2.20. B. Emergently admit the child to a hospital
The patient is currently suicidal with an explicitly stated plan with the most lethal and often-used means, for males, that results in suicide completion. He meets criteria for major depressive disorder with loss of interest in activities, depressed mood, decreased appetite, sleep and energy, and suicidal ideation. He should be emergently admitted to a hospital for safety until the acute risk of a suicide attempt has passed. While he will likely be started on an SSRI as well as psychotherapy in the hospital, the acuteness of the situation precludes waiting for either treatment modality to take effect. Given the information that the child and parents have already provided, no further evaluation in an ER is necessary. (180)

2.21. D. Disruptive mood dysregulation disorder (DMDD)
The boy is showing signs of DMDD. One of the most challenging aspects of making the diagnosis is the differential (185–186). Children with this presentation are often diagnosed with bipolar disorder. However, bipolar disorder consists of distinct mood episodes, as opposed to chronic irritability and moodiness. ODD, by definition, includes defiance to authority figures. Children with DMDD can have outbursts that are provoked by nonauthority figures as well. DMDD also requires that the outbursts be present in at least two settings, as opposed to just one for ODD. While DMDD outbursts can also result in physical harm to others, conduct disorder involves intentionally violating the rights of others by physical aggression or other means (189). Though children with intermittent explosive disorder also respond to a situation with aggression grossly disproportionate to the precipitating factor, after and between episodes, the episodes are discrete, with no aggression between them. (553)

2.22. C. 2.5 years
Normal separation anxiety typically peaks between 9 and 18 months of age and diminishes by around

2.5 years of age. This is in contrast to separation anxiety disorder, which can be diagnosed when normal separation anxiety is no longer developmentally appropriate, and anxiety significantly interferes with daily social and/or school functioning, if applicable. While children would be expected to have a flare of separation anxiety when introduced to a novel situation in which they are apart from their parents, such as starting school, this anxiety typically soon resolves. (194–195)

2.23. B. Suicidality
In October 2004, the FDA placed a "black-box" warning indicating that the use of certain antidepressants to treat major depressive disorder in adolescents may increase the risk of suicidal ideations and behaviors. In 2007, the FDA amended the black-box warning to state that depression carries an increased risk of suicide itself. To date, no childhood study of anxiety has found a statistically significant increase in suicidal thoughts or behaviors after treatment with an SSRI. (199)

2.24. B. Cognitive behavioral therapy (CBT)
The child is displaying symptoms of severe social anxiety, in that both social and occupational (school) functioning are disrupted. Evidence-based studies support the concurrent use of an SSRI and CBT. Though beta-blockers and buspirone have been used anecdotally in children for performance anxiety, no data support their efficacy. Interpersonal therapy is a treatment for major depressive disorder. Exposure and response prevention is the treatment of choice for obsessive–compulsive disorder. To date, randomized controlled clinical trials have shown no differences in symptom reduction in youth using benzodiazepines, though they are sometimes used for this purpose. (195, 198–200)

2.25. A. Cognitive behavioral therapy
Selective mutism is diagnosed when a child does not speak in certain situations, usually those of high stress such as school, but speaks normally in other, less-stressful situations. To that end, hearing is not an issue. The first-line treatment for school-aged children is cognitive behavioral therapy. SSRIs may be helpful for selective mutism, but this has not to date been borne out by the evidence. Family education can be beneficial, but it is not first line. Children with selective mutism may have delayed speech and language acquisition, but their speech is fluent, and speech therapy is not usually indicated. Beta-blockers have not been studied in selective mutism. (201–203)

2.26. B. Tourette
OCD in children is often comorbid with anxiety disorders, ADHD, and Tourette syndrome. The level of comorbidity among ADHD, OCD, and Tourette is high enough that the possibility of a shared genetic vulnerability is being studied. (204)

2.27. E. Chronic deterioration
The child's symptoms are consistent with childhood-onset schizophrenia, which is rare at this age and should be, as in adults, a diagnosis of exclusion. A younger age of onset is associated with a more chronic, severe course, with worse outcomes in cognitive and social domains than those of adult-onset schizophrenia, and increased severity of brain abnormalities. (207)

2.28. C. Marijuana
Multiple studies have now suggested a causative link between marijuana and schizophrenia, with others supporting an exacerbating effect of marijuana on schizophrenia (https://www.ncbi.nlm.nih.gov/pmc/articles/PMC7442038/). Other risks of chronic marijuana use include poor cognitive functioning, higher rates of motor vehicle accidents, impaired respiratory functioning, and increased risk for cardiovascular disease. (213)

2.29. C. Moderate
The man's intellectual deficits place him in the moderate range of intellectual disability. As expected, he is able to perform unskilled or semi-skilled tasks under appropriate supervision. Cognitive functioning, including speech, has not progressed beyond the third-grade level. An individual with mild intellectual disability would perform cognitively around the sixth-grade level, and would be expected to achieve minimal self-support. (94–95)

2.30. E. Seizures
Individuals with intellectual disability are more likely to have seizures than those in the general population. Alzheimer disease and hypotonia (in newborns) are found more in Down syndrome than in the general population. Decreased pigmentation of the substantia nigra, which can lead to Parkinson disease, is found in Rett syndrome. Ataxia is often found in adrenoleukodystrophy. (98)

2.31. E. Rubella
Cataracts, congenital heart defects, and microcephaly are symptoms of an infant born to a mother who was infected with rubella during the first trimester,

especially the first month, of pregnancy. Other symptoms include hearing difficulties and microphthalmia. Acquired rubella is the primary cause of intellectual disability caused by maternal infection. The other acquired infections are also causes of intellectual disability. (104)

2.32. D. <34
About 30% of children with autism spectrum disorder have intellectual disability, with 45% to 50% of those in the severe (IQ 20 to 34)-to-profound (IQ <20) range, making it the most common level of intellectual disability. An additional 30% of those with intellectual disability have IQs in the mild-to-moderate range. (124)

2.33. A. Speech therapy
The child shows symptoms consistent with autism spectrum disorder: restricted/fixed interests (the rocking horse), deficits in emotional reciprocity (poor engagement with parents), and an inability to adapt to change (insistence on the same food for every meal). Acquiring meaningful communicative language by ages 5 to 7 years will give her the best prognosis. As she is not deaf and has an IQ of 70, she will likely be able to make progress with verbal communication. Social skills training will likely be helpful, but is not the factor that leads to the best prognosis. Risperidone could be helpful for severe irritability. Neurofeedback is being studied for use in attention-deficit hyperactivity disorder (ADHD) and anxiety. CBT is being studied to help with anxiety, depression, and obsessive–compulsive disorder (OCD) in children with autism spectrum disorder. (127)

2.34. C. Norepinephrine reuptake inhibition
Atomoxetine is a norepinephrine reuptake inhibitor used in the treatment of ADHD. Clonidine and guanfacine are alpha-2 agonists. Bupropion inhibits reuptake of norepinephrine and dopamine. Modafinil is a dopamine reuptake inhibitor. Amphetamine facilitates dopamine release. (135)

2.35. D. Heroin withdrawal
Physical heroin withdrawal symptoms consist of nausea and vomiting, dilated pupils, sweating, anxiety, abdominal cramping, insomnia, diarrhea, and muscle aches. Symptoms begin a few hours after ingestion, peak 48 to 72 hours later, and last about a week, depending on chronicity of use. Cocaine intoxication also includes dilated pupils, increased heart rate, and hypertension, but also hyperthermia, so history in timing of symptoms is crucial for making the diagnosis. Similarly, MDMA intoxication can result in tachycardia and hyperthermia as well as fatigue and muscle spasms. LSD overdose can produce visual hallucinations and delusions. Alcohol withdrawal can include nausea, vomiting, sweating, and insomnia around 6 hours after the last drink. Symptoms 2 days afterward can include fever, heavy sweating, and hypertension, and delirium tremens in a chronic drinker. Given all of the similarities in this syndrome with other drug intoxication/withdrawal syndromes, the muscle aches and piloerection are distinguishing features. (213)

2.36. C. Alcohol
By senior year of high school, 92% of males and 73% of females have tried alcohol, making it the most often–tried substance. Less than half of high school seniors have tried marijuana and cigarettes, though the use of cigarettes is plummeting while the use of vaping is rising. Less than 20% have used inhalants. (212)

3

Neurocognitive Disorders

3.1. A 75-year-old woman in an assisted living facility becomes irritable several evenings a week about an hour after dinner, and questions where she is and how she got there. She has a standing order of as-needed quetiapine, which settles her and helps her sleep through the night. When she wakes in the morning, she is alert and oriented to person, place, and time, socializes easily with the staff and friends she has made, and does not recall much of her behavior from the night before. What neurotransmitter most likely plays the primary role in the patient's evening behaviors?

A. Acetylcholine
B. Dopamine
C. Ciprofloxacin
D. Glutamate
E. Serotonin

3.2. A 75-year-old woman is brought to the emergency department by her son, with whom she lives, due to intermittent periods of agitation, increased forgetfulness, and memory difficulties. Symptoms suddenly began 3 days ago and come and go with no apparent precipitating factors. Her son is especially concerned because she wandered out of the house last night looking for her husband who died 7 years ago. When her son asked her this morning where her husband was, she replied, "Son, you know he's been dead for 7 years!" She is diagnosed with hypertension, Alzheimer dementia, and diabetes, and takes hydrochlorothiazide (HCTZ), memantine, and metformin, all of which she has been out of for the last week due to a delay in the arrival of the mail-order medications. Examination shows a thin female who looks her stated age, in no acute distress. Vital signs are normal. O₂ saturation is 96% on room air. Complete blood count (CBC) shows leukocytosis, and urinalysis shows 2+ protein and moderate bacteria. What medication would most likely resolve this patient's symptoms?

A. HCTZ
B. Metformin
C. Metronidazole
D. Memantine
E. Haloperidol

3.3. One of the earliest and most prominent features of dementia is the decline of what function?

A. Attention
B. Memory
C. Executive function
D. Social cognition
E. Language

3.4. As opposed to delirium, what aspect of neurocognition remains intact in dementia?

A. Attention
B. Orientation
C. Memory
D. Consciousness
E. Social skills

3.5. An 82-year-old man presents to the primary care clinic along with his daughter for a routine visit. He last saw his primary care physician a year ago. He is diagnosed with coronary artery disease and atherosclerosis. He states that he is having problems remembering where he put his car keys and the names of his grandchildren, "but otherwise, my mind is as sharp as it ever was!" Vital signs are within normal limits. Physical examination reveals no acute abnormalities. After the doctor walks out of the room, the patient's daughter follows him and says "It's much worse than forgetting his car keys. I had to hide them at first, then had to disable the car, because it seems like once he turned 75 he started getting lost on the way home. He stayed like that for a while, then started forgetting his grandkids' names about a year ago. Then last month, he suddenly started developing headaches and said he felt dizzy." His memory has not gotten worse, but has not improved. What is the most likely diagnosis?

A. Vascular dementia
B. Delirium
C. Transient ischemic attacks
D. Alzheimer dementia
E. Normal aging

3.6. What is the average length of time until death once an individual is diagnosed with dementia of the Alzheimer type?

A. 3 years
B. 8 years
C. 13 years
D. 18 years
E. 23 years

3.7. Emergency medical services are called to the home of a 74-year-old man by his home health nurse who, upon arriving to work, discovered that he had fallen and was covered in urine and feces. She reports to the emergency medical technician (EMT) that she witnessed him passing out and falling to the ground after getting out of bed a week ago, and was able to get him back into the bed. She states that over the past 3 years he has had progressive difficulty remembering the names of his children and grandchildren, and that over the last month, he has been asking her to put the dog outside. When I tell him he does not have a dog, he points and says, 'The dog is standing right there! Put him outside!'" Despite getting 9 hours of sleep a night, he often seems drowsy, but then "perks up 10 minutes later, then gets sleepy again an hour later." She has been concerned about the way he walks. Temperature is 99.1 F, BP 110/70 sitting, 80/55 standing. Pulse is 80 sitting and 85 standing. Respirations 18. Cogwheeling rigidity is noted in his arms, along with a resting tremor. What is the most likely cerebral pathology?

A. Blanching of the substantia nigra
B. Pick bodies in the frontotemporal regions
C. Multiple subcortical white matter infarctions
D. Amyloid plaques in the cortex and hippocampus
E. Lewy inclusion bodies in the cerebral cortex

3.8. A person with an amnestic disorder is most likely to be able to correctly answer what mental status examination question posed to them?

   A. "Flag, ball, tree. Can you repeat those three words?"
   B. "What did you have for breakfast this morning?"
   C. "What is the name of this building?"
   D. "What is today's date?"
   E. "Where did you go yesterday?"

3.9. A 60-year-old man is brought to the outpatient clinic by his daughter, who reports that her father calls several times during the day. He is always surprised when she tells him that they had already talked earlier, after which he usually says that he wanted to ask her one more thing. When she is at his house, she notices that he asks her several times if she would like him to make her lunch, even though she has told him that she has already eaten. He then will tell her that he could not have asked that question already because she would have taken off her shoes if she had eaten. She first noticed the memory loss a couple years ago, and notes that it has gotten worse over the last year since his wife died and he has lived alone. She is concerned that he is not eating well, as his wife did all the cooking, and believes that he has lost 10 pounds since she died. She has been especially concerned because she has smelled alcohol on his breath a few times when she has visited him. He has hypertension and is on an angiotensin-converting enzyme (ACE) inhibitor, which she makes sure he takes daily. Blood pressure is 140/90. Other vitals are within normal limits. During the cognitive examination, he confidently gives incorrect answers to the three-word recall, even explaining the associations he made between the words in his mind to help him remember them. What is the most appropriate treatment for this patient?

   A. Selective serotonin reuptake inhibitor (SSRI)
   B. Thiamine replacement
   C. A cholinesterase inhibitor
   D. An increase in antihypertensive medication
   E. An N-methyl-D-aspartate (NMDA) receptor antagonist

3.10. A 66-year-old woman wakes from anesthesia following a round of electroconvulsive therapy (ECT) for chronic depression. The patient is most likely to demonstrate difficulty when asked which of the following questions to test memory?

   A. "What did you have for dinner last night?"
   B. "What are the names of your children?"
   C. "What is your birthdate?"
   D. "What were the three words I just asked you?"
   E. "Where do you currently live?"

3.11. A 14-year-old boy is brought to the emergency department (ED) by emergency medical services (EMS) after being unconscious for about 60 seconds. His parents report that he was playing football in the driveway with the neighborhood children when he and another boy collided, and he fell and hit his head on the pavement. He was not wearing a helmet. When he regained consciousness he was lethargic, which prompted them to take him to the ED. The child is fully awake, complaining of a headache, and looks confused. Neurologic examination is normal. Vital signs are within normal limits. When asked by his parents what he remembers about the accident, what is the most likely response?

   A. "Who are you people?"
   B. "I was playing football, got tackled, and fell and hit my head."
   C. "What accident?"
   D. "We were in the car and another car hit us."
   E. "Someone was running toward me, then I blacked out."

3.12. Cerebrovascular disease is most likely to cause amnesia when it affects the hippocampus and what other area of the brain?

   A. Medial thalamus
   B. Corpus callosum
   C. Suprachiasmatic nucleus
   D. Substantia nigra
   E. Arcuate nucleus

3.13. A 55-year-old woman is brought to the emergency department (ED) by EMS from a restaurant where she had been eating lunch with her best friend 15 minutes ago. The friend states that the patient suddenly looked confused and repeatedly asked where she was and how she got there, even though she was given the answers several times. Her friend, fearing that the patient was suffering from a stroke, called 911. In the ED, the friend tells the care team that the patient has no history of seizures or head injury, and has only been diagnosed with mild hypertension. Vital signs are normal. The patient is able to give her name and the name of her friend, but continuously has to be told that she is at the hospital. Consciousness is intact. Urine drug screen is negative, and comprehensive metabolic profile, CBC, head CT, and EKG reveal no abnormalities. Neurologic examination is normal. What is the most likely prognosis for her memory over the next 24 hours?

A. She will forget everyone but herself
B. Memory loss symptoms will wax and wane
C. She will regain past memories but not be able to form new ones
D. Memory loss will remain the same
E. She will make a complete recovery

3.14. As opposed to amnestic disorders, a person with dementia of the Alzheimer type would have impairment in what area of functioning?

A. Anterograde memory
B. Retrograde memory
C. Episodic memory
D. Semantic memory

3.15. The likelihood of benzodiazepines causing amnesia is increased with the addition of what substance?

A. Alcohol
B. Anticholinergics
C. Psychedelics
D. Barbiturates
E. Stimulants

3.16. A 34-year-old woman is at home talking with her spouse when she begins to make chewing movements, then stops talking and stares for about 30 seconds. Over the next 3 months, she has these episodes two to three times a week. She has no other medical or psychiatric conditions, and her only medication is that used to treat the described condition. What psychiatric abnormality is she most likely to experience between episodes?

A. Psychosis
B. Violent behavior
C. Personality changes
D. Manic symptoms
E. Depression symptoms

3.17. A 14-year-old boy is brought to a neurologist by his parents after experiencing several episodes during which he stops what he is doing and stares for several seconds. He is embarrassed afterward, and says he knew he was staring, "but I could not snap out of it." An EEG-captured event shows seizure activity over the temporal lobe. What is the most likely type of seizure he is experiencing?

A. Generalized seizure
B. Absence seizure
C. Simple partial
D. Complex partial
E. Psychogenic nonepileptic

3.18. A brain tumor that affects memory is most likely located in which region of the brain?

A. Parietal
B. Temporal
C. Occipital
D. Frontal
E. Cerebellum

3.19. A 23-year-male is driving too fast around a curve, loses control of the vehicle, and hits a tree. Though his body is held in place by his seatbelt, his head lurches forward, then slams back against the headrest, and he loses consciousness. When he awakens in the emergency department, he cannot recall the event. A head CT shows no acute bleeding and neurologic examination shows no focal deficits. He is diagnosed with a concussion and discharged with a neurology appointment in a week. What will be the most likely cognitive finding on neuropsychological testing?

A. Decreased information processing speed
B. Difficulty understanding spoken language
C. Impaired writing ability
D. Deficits in reading nonverbal cues
E. Impaired coordination between left and right hands

3.20. A 60-year-old man presents to a primary care physician with his wife due to a progression of weakness, unsteady gait, and loss of coordination over the last year. His wife adds that he has become irritable and neglectful of his duties at work as an assembly lineman and around the house, which is "so unlike him. He's always been the sweetest, most conscientious person I know." She adds that he occasionally appears to talk to his brother who died 5 years ago. He has had no medical care in the past 30 years. Vital signs are within normal limits. Physical examination reveals a well-developed, well-nourished male who appears slightly older than stated age. He has diminished lower extremity reflexes and vibration sense. Pupils are small and poorly reactive to light but react briskly to accommodation. What medication would be most helpful for this patient's condition?

A. Doxycycline
B. Penicillin
C. Radioactive iodine
D. Dolutegravir/rilpivirine
E. Acyclovir

3.21. A 55-year-old man is brought to the emergency department (ED) by EMS after being found in a park by passersby mumbling to himself and covered in watery feces. In the ED, the man mostly mumbles incoherently when asked questions, but is able to give his name and age. The EMS workers state that they have seen him for years sleeping under bridges and on park benches. Blood pressure is 90/60 and heart rate is 100. Temperature and respirations are within normal limits. Physical examination reveals a cachectic man with global wasting who looks older than his stated age. Neurologic examination is normal. A well-defined, pigmented, glossy rash is present on the dorsum of his hands and feet, and around his neck. Urine drug screen is negative, as is a head CT. Throughout the workup, his consciousness waxes and wanes. This patient's condition is caused by what vitamin deficiency?

A. A
B. B1 (thiamine)
C. B3 (niacin)
D. B12 (cyanocobalamin)
E. C

3.22. A 35-year-old man presents to his primary care physician with complaints of irritability, restlessness, difficulty concentrating, and insomnia over the past 2 months. He has not experienced these symptoms before, and has no medical illnesses and is on no medications. He works in construction, and notes that he has been working a lot of overtime over the past 9 months due to the recent demand for new houses. He adds that he has noticed some clumsiness and muscle pain as well, which are starting to interfere with his job. Blood pressure is 140/90. Other vital signs are within normal limits. BMI is 21. Physical examination reveals a well-developed, well-nourished male in no acute distress. Neurologic examination reveals no focal neurologic abnormalities. A complete metabolic panel shows no abnormalities. The patient's symptoms can be explained by chronic exposure to what toxin?

A. Lead
B. Mercury
C. Manganese
D. Arsenic
E. Toluene

ANSWERS

3.1. A. Acetylcholine
Sundowning is a type of delirium that occurs usually in elderly who have a diagnosis of dementia. The phenomenon is marked by confusion and behavioral changes. Though symptoms are often mitigated with an antipsychotic, which acts primarily on dopamine and, in some medications, serotonin, the primary neurotransmitter involved in delirium is thought to be acetylcholine. (226)

3.2. C. Metronidazole
The patient is displaying symptoms of delirium, including waxing and waning of consciousness, visual hallucinations, and impaired judgment. When possible, the underlying cause should be treated. In this case, the likely underlying cause is the urinary tract infection, as opposed to being off of HCTZ, memantine, and metformin for a week. Though haloperidol may temporarily alleviate the symptoms, it will not ultimately resolve them. (228)

3.3. B. Memory
Though dementia can affect many cognitive functions such as attention, executive function, social cognition, and language, memory is usually an early and prominent feature. (233)

3.4. D. Consciousness
Whereas, by definition, delirium involves a waxing and waning of consciousness, consciousness is preserved and remains clear in dementia. Deficits in attention, orientation, memory, and social skills can be present in both dementia and delirium. (233)

3.5. A. Vascular dementia
Memory problems to the extent that he gets lost driving home cannot be attributed to normal aging, as he is demonstrating significant impairment in functioning. The son does not report changes in consciousness, which rules out delirium. Though Alzheimer is the most common dementia, it is characterized by a gradual, progressive course of symptoms, as opposed to vascular dementia, in which symptoms typically occur in a stepwise fashion. Because he is not recovering between episodes, these are not transient ischemic attacks, after which function is regained. (236)

3.6. B. 8 years
Alzheimer dementia is a terminal illness, as the accumulation of plaques and tangles throughout the brain and the loss of brain tissue leads to progressive severity of impairment. Affected individuals lose the ability to swallow, which greatly increases the risk of aspiration pneumonia, dehydration, and cachexia. Other causes of death include pulmonary embolism and cardiovascular disease. The average life expectancy after diagnosis is 8 years. (238)

3.7. E. Lewy inclusion bodies in the cerebral cortex
Memory impairment with the presence of visual hallucinations, autonomic disturbances, and Parkinsonian symptoms (cogwheeling, resting tremor, bradykinesia) are symptoms of Lewy body disease. The Lewy inclusion bodies are found in the cerebral cortex. Parkinson disease, with its blanching of the substantia nigra, is not associated with visual hallucinations. Alzheimer disease, characterized by amyloid plaques in the cortex and hippocampus, also does not usually feature visual hallucinations. Subcortical white matter infarctions are the hallmark of Binswanger disease, also called subcortical arteriosclerotic encephalopathy, in which the main characteristic is psychomotor slowness. The Pick bodies are the pathognomonic sign of frontotemporal dementia, which is marked by personality and behavioral changes. (242–244)

3.8. A. "Flag, ball, tree. Can you repeat those three words?"
Short-term and recent memory are usually impaired in amnestic disorder, so a person likely would not be able to answer questions about what they ate that day or what activities they engaged in the day before. In severe amnestic disorder, orientation to place and time can be impaired. However, immediate memory remains intact, so a person can recall numbers or words right after they are said. The person would likely not be able to remember them for a 5-minute recall. (246)

3.9. B. Thiamine replacement
The amnesia is most likely due to poor nutritional deficiency and lack of thiamine in the diet, which is the cause of Korsakoff syndrome. This is often seen with chronic alcohol use. One of the hallmarks is confabulation, in which a person tries to cover up memory loss by filling in the gaps with a story, which can range from completely plausible to completely implausible. The proper treatment is to replace thiamine, which may lead to improvement after 3 months. Cholinesterase inhibitors and NMDA receptor antagonists can be useful for

Alzheimer dementia. An SSRI could be helpful if depression were thought to be the reason for the cognitive deficits. Better hypertension control could be helpful for vascular dementia. (246)

3.10. D. "What were the three words I just asked you?"

ECT is associated with anterograde amnesia for a few hours after a treatment. During this time, the patient may have difficulty forming new memories, and would therefore have trouble with a three-word recall. The patient would likely also have trouble remembering past events that occurred a few minutes before the treatment. (247)

3.11. C. "What accident?"

If a head injury results in amnesia, it will most likely be for the period of time leading up to the event and for the event itself. Therefore, the child is most likely simply not going to remember the accident. Confabulating a story (being in a car accident) would be most associated with Korsakoff syndrome. It is unlikely that he would forget his parents, who he has known all of his life. (247)

3.12. A. Medial thalamus

Cerebrovascular diseases which affect the bilateral medial thalamus are often associated with amnestic disorder. In addition to the hippocampus, lesions affecting the cerebellum, amygdala, and prefrontal cortex could also affect different types of memory. The suprachiasmatic nucleus is associated with circadian rhythm. The substantia nigra is associated with movement disorders such as Parkinson. Lesions affecting the corpus callosum can be associated with a myriad of dysfunctions. The arcuate nucleus regulates several functions of homeostasis. (247)

3.13. E. She will make a complete recovery

Transient global amnesia is marked by an abrupt onset of both retrograde and anterograde amnesia in the absence of delirium. Occasionally, the person may not be able to perform well-learned tasks. The vast majority of people make a complete recovery within 24 hours. (247)

3.14. D. Semantic memory

Dementia of the Alzheimer type leads to more severe loss of function and memory than amnestic disorder. While both can affect anterograde, retrograde, and episodic memory, amnestic disorders do not lead to loss of language, general knowledge (semantic memory), or praxis (the planning of movement to achieve a purpose). (248)

3.15. A. Alcohol

Benzodiazepines are the most commonly used prescription drugs that can cause amnesia. This effect is magnified when combined with alcohol, which can lead to anterograde and retrograde amnesia. (249)

3.16. C. Personality changes

The person in the scenario is having complex partial seizures, the most common type of seizure in adults. As she has repeated episodes, she can be diagnosed with epilepsy. The most common psychiatric manifestation between episodes is personality changes, though interictal psychoses, violence, and mood disorder symptoms can also occur. The presence of these interictal phenomena should lead to questions about medication side effects and compliance. (251)

3.17. C. Simple partial

Seizures are characterized as generalized if they affect the entire brain, and partial if the seizure activity occurs in a circumscribed area. Partial seizures are complex if they involve a change in consciousness and simple if consciousness is preserved. The seizures in this patient would therefore be described as simple partial. Though absence seizures can have a similar presentation, they involve brief disruptions of consciousness during which the person loses contact with the environment. Psychogenic nonepileptic seizures would not show up on an EEG. (249–251)

3.18. B. Temporal

A temporal lobe tumor could cause problems with memory loss and speech. A frontal lobe tumor could cause problems with personality and executive functioning. A parietal lobe tumor could cause problems with speaking and understanding and reading/writing. Occipital lobe tumors could cause problems with sight, and a cerebellar tumor could cause problems with coordination and dizziness. (253)

3.19. A. Decreased information processing speed

The most common type of head trauma is blunt force, in which motor vehicle accidents are the most common cause. As with many brain injuries due to head trauma, there is an initial period of posttraumatic amnesia. Afterward, cognitive symptoms can arise, the most common of which are decreased information processing speed, and other frontal lobe symptoms such as impaired attention, increased distractibility, and problems sustaining effort. Language disabilities can also occur. (254)

3.20. B. Penicillin

One of the reasons that physicians test for syphilis in new-onset personality and behavior changes is because neurosyphilis can lead to general paresis, which appears 10 to 15 years after the infection (but can occur at any stage of infection) and affects the frontal lobes. Executive functioning is disrupted, leading to symptoms such as poor judgment, irritability, and decreased care for self. Untreated neurosyphilis can also lead to tabes dorsalis, a condition in which the nerves in the dorsal columns of the spinal cord degenerate, leading to ataxia, poor coordination, weakness, and diminished reflexes. General paresis and tabes dorsalis can coexist. The Argyll Robertson pupil (small bilateral pupils accommodate to focus on a near object but react poorly to light) is specific for neurosyphilis. Treatment is with penicillin for 10 to 14 days to eradicate the *Treponema* infection, though some symptoms may be permanent. Doxycycline would be used to treat Lyme disease, which can cause impaired cognition, irritability, and nerve pain, but not a change in reflexes or pupils. Acyclovir is used to treat herpes simplex encephalitis, which also leads to personality changes, memory loss, and psychotic symptoms, and can include seizures, headaches, and focal neurologic deficits. Dolutegravir/rilpivirine is used to treat HIV, which untreated, can lead to HIV mild neurocognitive disorder and HIV-associated dementia. Clinical manifestations of neurosyphilis in a person with HIV infection may be more common. If this patient were also affected with HIV, he would likely be showing many more signs and symptoms of that infection. Radioactive iodine is used to treat hyperthyroidism, which can present with anxiety, irritability, and tremulousness, but not ataxia or the other neurologic symptoms exhibited by the patient. (255)

3.21. C. B3 (niacin)

Delirium, diarrhea, dermatitis, and dementia are four of the "five Ds" in pellagra, the disease caused by niacin deficiency (the fifth is death). Though relatively rare in developed nations, this disease can present in persons in conditions that can lead to chronic malnourishment, such as anorexia, alcohol abuse, and homelessness. Though the psychiatric manifestations of pellagra can be seen in other dietary deficiencies, the dermatitis is almost pathognomonic for pellagra. Scurvy, due to a deficiency of vitamin C, presents with delirium if untreated for a long time. B12 deficiency often presents with neurologic symptoms such as muscle weakness, unsteady movements, and numbness and tingling in addition to mental confusion. Thiamine deficiency leads to Wernicke–Korsakoff syndrome, which can present with delirium and dementia. Vitamin A deficiency does not have psychiatric manifestations. (261–262)

3.22. A. Lead

Lead can be found in solder, pipes, batteries, pottery, and roofing materials, among other substances, and can lead to slow poisoning in occupations such as auto repair, mining, and construction. The psychiatric manifestations of lead poisoning include difficulties with memory or concentration, mood symptoms, irritability, insomnia, and restlessness. Toxin exposure should be considered in new-onset psychiatric symptoms, especially when coupled with a predisposing history. These days, mercury poisoning can occur from contaminated fish or grain, and can also result in cognitive impairment, irritability, and depression. However, mercury poisoning includes neurologic signs such as visual field deficits and cerebellar ataxia. Manganese poisoning can also lead to irritability, but usually to somnolence, not insomnia, and can also be present in brick workers. Arsenic poisoning can cause altered mental status, but also a host of GI symptoms, such as vomiting, abdominal pain, and diarrhea, and can occur as a result of chronic exposure to herbicides. Toluene is a solvent found in substances including gasoline, glues, and paint, and chronic exposure over 5 to 10 years can lead to psychoorganic syndrome consisting of loss of concentration and memory, depression, and anxiety. It also leads to nerve, liver, and kidney damage. (262)

4

Substance Use and Addictive Disorders

4.1. A patient experiencing liver failure from alcohol, cravings to use again in spite of losing their job and marriage, and getting arrested for driving under the influence, would be classified as having which of the following alcohol disorders in the DSM-5?

A. Abuse
B. Addiction
C. Dependence
D. Intoxication
E. Use

4.2. The frequency of suicide in those with substance abuse is second only to which of the following psychiatric disorders?

A. Bipolar
B. Eating
C. Generalized anxiety
D. Major depressive
E. Panic

4.3. Which of the following pharmacologic agents is designed at helping tobacco dependence?

A. Acamprosate
B. Disulfiram
C. Levomethadyl acetate
D. Naltrexone
E. Varenicline

4.4. In the United States, which ethnic or racial group has the highest lifetime rate of substance use?

A. African Americans
B. American Indians
C. Asians
D. Caucasians
E. Hispanics

4.5. The locus coeruleus likely mediates the effects of which of the following drugs?

A. Amphetamines
B. Benzodiazepines
C. Cannabis
D. Nicotine
E. Opioids

4.6. Which range of blood alcohol concentration is considered to be the legal definition of intoxication in most states in the United States, as levels in this range have been shown to increase incoordination and cause errors in judgment.

A. 20 to 40 mg/dL
B. 40 to 60 mg/dL
C. 80 to 100 mg/dL
D. 200 to 250 mg/dL
E. >300 mg/dL

4.7. Which of the following signs or symptoms can be noted in alcohol withdrawal?

A. Bradycardia
B. Hypotension
C. Miotic pupils
D. Renal failure
E. Tremors

4.8. Long-term severe alcohol abuse can result in a seizure by lowering which of the following lab values?

A. Albumin
B. Ca
C. Creatinine
D. K
E. Na

4.9. A psychiatrist refers a middle-aged, alcoholic patient for a neurology evaluation after gait abnormalities were noted along with confusion and delusions. No signs of withdrawal are noted on examination and the patient does not appear acutely intoxicated and has mostly a linear thought process. Findings from the neurologist include normal vital signs, bilateral nystagmus, and pupils reacting unevenly to light. These findings are most consistent with which diagnosis?

A. Alcohol-induced psychotic disorder
B. Delirium tremens
C. Korsakoff syndrome
D. Unspecified alcohol-related disorder
E. Wernicke encephalopathy

4.10. A patient with heavy alcohol use reports all of the symptoms of a major depressive disorder. Which is the most appropriate initial treatment for most cases?

A. An atypical antipsychotic
B. A selective serotonin reuptake inhibitor
C. Education
D. Interpersonal psychotherapy
E. Naltrexone

4.11. A patient presents with alcohol dependence, fatigue, and insomnia, along with confusion noted on mental status examination. Reports of myoclonus and increased muscle resistance to movement were noted in the primary care doctor's notes. This patient should be tested for which of the following vitamin deficiencies?

A. Cyanocobalamin
B. D
C. Folic acid
D. Pantothenic acid
E. Thiamine

4.12. Which psychiatric diagnosis is one of the most common comorbid ones with alcohol-related disorders?

A. Anorexia nervosa
B. Antisocial personality
C. Attention-deficit hyperactivity
D. Autism spectrum
E. Schizophrenia

4.13. A patient with alcohol use disorder comes in for treatment for depression and insomnia. The psychiatrist highlights how impairing those symptoms are and then discusses the role that alcohol has played in these problems and that abstinence is possible. This approach is most in line with which of the following therapies?

A. Cognitive behavioral
B. Dialectical behavioral
C. Interpersonal
D. Motivational interviewing
E. Twelve step

4.14. Which of the following is the current standard treatment of choice for alcohol-related withdrawal seizures?

A. Anticonvulsants
B. Antipsychotics
C. Barbiturates
D. Benzodiazepines
E. Mood stabilizers

4.15. Aside from motivating the patient to remain abstinent, which of the following topics is most helpful to focus on initially during counseling for alcohol rehabilitation?

A. Causes of the disorder
B. Day-to-day life issues
C. Future plans
D. Social anxiety
E. Underlying depression

4.16. After detoxification for alcoholism, lingering level of anxiety and insomnia can best be initially treated with which of the following approaches?

A. An antidepressant
B. An antihistamine
C. A benzodiazepine
D. Behavior modification
E. Melatonin

4.17. Which of the following medical conditions is a contraindication to being on naltrexone for treating alcohol dependence?

A. Being on metronidazole
B. Continued use of alcohol
C. Coronary artery disease
D. Currently using opioids
E. Renal failure

4.18. Which of the following is the leading cause of preventable death in the United States?

A. Alcohol use
B. Car accidents
C. Gun violence
D. Suicides
E. Tobacco use

4.19. Even modest amounts of cannabis can have which of the following physical effects on the brain or body during intoxication?

A. Delayed reaction time
B. Depressed mood
C. Impaired long-term memory
D. Increased goal-directed activity
E. Physical tenseness

4.20. A cannabis-induced psychotic disorder is most commonly associated with which of the following premorbid psychiatric disorders?

A. Anxiety
B. Bipolar
C. Depressive
D. Eating
E. Personality

4.21. Apathy, low-energy, psychomotor retardation, and weight gain are often part of a syndrome associated with which of the following substances?

A. Barbiturates
B. Caffeine
C. Cannabis
D. Hallucinogens
E. Opioids

4.22. Synthetic THC's FDA approval in the United States is limited to a few medical conditions, including which of the following indications?

A. Chronic insomnia
B. Nausea in chemotherapy
C. Obstructive sleep apnea
D. Treatment-resistant back pain
E. Weight loss in anorexia nervosa

4.23. Which of the following medical risks can commonly occur with using higher dosages of cannabis?

A. Appetite suppression
B. Death
C. Diaphoresis
D. Mild bradycardia
E. Orthostatic hypotension

4.24. Which of the following signs or symptoms is common in opioid withdrawal?

A. Constipation
B. Hypotension
C. Lacrimation
D. Psychosis
E. Pupillary constriction

4.25. A patient presents to the ER after an overdose of an unknown substance. His pupils appear constricted, and he is sedated with slurred speech and has trouble focusing and answering questions. His vital signs are significant for bradycardia and hypotension and he reports being constipated. Which of the following medications would best reverse this overdose?

A. Flumazenil
B. N-acetylcysteine
C. Naloxone
D. Naltrexone
E. Varenicline

4.26. Which of the following is a main advantage of opioid substitution therapy?

A. Drowsiness is minimal.
B. Outpatient treatment is guaranteed.
C. Parental formulations are never needed.
D. There is no risk of dependence.
E. Treatment can be done quickly in 2 weeks.

4.27. Meperidine can interact with which of the following classes of psychiatric medications leading to agitation, seizures, coma, and death?

A. Benzodiazepines
B. Monoamine oxidase inhibitors (MAOIs)
C. SSRIs
D. Stimulants
E. TCAs

4.28. Suicide attempts and unintentional overdoses are often most lethal with which of the following substances of abuse?

A. Alcohol
B. Barbiturates
C. Benzodiazepines
D. Lysergic acid diethylamide (LSD)
E. Stimulants

4.29. Bath salts lead to a high by increasing levels of which of the following substances?

A. Catecholamines
B. Enkephalin
C. GABA
D. Glutamate
E. Oxytocin

4.30. An adolescent is brought to the ER after disrobing and shouting in the streets. Vital signs are significant for an elevated heart rate and low weight, along with a decreased respiratory rate. Neurologic examination is significant for dilated pupils and muscle weakness. Mental stats examination is significant for confusion with complaints of chest pain and the adolescent is profusely diaphoretic. Intoxication with what class of substances is most likely to have caused the above symptoms?

A. Alcohol
B. Barbiturates
C. Hallucinogens
D. Opioids
E. Stimulants

4.31. Bruxism and poor dentition can most directly be a result of abusing which of the following substances?

A. Clonazepam
B. Heroin
C. Ketamine
D. Methamphetamine
E. Psilocybin

4.32. A 50-year-old female with a past psych history significant for bulimia nervosa is interested in medication to help her quit smoking. Her medical history is significant for a heart attack in the past and most recently, she has been suffering from allergies and rashes. Which of the following medications would best be indicated to help her to quit smoking?

A. Bupropion SR
B. Nicotine inhaler
C. Nicotine patch
D. Polacrilex gum
E. Varenicline

4.33. Which of the following is a known risk of lysergic acid diethylamide (LSD) use?

A. Cerebrovascular events
B. Chronic hallucinations
C. Cross-tolerance with amphetamines
D. Hypotension
E. Liver failure

4.34. A patient in the ER for cardiovascular monitoring is being given supportive care for intoxication with an unknown substance. On examination, the patient is hypertensive and tachycardic. Nystagmus is noted along with increased salivation. The patient was found walking in the middle of the road and was biting himself and did not appear to be in pain. Which of the following is the most likely substance the patient took?

A. Alprazolam
B. Caffeine
C. Cannabis
D. Heroin
E. Ketamine

4.35. Which of the following substances can lead to flashbacks of the substance-induced experience even long after use?

A. Alcohol
B. Hallucinogens
C. Inhalants
D. Opioids
E. Stimulants

4.36. A patient presents to the emergency room with intense emotions after continued flashbacks of being intoxicated. The patient reports feeling confused, as the last reported substance use was many weeks ago. The patient describes flashbacks of different experiences including seeing flashes of color, seeing trails of images moving, and hearing sounds. Before diagnosing this patient with a substance-related disorder, which of the following medical or psychiatric diagnoses should be ruled out first?

A. Asthma
B. Borderline personality disorder
C. Hepatic failure
D. Migraines
E. Schizophrenia

4.37. A patient presenting to the ER with psychosis and agitation is refusing PO intake. The patient reports muscle pain and trouble walking after receiving treatment for PCP intoxication. Which of the following medical conditions has most likely occurred from the treatment?

A. A dystonic reaction
B. Convulsions
C. Hallucinogen-persisting perception disorder
D. Rhabdomyolysis
E. Serotonin syndrome

4.38. A patient is brought to the ER with aggression and amnesia. Examination is significant for nystagmus and decreased reflexes, malodorous breath, and a rash around the nose and mouth. These findings are most consistent with intoxication from which of the following substances?

A. Alcohol
B. Benzodiazepines
C. Hallucinogens
D. Opioids
E. Inhalants

4.39. Which of the following substances of abuse can cause a type of leukoencephalopathy showing diffuse cerebral, cerebellar, and brainstem atrophy on CT or MRI?

A. Barbiturates
B. Hallucinogens
C. Inhalants
D. Simulants
E. Steroids

ANSWERS

4.1. E. Use
In the past, various DSM terms have been used to refer to those with substance abuse. Alcohol/substance dependence and abuse were terms used in previous DSM editions. The word addiction or addict is not an official medical term. Substance use disorder is a DSM-5 term referring to prolonged use and abuse of a substance and the specific substance should be specified. Criteria include two or more physiologic symptoms, symptoms of addition, and/or psychological sequelae of use for a period of 12 months, leading to psychosocial impairment. Some symptoms include tolerance, withdrawal, cravings, using more than intended, difficulty stopping, etc. along with those mentioned above such as using in spite of health problems or adverse social or occupational consequences. Substance intoxication is the diagnosis used to describe specific signs or symptoms from recent exposure to the substance. (1, 2)

4.2. D. Major depressive
Approximately ⅓ to ½ of those with opioid abuse or dependence and about 40% of those with alcohol abuse or dependence meet criteria for a major depressive disorder. Those with substance use alone are 20 times more likely to die by suicide than the general population, with a total of around 15% of those with alcohol abuse or dependence committing suicide. The frequency of suicide in substance use is only secondary to that in major depressive disorder. (272)

4.3. E. Varenicline
Along with nicotine delivery devices and bupropion, varenicline can help with tobacco dependence. Acamprosate, disulfiram, and naltrexone can help with alcoholism. Levomethadyl acetate can help with heroin addiction. (273)

4.4. B. American Indians
In the United States, the highest lifetime rate of substance use is among American Indians or Alaska Natives. Caucasians have higher rates compared to African Americans. (274)

4.5. E. Opioids
The locus ceruleus, the largest group of adrenergic neurons, is thought to mediate the effects of the opiates and opioids. The dopaminergic neurons in the ventral tegmental area (VTA) are involved with the sensation of reward and may represent a mediation of the effects of amphetamines and cocaine. (274)

4.6. C. 80 to 100 mg/dL
The legal definition of intoxication in most states in the United States is a blood alcohol concentration of 80 to 100 mg ethanol per deciliter, or 0.08 to 0.10 g/dL. At levels between 80 and 200 mg/dL, typically incoordination is increased and judgment errors are more likely to occur, along with mood instability and a deterioration in cognitive status. Levels of 20 to 30 mg/dL can lead to slowed motor performance and decreased ability to think. Levels of 30 to 80 mg/dL can lead to increased motor and cognitive problems. Nystagmus, slurred speech, and blackouts can occur at levels between 200 and 300 mg/dL and above 300 mg/dL vital signs are impaired and death can occur. (276)

4.7. E. Tremors
Classic signs of alcohol withdrawal include irritability, nausea, vomiting, and autonomic hyperactivity, including sweating, facial flushing, mydriasis, tachycardia, and hypertension. An alcohol withdrawal tremor can look like either a physiologic tremor (i.e., continuous, high amplitude, more than 8 Hz) or a familial tremor (i.e., bursts of activity, slower than 8 Hz). (276)

4.8. E. Na
Seizures in long-term alcohol abuse can be caused by hyponatremia, as well as by hypoglycemia and hypomagnesemia. (276)

4.9. E. Wernicke encephalopathy
Wernicke encephalopathy is an acute neurologic disorder presenting as ataxia (mostly gait), vestibular dysfunction, confusion, and ocular motor abnormalities including nystagmus, gaze palsy, anisocoria (unequal pupil size), etc. Most remit whereas some progress to Korsakoff syndrome, consisting of anterograde amnesia and often confabulation. Symptoms of delirium tremens include confusion and hallucinations though also autonomic findings would be noted including tachycardia, diaphoresis, fever, etc. Alcohol-induced psychotic disorders consist of hallucinations or delusions in the context of heavy drinking or withdrawal. Unspecified alcohol-related disorder is the DSM-5 term for alcohol-related disorders not meeting criteria for any other diagnoses. (277)

4.10. B. Education
Most alcohol-induced depressions, even severe, resolve within a few days to a month of abstinence without treatment. Typically, education and cognitive behavioral therapy (CBT) are the initial appropriate treatment options and there should be a 2- to 4-week trial of abstinence, education, and CBT before initiation of antidepressants. (278)

4.11. E. Thiamine
Patients with a history of heavy alcohol use and the above symptoms should be checked for a thiamine deficiency (vitamin B1). Thiamine deficiency can cause pellagra and when it gets to the point of alcoholic pellagra encephalopathy with features of Wernicke–Korsakoff, often there is no response to thiamine treatment. Symptoms of alcohol pellagra include general symptoms such as fatigue, anorexia, insomnia, irritability, etc. along with physical findings noted above such as myoclonus and oppositional hypertonia. Confusion seen with thiamine deficiency can range from mild all the way to a severe delirium. (279)

4.12. B. Antisocial personality
Antisocial personality disorder, along with other substance-related disorders, mood and anxiety disorders are among the most common comorbid conditions with alcohol use disorders. Antisocial personality disorder is particularly common and often precedes the alcohol disorder. Mood disorders are present in around 30%–40% of those with alcohol use disorders. Anxiety disorders are also commonly found in those with alcohol use disorder, at a comorbidity around 25%–50%. (280)

4.13. D. Motivational interviewing
The above approach is most in line with motivational interviewing. This can help the patient to recognize the adverse consequences of drinking and be motivated to stop. The therapist should explore the adverse consequences of alcohol with the patient in a persistent but nonjudgmental manner. (281)

4.14. D. Benzodiazepines
After having a neurologic evaluation to rule out a comorbid or nonalcohol-related cause of the seizure, benzodiazepines (i.e., lorazepam, chlordiazepoxide, diazepam, etc.) are the treatment of choice that should be used for managing alcohol-related withdrawal seizures. Anticonvulsants are not thought to offer additional benefits. Any CNS depressant such as benzodiazepines, barbiturates, or alcohol can help minimize alcohol withdrawal, though benzodiazepines are thought to be safer and offer better control of the withdrawal symptoms. While carbamazepine at a dose of 800 mg daily has been shown to be as effective as benzodiazepines with less abuse potential and is being used more often now, currently the standard is still a benzodiazepine. (281)

4.15. B. Day-to-day life issues
Treatment for alcohol rehab should be the same regardless of the setting. Initial counseling for the first few months should focus on day-to-day life stressors and helping the patient to function and maintain abstinence. Psychotherapy to get at the root cause of the disorder (i.e., no single event is the sole cause of alcoholism), focusing on depression that caused it (i.e., often it is the other way around, the alcohol contributed to the mood disorder), or insight-oriented therapy that can provoke anxiety can get in the way of abstinence and is not indicated within the first 3 to 6 months of treatment. (282)

4.16. D. Behavior modification
After detoxification, unless the patient has an independent psychiatric disorder, an antidepressant or antianxiety medications should not be prescribed. Behavior modification and reassurance are the best approaches to treat residual anxiety and insomnia, as the effect of these medications may be short term and put the patient at risk to escalate the dose. The patient should be counseled that lingering sadness and mood swings can occur for a few months when abstinence begins and that behavioral therapy and continued abstinence are most effective. (283)

4.17. D. Currently using opioids
Contraindications to using naltrexone include currently using opioids or withdrawing from opioids, or an anticipated need for opioid medications. Liver failure or hepatitis is also a contraindication for use. The other contraindications listed are for alternative medications used to treat alcohol dependence including acamprosate (i.e., severe renal impairment) or disulfiram (i.e., use with alcohol or metronidazole, coronary artery disease, or a severe myocardial infarction). (284)

4.18. E. Tobacco use
Tobacco use is the leading cause of preventable death in the United States, followed by poor diet/physical inactivity, and the third leading cause is alcohol use, which accounts for 10% of deaths among all working adults, and contributes to 25% of all suicides and 31% of automobile fatalities. (285)

4.19. A. Delayed reaction time
Cannabis intoxication can impair cognition and performance and result in impaired reaction times and perceptions, along with motor coordination issues. During a classic cannabis "high," many experience mild euphoria and relaxation, not tenseness. Depression can be a symptom of cannabis withdrawal. Short-term memory impairment is common along with difficulty sustaining goal-directed mental activity. (288)

4.20. E. Personality
While transient paranoia is common with cannabis use, a cannabis-induced psychotic disorder is rare and is typically associated with a pre-existing personality disorder. Unlike hallucinogens, cannabis use is rarely associated with an adverse psychological reaction. (289)

4.21. C. Cannabis
Amotivational syndrome can be seen with cannabis use. It is unclear if the amotivation symptoms are directly an effect of the cannabis use versus traits of those who use cannabis heavily. Symptoms include apathy, anergia, and weight gain, with a slothful appearance. (289)

4.22. B. Nausea in chemotherapy
The FDA has approved dronabinol, a synthetic form of THC, for treatment of chemotherapy-related nausea and vomiting. While it is also approved for anorexia-related weight loss in HIV, it is not approved for weight loss due to other medical or psychiatric conditions including anorexia nervosa. Dronabinol is being studied as a treatment for obstructive sleep apnea, though is not yet approved. Other countries have approved other synthetic THC versions to help with neuropathic pain and multiple sclerosis. (290)

4.23. E. Orthostatic hypotension
Orthostatic hypotension is thought to be a common side effect from high doses of cannabis. Other common side effects include increased appetite, dry mouth, and a mild tachycardia. There are no documented cases of death from cannabis intoxication, though the greatest risk with chronic use is of chronic respiratory disease and lung cancer. (291)

4.24. C. Lacrimation
Lacrimation, along with piloerection (goosebumps), rhinorrhea, yawning, and muscle cramps are all possible symptoms of opioid withdrawal. Diarrhea rather than constipation can be a symptom of opioid withdrawal as well. Changes in vital signs in opioid withdrawal include hypertension, tachycardia, hypothermia, or hyperthermia. Pupillary dilation is noted in opioid withdrawal, not pupillary constriction. Psychotic symptoms including hallucinations can be a sign of delirium tremens in alcohol withdrawal. (292)

4.25. C. Naloxone
The above signs and symptoms are consistent with opioid intoxication. Naloxone is a short-acting intravenous medication that can reverse opioid overdoses. Often repeat doses are needed given the duration of action is short compared to the long half-life of many opioids. Naltrexone is a long-acting agent that is used after detox to help prevent a relapse. N-acetylcysteine is used in Tylenol overdoses. Flumazenil is used to reverse benzodiazepine overdoses. Varenicline is used to treat nicotine dependence. (293)

4.26. A. Drowsiness is minimal
Opioid substitution therapy, including methadone and buprenorphine, can eliminate the need to use opioids in illegal and injectable forms, minimizing HIV and hepatitis risk. Other positives include that they cause minimal euphoria and drowsiness and can help the patient to engage in employment instead of criminal activity to obtain the opioid. These agonists are utilized for both inpatient and outpatient detoxification and buprenorphine comes in a parenteral form. They do still carry risks of dependence and abuse. The combination of buprenorphine plus naloxone can help decrease the risk of diversion and abuse. Often, a period of at least 4 weeks is needed with demonstration of stabilization prior to lowering the dose of the agonist. (295–296)

4.27. B. MAOIs
An idiosyncratic drug interaction between meperidine, an opioid, and MAOIs (monoamine oxidase inhibitors) can result in autonomic instability, agitation, seizures, coma, and death. These two medications should never be given together. (297)

4.28. B. Barbiturates
Barbiturates are lethal in overdose because they lead to respiratory depression. They are a common cause of fatal drug overdoses, especially in children when found in medicine cabinets. They lead to coma, respiratory arrest, cardiovascular failure, and death. In contrast, the benzodiazepines when taken alone have a large margin of safety due to less respiratory suppression. However, most lethal overdoses occur when benzodiazepines are combined with other sedatives, including alcohol. (299)

4.29. A. Catecholamines
Bath salts release a variety of chemicals including cathinone and cathine. Similar to the mechanism of action of cocaine, the cathinones increase synaptic catecholamine levels by inhibiting dopamine, serotonin, and norepinephrine reuptake transporters. (303)

4.30. E. Stimulants
The above signs and symptoms are classic for stimulant intoxication, along with others such as euphoria, dangerous sexual behavior, and possible mania. Alcohol, barbiturates, and opioids are sedatives. Pinpoint pupils are associated with opioid intoxication. (304)

4.31. D. Methamphetamine
With intranasal use, methamphetamine can cause vasoconstriction which can lead to mucosal alteration and bruxism (tooth grinding), resulting in poor dentition, also referred to as "meth mouth." (307)

4.32. D. Polacrilex gum
Nicotine replacement therapies double the rates of cessation. Nicotine polacrilex gum would be a good choice for this patient since the other medications are contraindicated given her medical and psychiatric history. Bupropion, an antidepressant medication is contraindicated in those with a history of bulimia (or anorexia nervosa), due to increased risk of seizures. Varenicline can relieve cravings and withdrawal. It has a small but increased risk of causing cardiovascular events in those with pre-existing disease. Nicotine patches should be avoided in this patient as rashes are common adverse side effects. Nicotine nasal spray should also be avoided in this patient as it can cause watery eyes and coughing in up to 70% of patients. (310)

4.33. A. Cerebrovascular events
LSD can cause death via cardiac or cerebrovascular pathology given it is a sympathomimetic, which can lead to hypertension, as well as hyperthermia. There is no evidence that LSD can cause chronic psychosis, though it can lead to chronic depression and anxiety. While cross-tolerance between certain hallucinogens can develop, it is not found to develop between LSD and amphetamines. (319)

4.34. E. Ketamine
Ketamine, a dissociative anesthetic agent, causes cardiovascular stimulation. Findings on examination include tachycardias and hypertension along with increased salivation and nystagmus. Dystonic reactions can also be seen. A common complication is a lack of concern for the environment and personal safety. (320, 321)

4.35. B. Hallucinogens
Long after ingesting hallucinogens, flashbacks of the symptoms can be experienced in 15% to 80% of users, known as hallucinogen-persisting perception disorder. DSM-5 criteria include reexperiencing symptoms following cessation of use, causing significant distress or functional impairment. Complications of this disorder can include major depression and suicidal ideation, along with panic disorder. (322)

4.36. D. Migraines
The patient described above has hallucinogen-persisting perception disorder. Migraines and seizures can lead to flashback-like experiences and are important medical conditions that should be ruled out prior to diagnosing this disorder. Posttraumatic stress disorder can also cause flashbacks and should be ruled out. (322)

4.37. D. Rhabdomyolysis
Trapping ionized PCP via urinary acidification has been used for treatment of PCP intoxication. This strategy is no longer recommended because metabolic acidosis can lead to rhabdomyolysis and result in renal failure. Trapping ionized PCP in the stomach via NG suction is also not recommended due to induction of electrolyte imbalances. Administration of charcoal is now the treatment of choice for PCP intoxication. (324)

4.38. E. Inhalants
The diagnostic criteria for inhalant intoxication include a maladaptive behavioral change and at least two physical symptoms. Behavioral changes can include apathy, impaired judgment or functioning, or aggression. Physical symptoms include nausea, anorexia, nystagmus, diplopia, and decreased reflexes. Rashes around the nose and mouth and an unusual breath odor, along with findings of residue on the hands, face, or close, are all signs of inhalant abuse. (326)

4.39. C. Inhalants
Chronic inhalants can cause many dangerous medical complications, including death. Chronic inhalant use can lead to a leukoencephalopathy showing diffuse cerebral, cerebellar, and brainstem atrophy on neuroimaging. (327)

5

Schizophrenia Spectrum and Other Psychotic Disorders

5.1. A 21-year-old man is brought to the mental health center by his father, who states that the patient had been withdrawing from family and friends over the past 6 months to the point that he sits in his room all day watching TV. He was fired from his job 3 days ago as a food delivery driver after he sat behind the wheel of his car in a customer's driveway for 2 hours until his father got him on the phone and convinced him to drive home. The patient and his father are asked to wait in the waiting area for the first available doctor. The father sits and the patient stands. Two hours later when the doctor comes, the patient is standing in the exact same position. The father states that his son has not said anything for the last 24 hours, but will follow commands. Vital signs are within normal limits. Comprehensive metabolic panel, heavy metals, urine drug screen, lumbar puncture, and head CT are all negative. This patient is most likely to experience hallucinations of what sensory modality?

A. Auditory
B. Gustatory
C. Olfactory
D. Tactile
E. Visual

5.2. What is the leading cause of premature death in people with schizophrenia?

A. Suicide
B. Heart disease
C. Homicide
D. Accidents
E. Metabolic syndrome complications

5.3. A 35-year-old woman presents to the outpatient clinic with a complaint of hearing three voices talk about how bad she is and "all of the horrible things I've done throughout my life" for the past 4 days. She is distressed because "the voices had gotten much better for a couple of weeks, and I didn't feel as down, so I thought I was finally cured." She states that she has heard the voices of and on, more days than not, for the past 10 years and that she was hospitalized for a suicide attempt 9 years ago. At the time, "I felt lower than I usually do. I didn't get out of bed because I was too tired, even though I slept all day. I didn't eat and didn't want to do anything. The voices were even worse, then." She was started on medication, "but I don't remember what it was. I never filled the prescription." She has been intermittently homeless because she cannot keep a job due to voices distracting her at work, frequent bouts of depression, and "I don't want to be around people anyway." She makes poor eye contact, and affect is flat. Mood is "down and frustrated." Speech is normal rate, volume, and tone. She endorses current auditory hallucinations. What is the most likely diagnosis?

A. Schizophrenia
B. Schizophreniform disorder
C. Major depressive disorder with psychotic features
D. Schizoaffective disorder
E. Brief psychotic disorder

5.4. A 50-year-old woman is brought to the emergency department by law enforcement after being found outside of a local television news anchor's house. She states that she went to his house because she "knows" he loves her, "but he's too afraid to let me know," despite him telling her he is happily married and taking out a restraining order on her. "I wanted to give him the opportunity to say he loves me without embarrassing him in front of other people." She states that she knew he would be her husband 3 years ago when she first saw him on TV. She continues to work as a paralegal, but is afraid now that her job is in jeopardy due to the trespassing charge. She has been reprimanded at work because she tells clients about his love for her. She states that she feels depressed and frustrated because he "won't admit the truth." What is the most likely diagnosis?

A. Schizophrenia
B. Schizoaffective disorder
C. Delusional disorder
D. Schizotypal personality disorder
E. Major depressive disorder with psychotic features

5.5. A 55-year-old man is brought to the emergency department by his parents, with whom he lives. They state that he attacked them an hour ago "out of the blue. He's never done that since he was first diagnosed with schizophrenia 35 years ago." They were all eating lunch together as they do every day at noon, when the patient suddenly got up and lunged at his father with a knife. His mother was able to talk him down and convince him to come to the hospital. The patient states that he has heard voices talking to each other since before he was diagnosed, but has never had visual hallucinations. However, that evening he saw his father "transform into a vampire," and felt that he had to stab him through the heart. He is worried that something similar may happen again, as are his parents. He has been on a nightly does of olanzapine for the past two years. What should the next step be in the evaluation and management of this patient?

A. Administer an intramuscular antipsychotic
B. Consult the hospital psychiatrist
C. Perform a medical workup
D. Admit the patient to an inpatient psychiatric facility
E. Contact the patient's outpatient psychiatrist

5.6. A 65-year-old woman is brought to the emergency department by her son who states that his mother has lived at home alone since the death of her husband 6 years ago. He reports that she seemed to adjust well and spent time with friends and family until about a year ago, when she started to stay more to herself in the house, and eventually stopped going to all functions. She used to work as a chef and would cook elaborate meals for herself that would sustain her for several days. This morning, she called him to say that all of the food in the house was poisoned, and that she needed him to bring more. After driving 6 hours to check on her, he found her house to be malodorous, with mold in the unplugged refrigerator, her hair matted, and with foul body odor. He notes that she looks like she has lost 30 pounds in the last year. When he presented her with the fresh food, she exclaimed, "This is poison! You're trying to poison me, too!" Temperature is 98.8 F, pulse 104, BP 90/60, and respirations 16. Physical examination reveals a thin, malodorous female in no acute distress. UDS is negative. Comprehensive metabolic profile shows increased sodium. Urine specific gravity is high. Head CT is negative, as is urine drug screen. She is started on IV fluids for dehydration. What is the most appropriate disposition?

A. Discharge to home with a home health aide
B. Discharge to an assisted living facility
C. Discharge to her son's home
D. Admission to the hospital
E. Discharge to home with a next-day psychiatry appointment

5.7. A 37-year-old woman notices that she has been having difficulty sitting still at work at her job at a call center and at home for the last week. She was discharged from an inpatient psychiatric facility 2 weeks ago with a diagnosis of schizoaffective disorder. During the 2-week hospitalization, she was started first on risperidone, which led to lactation, then was switched to haloperidol. She has no current problem with neck stiffness, but feels an urge to move her legs and walk around. Because of her productivity quota at work she does not get up to walk, but instead crosses and uncrosses her legs constantly. She has the same problem at night, with the restlessness interfering with her sleep, so she gets up and walks around for relief. What medication is the first-line treatment for these symptoms?

A. Ropinirole
B. Benztropine
C. Propranolol
D. Trihexyphenidyl
E. Valbenazine

5.8. A 35-year-old man complains of finger and tongue movements that have been getting rapidly worse over the last 3 months. The movements have been present over the last 10 years, since he was diagnosed with schizophrenia and started on fluphenazine. Movements are now to the point that he has trouble holding a cup to drink. Over the years, the fluphenazine has been lowered to the most effective dose, which is still moderately high. He has been through adequate trials of valbenazine, deutetrabenazine, benztropine, and alprazolam, all of which were ineffective. An abnormal involuntary movement scale (AIMS) assessment places the movements in the severe range. What is the most appropriate treatment for this patient?

A. Change to haloperidol
B. Attempt a slower and more gradual decrease of fluphenazine
C. Begin tetrabenazine
D. Change to aripiprazole
E. Change to clozapine

5.9. A 35-year-old woman is being discharged later in the day from her second hospitalization due to an acute psychotic episode. She was brought to the hospital 8 days ago after passersby called the police because she was yelling at women on the street, accusing them of sleeping with her husband when he was a baby. During the initial hospitalization 2 years ago, she was started on quetiapine and was stable enough that she could return to work in hotel maintenance. She stopped taking the medication a year later because "I was doing fine. I didn't need it anymore." She was restarted on the quetiapine during this hospitalization, and required a 20% higher dosage to regain stability. During the discharge planning meeting, she asks the physician, "How long do I have to stay on this drug? I don't want to be on medication forever." How should the physician respond?

A. "You should stay on the medication for at least 2 years, then get reassessed to see if you can stop it."
B. "You should stay on the medication for 1 year, then go back down to your previous dose."
C. "You should stay on the medication for at least 5 years, then get reassessed to see if you can stop it."
D. "That can be assessed on a regular basis. Perhaps you will be able to come off of it someday."
E. "You should stay on the medication indefinitely because you're likely to have another episode if you don't."

5.10. A 43-year-old man is emergently admitted to an inpatient psychiatric facility for the fifth time in 12 months after EMS was called to his parents' house due to him running naked in living room and overturning furniture. When told to stop, he ran outside and started pulling up clumps of grass out of the lawn. He was first diagnosed with schizophrenia at age 22, and has been treated with haloperidol, fluphenazine, aripiprazole, aripiprazole lauroxil, and paliperidone. He is currently on paliperidone palmitate every month. The previous medications have either been ineffective or partially effective at maximum doses. His parents assure the admitting physician that they made sure he took his oral medication daily, and that they take him to follow-up appointments. "No medicine has worked for him for long." He has mild hypercholesterolemia. Comprehensive metabolic panel is within normal limits. What should be the next step in his medication regimen?

A. Augment with an oral first-generation antipsychotic
B. Change to a first-generation long-acting injection
C. Change to clozapine
D. Change to the 3-month formulation of paliperidone palmitate
E. Augment with a first-generation long-acting injection

5.11. Patients who show any improvement on an antipsychotic should remain on that medication to monitor for further improvement for at least what length of time?

A. Four weeks
B. Six weeks
C. Three months
D. Six months
E. One year

5.12. CT scans of patients with schizophrenia consistently show what neuroanatomical abnormality?

   A. Decreased number of D2 receptors in the caudate
   B. Enlarged ventricles
   C. Increased white matter in the thalamus
   D. Enlarged amygdala
   E. Decreased density of D2 receptors in the nucleus accumbens

5.13. What laboratory test must be monitored in patients taking clozapine in order for them to continue receiving the medication?

   A. Complete blood count with differential
   B. Comprehensive metabolic panel
   C. Lipid profile
   D. Hemoglobin A1c
   E. Liver function tests

ANSWERS

5.1. A. Auditory
The patient is displaying classic symptoms of catatonia, which were preceded by a several-month history of withdrawing from family and friends. Given the history, his age, his current presentation, and the negative extensive medical workup, he most likely has a schizophrenia spectrum disorder, in which auditory, then visual hallucinations, are most common by far. Gustatory, olfactory, and tactile hallucinations, especially in the absence of auditory and or visual hallucinations, may indicate that further workup is needed. (338–339)

5.2. A. Suicide
Suicide is the leading cause of premature death in people with schizophrenia, with 5% to 6% dying by suicide, according to the DSM-5-TR. The biggest risk factor is the presence of a major depressive episode, with command hallucinations and drug abuse also playing significant roles. Metabolic syndrome complications can occur as a result of treatment with second-generation and later antipsychotics but is not the leading cause of premature death. While people with schizophrenia are more likely to be the victim of homicide than to commit an act of homicide, both are much less common than suicide. Accidents are the leading cause of premature death in young children, and occur more often in adults with schizophrenia than in the general population, but are not the leading cause of premature deaths in adults. Heart disease is the leading cause of death in the United States for everyone. (339)

5.3. D. Schizoaffective disorder
The most likely diagnosis is schizoaffective disorder. She reports a steady baseline of symptoms of schizophrenia, including persistent auditory hallucinations most days, and displays negative symptoms of poor eye contact and flat affect. In addition, she has endorsed enough symptoms to have met criteria for major depressive disorder in the past, and usually has somewhat of a depressed mood. Though schizophrenia can have a mood component with it, given that she meets full criteria for both schizophrenia and depression, schizoaffective disorder is still the better diagnosis. In major depressive disorder with psychotic features, once the depression remits, so should the psychosis, but her psychotic symptoms are almost ever-present. Schizophreniform disorder lasts less than 6 months. Though the most recent hallucinations have been present for only 4 days, this is in the context of a 10-year history of hallucinations. (342)

5.4. C. Delusional disorder
What separates delusional disorder from a psychotic disorder such as schizophrenia or schizoaffective disorder is that the delusion is nonbizarre, and that there could possibly have been a kernel of truth at the beginning of the delusion. Also, aside from the impact of the delusions or its ramifications, function is not markedly impaired. (It's *possible* that the TV anchor could be in love with her, vs. being virtually impossible that aliens are contacting her through the radio.) Major depressive episodes are episodic, and the psychotic features would likely be more out of touch with reality. Individuals with schizotypal personality disorder usually are loners, prefer to keep to themselves, and have few, if any, close relationships. (345–346)

5.5. C. Perform a medical workup
Though it is tempting to assume that the patient's presenting problems are due to an exacerbation of schizophrenia, given that he is displaying new, uncharacteristic behaviors and new psychotic symptoms (visual vs. auditory hallucinations), a medical workup is warranted. A long-standing diagnosis of schizophrenia does not preclude someone from having a medical cause of psychotic symptoms, such as substance intoxication, infections, metabolic issues, etc., so the same medical workup should be done as if the person did not have a schizophrenia diagnosis. (347)

5.6. D. Admission to the hospital
The patient is acutely psychotic, and is a danger to herself due to neglect, as evidenced by poor hygiene so chronic that her hair is matted, dehydration, and weight loss. Until the psychosis clears and her baseline can be determined, she needs to be hospitalized for her own safety, whether on a psychiatric inpatient unit for psychosis or a medical unit for further workup to determine diagnosis. Given that she lives alone, if she does not return to presymptomatic functioning, the family and a social worker should meet to discuss disposition options, including living with her son, living at an assisted living facility, or living at home with a home health aide, depending on the severity of her residual symptoms and efficacy of treatment. (351)

5.7. C. Propranolol
The woman is suffering from akathisia, a feeling of restlessness and needing to move, especially in the legs. This is most often caused by antipsychotics, usually those of the first generation, such as haloperidol. Treatment is first to try to decrease or stop the offending agent. If that is not feasible, then the next is

to use a beta-blocker such as propranolol. Ropinirole is used for restless legs syndrome. Though the symptoms are largely the same, they typically occur in the evening or nighttime, as opposed to all day. Benztropine is used for the stiffness of extrapyramidal symptoms. Trihexyphenidyl is used for sialorrhea, and valbenazine for tardive dyskinesia. (351)

5.8. E. Change to clozapine
The patient is displaying severe tardive dyskinesia, which is not unexpected given a 10-year history of being on a first-generation antipsychotic starting at a relatively young age. The treatment of choice is to decrease the offending agent. However, for him, this cannot be done without risking an exacerbation. The next treatment is to change to a second-generation antipsychotic, if possible. Given the severity of his movements, he needs to change to clozapine, as that is both a second-generation antipsychotic and is effective in reducing severe tardive dyskinesia. Given that he has already been on two vesicular monoamine transport-2 (VMAT-2) inhibitors, and due to the severity of his movements, it is reasonable to guess that trying a third (tetrabenazine) also will not be effective. He should not be changed to another first-generation antipsychotic (haloperidol). Though aripiprazole is a second-generation antipsychotic, the severity of the movements again makes clozapine a better choice. (354)

5.9. E. "You should stay on the medication indefinitely because you're likely to have another episode if you don't."
The patient has now had two acute psychotic episodes with a diagnosis of schizophrenia. Furthermore, her interepisode functioning is high enough that she is able to maintain a job. Given those factors, most experts recommend that consideration be given for indefinite treatment. (354)

5.10. C. Change to clozapine
The patient has adequately tried and failed over four different first- and second-generation antipsychotics, in both oral and long-acting injectable forms. Given that his parents are diligent about making sure he takes his oral medications and taking him to appointments, clozapine should be the next consideration. Changing to a longer-acting form of a medication he is currently not doing well on is likely to be just as ineffective, especially since he has already been on both first-generation antipsychotics that are available as a long-acting injection. He should try what is considered the most effective antipsychotic as monotherapy before combining two antipsychotics. (354)

5.11. C. Three months
An adequate trial of an antipsychotic medication is 4 to 6 weeks at an adequate dose. If the patient shows improvement, they should remain on that medication for at least 3 and up to 6 months, as improvements can continue to occur over that length of time. (355)

5.12. B. Enlarged ventricles
Enlarged third and lateral ventricles are a consistent finding in the brains of individuals with schizophrenia. Many structures, such as those of the limbic system (amygdala, hippocampus, and parahippocampal gyrus) and the thalamus are reduced in size. However, there is an increase in the D2 receptor density in the caudate, putamen, and nucleus accumbens. (358)

5.13. A. Complete blood count with differential
Though rare, the 0.3% incidence of agranulocytosis in patients taking clozapine is enough to mandate weekly complete blood counts with differential for the first 6 months, biweekly for the next 6, then monthly. If one lab draw is missed, the pharmacy will not dispense the next dose of the medication, and the monitoring schedule resets. A comprehensive metabolic panel, or at least a basic one, lipid profile, and A1c are important for monitoring metabolic side effects. Clozapine is not known to affect the liver. (354)

6

Bipolar Disorders

6.1. According to the DSM-5-TR, what is a criterion that distinguishes a manic from a hypomanic episode?

A. Length of the episode
B. Number of symptoms
C. Level of impairment during a depressive episode
D. Insidious versus gradual onset
E. The need for hospitalization

6.2. A 30-year-old woman presents to her primary care physician with a chief complaint of "mood swings. Some days I'm up, and some days I'm down." She states that she has periods during which she does not "feel like doing anything. I don't want to go to work, but I do anyway, and still do a good job." During those times, she does not want to spend any more time with people than she has to, and will come home and "mindlessly watch TV, but I'm not really paying attention to it." She has lost some friends because "I drop off the face of the earth except for work." These symptoms last for a few weeks to a few months at a time. She denies changes in sleep or appetite, feeling guilty or worthless, or ever having suicidal ideation. Other times, "I'm up and ready to go, and feel like I can be the life of the party. I dress better, I feel better, I'm more productive at work, sometimes to the point that I almost overlook some details in order to finish a task." During those times, which last at least several weeks, she stays up later than usual, getting about 3 hours of sleep rather than her usual 8, "and I'm not tired the next day. It actually feels pretty good!" She has never seen a therapist or a psychiatrist or been hospitalized, has no chronic medical illnesses, takes no medications and denies drug use. Vital signs are normal and physical examination is noncontributory. What is the most likely diagnosis?

A. Persistent depressive disorder
B. Borderline personality disorder
C. Cyclothymia
D. Bipolar II disorder
E. Bipolar I disorder

6.3. A 21-year-old college student is brought to the emergency department by his friends who are concerned that he has stayed up for 3 days straight and "talks so much that he doesn't make any sense." They state that he started seeming "real hyper" about a week ago, and since then "went into god mode." They state that he thinks he knows more than anyone on campus and talks at length about different subjects, "even though it's obvious he has no idea what he's talking about." He stays up all night "writing what he says is a new quantum physics textbook, even though he's a history major." He has overdrawn his credit card from buying multiple 3D printers and materials which he says he needs to "print out a scale model of the universe." He and his friends say that the patient does not use drugs. He has had no prior episodes, and no chronic medical or psychiatric conditions. UDS is negative. The patient is admitted to the hospital for a week and stabilized on medication. On the day of discharge, he asks how long he needs to stay on medication. What is the most accurate reply?

A. At least 1 month
B. At least 3 months
C. At least 6 months
D. At least 1 year
E. Indefinitely

6.4. What factor predicts a better prognosis for a patient with bipolar I disorder?

A. Male gender
B. Advanced age of onset
C. Depressive features
D. Interepisode depressive features
E. A longer duration of manic episodes

6.5. A 32-year-old woman is brought to the emergency department by her husband after he found her jogging naked down the street in their neighborhood in the middle of the night because she "says she felt like she needed to exercise right then." He reports that she has a 10-year history of bipolar disorder, and that she does well "except when she is off her medications. We were gone on vacation for 2 weeks and forgot them. We thought she'd be fine for that amount of time. As soon as we got home 2 days ago, she took her lithium, but I guess it was too late." He notes that she started wanting to spend more and more money on drinks and expensive jewelry and souvenirs while they were away. The patient tells the emergency department all about the vacation, barely stopping to take a breath. They both report that she has not slept more than 4 hours since returning. What is the most appropriate disposition?

A. Admission to an inpatient psychiatric hospital
B. Discharge with follow-up the next day with her psychiatrist
C. Admission to a partial hospital program
D. Admission to an intensive outpatient program
E. Discharge with a prescription for a sedative

6.6. What is the most evidence-based medication for acute bipolar depression?

A. Lithium
B. Fluoxetine
C. Olanzapine
D. Quetiapine
E. Brexpiprazole

6.7. A 45-year-old woman is brought by EMS to the emergency department following an acute suicide attempt by overdose on acetaminophen. She states that she has been depressed for the last several months to the point that she has lost her job because "I can't get out of bed." She is now worried that she soon will not have the money to care for her daughter. "I'm a single mother. My daughter deserves to have someone who can care for her, and that's not me." She was diagnosed with bipolar disorder 15 years ago, and has been on trials of valproate, olanzapine, carbamazepine, and lithium. However, she had trouble remembering to take the medications daily. Mania has been well controlled over the last 2 years with paliperidone palmitate monthly. However, she still has breakthrough episodes of depression, and says that she sees no other way out for herself or her daughter than suicide. She has not had a previous suicide attempt, stating that she has never felt this hopeless before. She is emergently admitted to the hospital. Following medical stabilization, what is the most appropriate treatment?

A. Lithium
B. Quetiapine
C. Electroconvulsive therapy
D. Valproate
E. Lamotrigine

6.8. A 21-year-old college student presents to the student health center with complaints of depressed mood, decreased appetite, and poor concentration for the last week. She has been attending class, but once lecture concludes, goes straight to her room, studies, and does not spend time with her friends. She denies suicidal ideation and has had no prior suicide attempts. She was diagnosed with bipolar II disorder 6 months ago during a hypomanic episode and was started on valproate. She is also diagnosed with hypothyroidism for which she is on thyroid replacement therapy. She states that she has been unhappy with the valproate, which is leading to weight gain and contributing to the depression. What is the most appropriate treatment?

A. Lithium
B. Quetiapine
C. Aripiprazole
D. Fluoxetine
E. Lamotrigine

ANSWERS

6.1. E. The need for hospitalization
The main differences between manic and hypomanic episodes are no marked impairment in functioning and no need for hospitalization in the latter. However, a person with bipolar II disorder can have marked impairment and need hospitalization during the depressive episode. The number of symptoms needed to diagnose a manic or hypomanic episode is the same. There is no difference in episode length or onset. (368)

6.2. C. Cyclothymia
This patient exhibits symptoms of both depression and hypomania, but does not meet full criteria for either. Because there are some manic symptoms, she cannot be diagnosed with a unipolar depressive disorder. The manic symptoms do not appear to cause marked problems with social or occupational functioning, so she cannot be diagnosed with bipolar I. The depressive symptoms have led to problems with social functioning. However, she does not endorse enough symptoms to meet criteria for major depressive disorder, which also eliminates bipolar I. The diagnosis that most fits is cyclothymia. Though she starts by saying her moods are up and down over a period of days, she later clarifies that the distinct moods last for weeks or months at a time. Mood swings in borderline personality disorder often occur over hours to days. (369)

6.3. B. At least 3 months
An untreated manic episode lasts about 3 months, so he should be on the medication for at least that amount of time. However, given that he has had one full-blown manic episode, he has a 90% chance of having another, so many clinicians would be hesitant to discontinue medication after that length of time. (371)

6.4. B. Advanced age of onset
While not protective, several factors predict a better outcome in patients with bipolar I disorder. Among them is an advanced age of onset. Others are a short duration of manic episodes, few suicidal thoughts, and few coexisting psychiatric or mental health problems. Conversely, male gender, depressive features, and interepisode depressive features are all factors that predict a poor outcome. (372)

6.5. A. Admission to an inpatient psychiatric hospital
This patient is floridly manic and putting herself in danger (jogging naked in the middle of the night). The increase in alcohol use is also concerning. She needs acute hospitalization for medication that will break the manic episode as quickly as possible. Rapid titration of medications should be done in a secured medical environment for her safety, and discharge to home, even with a follow-up the next day, would not achieve that. She would also not be in a secure environment in an intensive outpatient or partial hospitalization program. (372)

6.6. D. Quetiapine
Unlike acute monopolar depression, in which an SSRI would most likely be the first line of treatment, in bipolar depression, atypical antipsychotics have shown the most efficacy. Of those medications, quetiapine has the most evidence. Lithium has only limited evidence for bipolar depression. Though olanzapine has positive studies or efficacy, it does not have the best evidence. Brexpiprazole is used as an adjunct for unipolar, not bipolar, depression. (373)

6.7. C. Electroconvulsive therapy
This patient is in the midst of a severe bipolar depression, has made a potentially lethal suicide attempt and is still actively suicidal, which constitutes an acute medical emergency. For those reasons, and because her history has shown that oral medication compliance is difficult for her, electroconvulsive therapy is warranted. If that were not an option, quetiapine would be the medication of choice, as it has the best evidence for bipolar depression. Though lamotrigine also has evidence, the acute nature of the depression would preclude using a medication that will take weeks to titrate. Lithium has limited evidence for bipolar depression, and valproate is indicated for acute mania. (374)

6.8. E. Lamotrigine
Though lithium could be a viable option for long-term treatment, it has not shown much efficacy in acute bipolar depression. In addition, a prior diagnosis of hypothyroidism would make lithium a less attractive option given its propensity to cause hypothyroidism. Also to be avoided, if possible, is a medication that can lead to weight gain, which eliminates most atypical antipsychotics. Fluoxetine and other antidepressants are less effective for bipolar depression than for monopolar depression. Lamotrigine is effective for acute bipolar depression and not likely to lead to weight gain. Given that she is still somewhat functioning and is not presenting with a level of depression that would constitute a medical emergency, such as having active suicidal ideation, lamotrigine is an optimal choice. (375)

7

Depressive Disorder

7.1. What is the most common symptom reported by patients with depression?

A. Difficulty sleeping
B. Decreased energy
C. Poor appetite
D. Poor concentration
E. Suicidal ideation

7.2. A 25-year-old man returns to the mental health center after having been prescribed a selective serotonin reuptake inhibitor (SSRI) for the past 6 weeks. He states that he is now able to focus much better in his law school classes. His mood has improved to the point that he does not "feel like there's always a dark cloud over my head." He reports increased energy, which he attributes to getting 7 hours of sleep a night "for the first time in years," and to "finally being hungry enough to eat as much as everyone else." He ends by saying "I thought everyone felt the same way I did. I didn't realize I could feel good most of the time. I had just felt so bad for so long." What is the most likely diagnosis?

A. Persistent depressive disorder
B. Major depressive disorder
C. Bipolar disorder
D. Generalized anxiety disorder
E. Cyclothymia

7.3. A 70-year-old woman presents to the primary care physician with complaints of difficulty concentrating over the last 4 weeks. "My brain is in a fog. I'm having trouble remembering things as well." She worries that she is showing signs of Alzheimer dementia, "like my father did before he died." She states that she used to do crossword puzzles daily to stay sharp, "but now I can't even finish one, so I've lost interest." She reports difficulty getting to sleep, which she attributes to anxiety about "forgetting things and losing my mind." She notes that she has lost about 4 pounds over the last month due to decreased appetite. She has no chronic medical illnesses and takes no medications. Vital signs are within normal limits. Physical examination reveals no abnormalities. Urinalysis, urine drug screen, complete blood count, and comprehensive metabolic panel are all within normal limits. What is the most likely diagnosis?

A. Dementia of the Alzheimer type
B. Generalized anxiety disorder
C. Major depressive disorder
D. Vascular dementia
E. Normal aging

7.4. Patients with depression are most likely to abuse what substance?

A. Alcohol
B. Benzodiazepines
C. Cocaine
D. Cannabis
E. Amphetamines

7.5. A 70-year-old man presents to the primary care physician with a complaint of weight loss. He lost his wife of 45 years 5 months ago, "and I haven't been the same since. I can't stop crying and thinking about her. The only thing that helps is knowing that when the good Lord calls me home, we'll be together in heaven." He lives alone and has no children or immediate family nearby. He states that during the day he is either in the bed sleeping or watching television, "but I just have it on. I'm not paying attention to it. It can't keep my attention anymore." He goes out to get groceries occasionally, "but I'm not hungry." He notes that his pants are now too big. He used to talk with some friends, "but I don't feel like doing that anymore. It takes too much out of me." Physical examination reveals an emaciated man who looks older than his stated age. The electronic medical record shows that he last lost 30 pounds since his visit 1 year ago, and that his BMI is now 16, down from 21. What is the most appropriate management?

A. Referral to a psychiatrist
B. Starting antidepressant therapy
C. Referral to a grief counselor
D. Inpatient hospitalization
E. A social work consult

7.6. A 34-year-old woman is diagnosed with major depressive disorder for the first time and started on an SSRI. After 8 weeks on a medium dosage of the medication, she states that she feels "about 50% better. I'm going to work every day, but it's still hard to concentrate and I feel a little 'blah'." Prior to starting treatment, she was in danger of losing her job because she stayed at home in bed for 3 weeks. She is on no other medications and has no other illnesses. What is the most appropriate next step in treatment?

A. Continue current management
B. Augment with an antidepressant of a different mechanism
C. Increase the dose of the current medication
D. Begin ketamine treatment
E. Change medication to another antidepressant

7.7. A 25-year-old woman who has been treated with antidepressant therapy as an outpatient for the last 3 months now reports that she is "back to myself." She states that her mood is usually an "8 or 9 out of 10, like I was before I got depressed." She denies difficulty with energy, concentration, sleep, or appetite, all of which were impaired during the major depressive episode, her first, which lasted for 2 months before she began treatment. She denies ever having suicidal ideation. Now that she feels better, she wishes to stop the medication. What is the most appropriate next step in treatment?

A. Start a 1- to 2-week taper now
B. Begin a 1- to 2-week taper in 6 months
C. Taper the mediation over the next 6 months
D. Continue the medication at a lower dose for 6 months, then reassess
E. Begin a 1- to 2-week taper in 12 months

7.8. During a therapy session for a 19-year-old man with major depressive disorder, he recalls a time 2 years ago in which his mother told him that she was disappointed in his grades at school. "Since then, I've felt that I always let everyone down and that I'm a failure at everything." The therapist challenges the patient's belief that he is no good at anything, and helps him develop a more realistic view of his abilities. This is an example of what type of psychosocial therapy?

A. Cognitive behavioral
B. Behavior
C. Interpersonal
D. Psychoanalytically oriented
E. Family

7.9. Studies have consistently shown that a substantial minority of patients with depression have an increase in what physiologic chemical?

A. GABA
B. Cortisol
C. Brain-derived neurotrophic factor (BDNF)
D. Prolactin
E. Growth hormone

7.10. Structural image studies show reduced volume in what brain structure in elderly patients with depressive disorders?

A. Hippocampus
B. Thalamus
C. Basal ganglia
D. Periventricular areas
E. Hypothalamus

7.11. What life stressor is most often associated with the development of depression?

A. Loss of a job
B. Sexual abuse
C. Loss of a parent or spouse
D. Chronic homelessness
E. Divorce

7.12. A 44-year-old woman during her first therapy session for depression recounts that at age 7, she was removed from her parents and placed in foster care due to their drug use. At age 16, she was doing well in school and at home until her foster mother died. When she was 35, she lost her job of 10 years due to the company's financial problems and resultant bankruptcy. A month ago, she lost her job of 8 years due to a global economic downturn. "Why even try? No matter what I do, I keep getting knocked down." According to the learned helplessness theory of depression, what should be the goal of treatment for this patient?

A. Working through feelings of abandonment by her birth and foster mothers
B. Helping her develop a more positive sense of self
C. Examining cognitive distortions about the likelihood of future untoward events
D. Helping her see that her depression is adaptive to the environmental stressors
E. Assisting her with learning a sense of control and mastery of the environment

ANSWERS

7.1. B. Decreased energy
The most common complaint of patients with depression is reduced energy (97%). About 80% report difficulty sleeping. Eighty-four percent report poor concentration. Many patients have decreased appetite. About 66% have suicidal ideation. (379)

7.2. A. Persistent depressive disorder
Though this patient is reporting being happy, it is in the context of not feeling as sad, as opposed to grandiosity. There is no history of mania, so bipolar disorder and cyclothymia would not be diagnosed. Though generalized anxiety disorder can present with difficulty concentrating and difficulty sleeping, he does not mention anxiety. He reports feeling depressed almost all of the time, which is more consistent with persistent depressive disorder than major depressive disorder, which has discrete episodes. (382)

7.3. C. Major depressive disorder
Given the patient's relatively sudden and acute onset of cognitive difficulties, it is unlikely that she has Alzheimer dementia, or that this is normal aging, both of which would be much more gradual. She has some symptoms of generalized anxiety disorder, such as difficulty with concentration and poor sleep, attributed to worrying. However, it would be uncommon, though not impossible, for it to present for the first time in the eighth decade (median age is in the 30s). Vascular dementia could present with acute problems in cognition, but is less likely as she has no history of cardiac or other health problems. Another explanation for her symptoms of poor concentration, loss of interest in crossword puzzles, difficulty sleeping, and decreased appetite is major depressive disorder. If depression profoundly affects cognition in the elderly, it is sometimes referred to as "pseudodementia." Once the depression is treated, prior cognitive functioning should return. (385)

7.4. A. Alcohol
While patients with a depressive disorder at times turn to stimulants such as cocaine and amphetamines, or to cannabis for relief of depression, alcohol use disorder frequently coexists in both major depressive disorder and bipolar I disorder, with a stronger association with depression in women than in men. People also sometimes use alcohol in a futile attempt to relieve depression. (386)

7.5. D. Inpatient hospitalization
Though the death of his wife was likely the cause of his current symptoms, he still meets criteria for major depressive disorder. The most concerning aspect is his nutritional status. Though he does not appear suicidal, he is in medical danger due to self-neglect from lack of appetite, confirmed by subjective report and objective measures of his weight and clothes. He needs to be hospitalized to begin treatment and refeeding. During hospitalization, the other measures, such as a psychiatric and social work referral and grief counseling, can be initiated. (388)

7.6. C. Increase the dose of the current medication
The goal in treatment of major depressive disorder is remission, not reduction of symptoms. As this patient has been on the same dose of the SSRI for 8 weeks, it is unlikely that she will experience significant further improvement. The next step is to increase the dosage of the medication, as it has been somewhat helpful. If the dose increase yields no further improvement, then augmentation with another antidepressant of a different mechanism, such as a norepinephrine dopamine reuptake inhibitor, as opposed to changing medications, would be indicated given that she has some proven benefit from the current medication. Ketamine is used for treatment-resistant depression. Given that this is the patient's first medication trial, she should not yet be considered treatment resistant. (390)

7.7. B. Begin a 1- to 2-week taper in 6 months
Given that the patient has experienced only one episode of major depression, which did not warrant inpatient hospitalization or did not involve suicidal ideation, she is a candidate for an attempt at medication discontinuation. An antidepressant that has led to complete remission of symptoms should be maintained for at least 6 months after remission, after which it can be tapered over 1 to 2 weeks, depending on the half-life of the medication. If she were on her second or more episode of major depression, or this episode was severe, then maintenance dosing should be considered. (390)

7.8. A. Cognitive behavioral
A cognitive behavioral therapist examines a person's automatic thoughts ("I'm no good at anything"), cognitive distortions (generalization), and other maladaptive beliefs and helps them develop more realistic attributions and ways of thinking. Behavior therapy usually involves operant conditioning, such

as punishment and reinforcement, to shape patient responses and interactions. Behavior therapy does not have many studies supporting its use in major depressive disorder. Interpersonal therapy focuses intently on relationships and how dysfunctional relationships can perpetuate depression. Though the patient talks about his mother in this example, his distress is centered on his feelings of failure, as opposed to his relationship with her. Psychoanalytically oriented therapy focuses on the relationship between therapist and patient, with the goal of bringing about change in the patient's personality structure. Family therapy involves working with multiple family members, as opposed to just mentioning a family member during a session. (392)

7.9. B. Cortisol
Several decades of testing of cortisol levels in depressed patients have shown a hyperactive hypothalamic–pituitary–adrenal axis, which leads to increased plasma, salivary, and urinary free cortisol levels, likely due to increased neurons in the hypothalamus. GABA, BDNF, and growth hormone are all decreased in major depression. A change in prolactin level has not been found. (394–395)

7.10. A. Hippocampus
The increased cortisol, which occurs due to increased corticotrophin-releasing hormone from the hypothalamus, damages the hippocampus, which normally inhibits hypothalamic–pituitary–adrenal (HPA) axis activity. Therefore, in contrast to an increased number of neurons in the hypothalamus in an individual under stress, there is a resultant decrease in hippocampal volume in image studies. This then can set up a feedback loop in which the HPA axis is further activated, which propagates the neuronal hippocampal loss due to the increased amount of cortisol. The basal ganglia and periventricular regions, like the thalamus, also show hyper- versus hypointensities in structural images. (395–397)

7.11. C. Loss of a parent or spouse
The life event most associated with the development of depression or the onset of a depressive episode is the loss of a parent before age 11 or the loss of a spouse, respectively. Unemployed persons are more likely to report depression than persons who are employed. (398)

7.12. E. Assisting her with learning a sense of control and mastery of the environment
The psychosocial theory that best fits this patient's circumstances is that of learned helplessness. She has been buffeted by several events out of her control and therefore, according to learned helplessness behaviorists, needs to learn that she has some environmental control in order to alleviate her symptoms of depression. Working through abandonment feelings and developing a more positive sense of self would be in line with a psychodynamic theory of depression. Examining cognitive distortions would be a goal of treatment from a cognitive theory, and seeing depression as adaptive would be expected from a therapist subscribing to evolutionary theory. (399–400)

8

Anxiety Disorders

8.1. A 14-year-old boy is brought to the outpatient psychiatrist by his parents because of a fear of dogs and thunderstorms. When he encounters one of them he starts breathing heavily, sweating, complaining of chest pain, and feeling dizzy. As they live in an area frequented by storms, he has "a panic attack" three or four times a week. The first time the symptoms occurred 3 months ago, his parents took him to the emergency department out of fear that he was having a heart attack. The workup was negative, and he was given an antianxiety agent to take on as-needed basis, which they have been refilling through his primary care physician. Since then, he has always carried the medication with him and insists on returning home if he realizes he does not have it. The school nurse has a supply of the medication in case he needs it. He avoids sleepovers out of fear of being embarrassed in front of his peers if he encounters one of the stressors. What is the most likely diagnosis?

A. Specific phobia
B. Panic disorder
C. Agoraphobia
D. Generalized anxiety disorder
E. Social phobia

8.2. The disruption of sleep is a core feature in what anxiety disorder?

A. Specific phobia
B. Panic disorder
C. Agoraphobia
D. Generalized anxiety disorder
E. Social phobia

8.3. Panic attacks, on average, last what length of time?

A. 1 to 5 minutes
B. 10 to 15 minutes
C. 20 to 30 minutes
D. 45 to 60 minutes
E. 60 to 90 minutes

8.4. A 38-year-old investment banker has recently earned a promotion that now involves giving oral weekly updates to the senior staff of the company. She has always been afraid of speaking in public, and would experience insomnia and gastrointestinal (GI) upset the night before she had to give a speech in school. She has been told that her first presentation will occur in 1 week, and calls her primary care physician for "anything that can help me get through this." What is the most appropriate pharmacologic management?

A. Begin a selective serotonin reuptake inhibitors (SSRI)
B. Begin a prn beta-blocker
C. Begin a prn benzodiazepine
D. Begin a prn benzodiazepine and concurrent SSRI
E. Begin a prn beta-blocker and concurrent SSRI

8.5. A 40-year-old woman presents with her wife to the psychiatric outpatient clinic with a chief complaint of, "I need to be okay with driving again. This is hampering my job, my social life, my home life, and is no way to live." She states that, 3 months ago, she was driving alone down a busy road when she was sideswiped by another vehicle. Neither driver was injured during the accident. However, her vehicle was damaged to the point that it could not be immediately driven, so she was given a loaner car at the shop while hers was being repaired. When she pulled out of the car repair shop parking lot, she was overcome by an intense wave of fear and pulled over and called her wife to take her home. Since then, she has experienced the same fear when attempting to drive, and either depends on her wife or a ride-sharing service for transportation. She does not want to use medication "because I don't want to depend on a pill." What should be the first step in psychotherapy for this patient's condition?

A. Teaching relaxation techniques
B. Visualization of getting into a car
C. Discussing the reasons she would like to drive
D. Having her drive within the office parking lot
E. Accompanying her on a short drive.

8.6. A 39-year-old man presents to the psychiatric outpatient clinic after experiencing his fifth episode of heart racing, sweating, dizziness, and shortness of breath in the last 3 weeks. He works as a chef and states that the first time the symptoms occurred a month ago, he was working a double shift at his restaurant. He said nothing about it and waited until the symptoms resolved on their own, which took about 20 minutes. He felt that he may have become overstressed and did not think much of it until it happened again 3 days later. He has had three more episodes in the past month. He went to the emergency department (ED) after the third and fourth episodes out of concern about having a heart attack, and was told, after an extensive cardiac workup, that his heart was fine. He is worried that he will lose his job if the episodes continue. He has never been on medications and has no chronic medical illnesses. Vital signs are temperature 98.0F, BP 150/90, pulse 95, and respirations 18. The evaluation should include a workup for what medical condition?

A. Diabetes
B. Lupus
C. Syphilis
D. Hyperthyroidism
E. Pancreatic cancer

ANSWERS

8.1. A. Specific phobia

Though the child shows the same symptoms as those of a panic attack, and may indeed be having full-blown panic attacks, he cannot be diagnosed with panic disorder, as the attacks are not unexpected. Because there are circumscribed triggers, specific phobia is the most likely diagnosis. He continues to leave the house and go to school, thus removing agoraphobia as a diagnosis. The fears are circumscribed and limited to the two stressors, which eliminates generalized anxiety disorder. Though he avoids some social situations due to being embarrassed if he were to have a panic attack in front of his peers, he would not be diagnosed with social anxiety, as the root cause of the fear is the specific triggers, as opposed to the social situation itself. (403–406)

8.2. D. Generalized anxiety disorder

Though someone experiencing a panic attack during the night would most likely experience a disruption in sleep, as would someone who encountered the trigger of a specific phobia at night, only for generalized anxiety disorder is sleep disruption a criterion in and of itself. Likewise, someone with a fear of being embarrassed in a social situation that was severe enough to warrant a diagnosis of social anxiety disorder may lose sleep the night before such a situation would occur, such as giving a speech in class the next day. (405)

8.3. C. 20 to 30 minutes

Panic attacks typically begin with physiologic symptoms of sweating, tachycardia, shaking, and shortness of breath, as well as psychological symptoms of impending doom and a feeling that something is wrong. These symptoms usually peak in about 10 minutes before resolving over the period of the next 10 to 20 minutes, for an average total length of 20 to 30 minutes. (406)

8.4. D. Begin a prn benzodiazepine and concurrent SSRI

Though beta-blockers (specifically propranolol) are often used for social anxiety disorder, the evidence for its use is scant, and SSRIs are still considered first-line treatment. Normally, the patient would be started on an SSRI alone and told that it will take the standard few weeks for it to become effective. In this case, the patient's job is dependent on her performance in the next few days, so she cannot wait several weeks. Therefore, it would be acceptable to start on a benzodiazepine for immediate relief, with the understanding that it will only be used while the SSRI takes effect, after which it will be discontinued. (407)

8.5. A. Teaching relaxation techniques

The patient is suffering from a specific phobia, that of driving. The treatment of choice is graded exposure, in which the patient would be reintroduced to the elements of driving. For example, she could begin with visualizing herself behind the wheel of a car or holding the car keys in her hand and eventually progress to driving in a self-contained area, such as the office parking lot, with the end goal of fully driving by herself. One of the cornerstones of graded exposure is first learning how to deal with the anxiety that the exposures will inevitably cause. For that reason, learning relaxation techniques would be the first step in graded exposure therapy. This patient has already stated her reasons for wanting to drive, so going through those again is not likely to yield much, if any, benefit. (408)

8.6. D. Hyperthyroidism

Many medical disorders, such as hypo- or hyperthyroidism, hyperparathyroidism, and pheochromocytomas, can have symptoms that resemble panic attacks. This patient increased heart rate and hypertension, which are signs of hyperthyroidism. Episodic hypoglycemia associated with insulinomas, but not diabetes in general can cause symptoms that mimic panic attacks. Pancreatic cancer can lead to a feeling of doom and anxiety, but not usually panic attacks. Syphilis and lupus are not known to cause panic attacks. (406)

Obsessive-Compulsive and Related Disorders

9.1. Which of the following types of obsessions is most commonly associated with obsessive–compulsive disorder (OCD)?

A. Contamination fears
B. Counting
C. Pathologic doubt
D. Sexual acts
E. Suicidal thoughts

9.2. Which pattern of body concern is most often associated with body dysmorphic disorder?

A. Concern about multiple different areas of the body
B. Emphasis on the thighs and stomach
C. Focus on body symmetry
D. Intense preoccupation with weight and shape concerns
E. Possessing good insight about their actual versus desired appearance

9.3. A child presents to the hospital with severe emaciation and parents report significant restricting behaviors. This child denies body image concerns though parents report that she has visible mealtime anxiety. She refuses to talk more when asked about her eating and just stares blankly ahead. She reports some school worries though parents confirm she sleeps and focuses well. Physical examination is noteworthy for a palpable abdominal mass. She ends up being transferred to the intensive care unit (ICU) for extremely low hemoglobin and hematocrit and there is a concern that she is bleeding out. Which of the following is most likely the underlying diagnosis?

A. Anorexia nervosa
B. Generalized anxiety disorder
C. Major depressive disorder-
D. Trichotillomania
E. Unspecified psychotic disorder

9.4. The most common demographic group to be affected by olfactory reference syndrome includes which of the following?

A. Elderly, single females
B. Married, middle-aged males
C. Married, middle-aged females
D. Middle-aged, single females
E. Young, single males

9.5. Obsessive–compulsive disorder (OCD) symptoms from a neurologic cause, such as basal ganglia disease, are more likely to have which type of onset in which demographic group?

A. Insidious onset in a middle-aged person
B. Insidious onset in an elderly person
C. Insidious onset in younger individuals
D. New-onset symptoms in middle-aged individuals
E. New-onset symptoms in older individuals

9.6. Damage to which brain region can cause excessive hoarding?

A. Cingulate cortex
B. Frontal lobe
C. Hippocampal lobe
D. Parietal cortex
E. Temporal lobe

9.7. Which of the following criterion is required for making a diagnosis of trichotillomania, or hair-pulling disorder, according to International Classification of Diseases, Tenth Revision (ICD-10), but is not a part of the DSM-5 criteria?

A. Anxiety that precedes and is relieved by the hairpulling
B. Hairpulling despite repeated attempts to change
C. Impairment in social functioning
D. Pulling out hair from more than one site of the body
E. Recurrent pulling resulting in hair loss

9.8. A patient chooses to wear a wig after repeatedly pulling their hair out. The patient is unable to stop, as it is reported to alleviate significant anxiety at the moment. Which of the following psychiatric disorders is most commonly comorbid with this condition?

A. Attention deficit hyperactivity disorder
B. Anorexia nervosa
C. Excoriation disorder
D. Schizophrenia
E. Substance use disorder

9.9. A patient presents with struggles falling asleep due to constant checking of the locks in the home and having to tap on all of the windows 10 times in multiples of 10. Examination is notable for frequent eye blinking and throat clearing. The patient is still struggling after being on sertraline 200 mg PO daily for 3 months. In this scenario, there is the most evidence base to support the use of which of the following psychiatric medications as adjunctive treatment for this disorder?

A. Aripiprazole
B. Clomipramine
C. Lamotrigine
D. Memantine
E. Olanzapine

9.10. Both therapy and medication for obsessive–compulsive disorder (OCD) can correct abnormalities in functioning in which of the following brain pathways?

A. Corpus callosum
B. Corticospinal and corticobulbar tracts
C. Cortico-striatal-thalamic-cortical
D. Dorsal column–medial lemniscus pathway
E. Retinohypothalmic tract

ANSWERS

9.1. A. Contamination fears
The most common pattern in OCD is an obsession of contamination, which is often followed by washing or compulsive avoidance of the contaminated object. Pathologic doubt is the second most common obsession seen in OCD, often followed by checking compulsions. The third most common pattern in OCD is intrusive obsessional thoughts without compulsions. (415)

9.2. A. Concern about multiple different areas of the body
The most common concern in patients with body dysmorphic disorder involves the face and head and can also include the skin, nose, and hair. Most patients with body dysmorphic disorder worry about five to seven different body areas. Only about a quarter of patients are concerned with symmetry of their appearance, and only about a quarter of patients have reasonable insight. Weight- and shape-related concerns of other body areas, such as the thighs and stomach are more consistent with body dysmorphia from an eating disorder. (416)

9.3. D. Trichotillomania
While the patient above presents with some features of anorexia, the physical examination findings of a palpable abdominal mass point toward a bezoar. Most likely she is pulling and eating her hair (trichophagia) after pulling it out (trichotillomania), which is leading to an intestinal obstruction. Medical complications of trichophagy include trichobezoars, intestinal obstruction, and malnutrition. (418)

9.4. E. Young, single males
Olfactory-reference syndrome involves the preoccupation of having the false belief that one has an offensive body odor. It is most commonly found in young, single males, with an average age of onset of 25 years old. (419)

9.5. E. New-onset symptoms in older individuals
When OCD develops before the age of 30 years and new-onset symptoms in older individuals occur, concern should be raised for a potential neurologic disease. This can include disorders such as Sydenham chorea and Huntington disease. (420)

9.6. A. Cingulate cortex
Hoarding can be common with certain genetic conditions including Prader–Willi syndrome and Alzheimer disease. Damage to the anterior ventromedial prefrontal cortex along with the cingulate cortex can lead to heavy hoarding behaviors. (421)

9.7. A. Anxiety that precedes and is relieved by the hairpulling
Per ICD-10 criteria for trichotillomania, all that is required for a diagnosis is the notice of hair loss due to hair-pulling behavior and hair-pulling behavior that is preceded by increased anxiety that is relieved by the hairpulling. For the DSM-5 criteria, there must also be recurrent hairpulling resulting in hair loss, along with repeated attempts to change the behavior, an impairment in functioning, or the behavior leading to significant distress. (422)

9.8. C. Excoriation disorder
The patient described in the vignette has hair-pulling disorder, or trichotillomania. The most common comorbidity with it is excoriation disorder. Other common comorbidities include obsessive–compulsive disorder (OCD). More than half of those with excoriation disorder have another psychiatric disorder, most commonly a mood or anxiety disorder. (423, 424)

9.9. A. Aripiprazole
Both risperidone and aripiprazole are best supported as adjunctive treatment for obsessive–compulsive disorder (OCD) when patients fail to respond fully to selective serotonin reuptake inhibitors (SSRI) trials. High doses of SSRIs for at least 12 weeks should be utilized first. Though conflicting data, some show that the atypical antipsychotics are particularly useful when tics are comorbid with the OCD. Response to the atypical antipsychotics is typically quick (i.e., 4 weeks). Memantine and lamotrigine are experimental agents that might be promising in the future, along with other meds such as riluzole, ketamine, and NAC. (424)

9.10. C. Cortico-striatal-thalamic-cortical (CSTC)
It is thought that CSTC pathway plays a role in contributing to the cognitive–affective impairments in OCD, with abnormal activation and inhibition. These impairments result in cognitive inflexibility and alteration in the habit system and contribute to motor impulsivity. Medication treatment and cognitive behaivoral therapy (CBT) have been shown on imaging studies to normalize the functional alterations in the CSTC pathway in OCD. (426)

10

Trauma- and Stressor-Related Disorders

10.1. A patient was just diagnosed with breast cancer and seeks help from a psychiatrist after experiencing 2 months of depressed mood and anxiety. She has missed many days of work and has stopped going to her favorite weekly art class. She reports still eating and sleeping well and denied any suicidal thoughts. Which of the following is her most likely diagnosis?

A. Acute stress disorder
B. Adjustment disorder
C. Major depressive disorder
D. Posttraumatic stress disorder (PTSD)
E. Unspecified anxiety disorder

10.2. In addition to negative mood, two symptoms from which of the following criteria must be met for a diagnosis of posttraumatic stress disorder (PTSD)?

A. Arousal alterations
B. Avoidance
C. Different traumas
D. Dissociative
E. Intrusions

10.3. A lack of specificity in which criteria is a potential challenge in diagnosing someone with an adjustment disorder?

A. Age of onset
B. Avoidance and hyperstartle symptoms
C. Psychosocial consequence descriptions
D. Symptom presentation time frame
E. The stressor and severity descriptions

10.4. A diagnosis of posttraumatic stress disorder (PTSD) can only be made if which of the following criterion is met?

A. Anxiety and depression are present
B. Constant symptoms exist without fluctuations
C. Symptom presentation arises rapidly
D. Persistent symptoms exist for at least 1 month
E. Two avoidance symptoms are met

10.5. A patient was robbed getting into her car. Three months later she presents with ongoing nightmares, flashbacks, trouble sleeping and focusing. She is overwhelmed with fear and anger and can no longer bring herself to drive. Which medication has the most robust evidence to help with this diagnosis?

A. Topiramate
B. Paroxetine
C. Prazosin
D. Risperidone
E. Venlafaxine

10.6. Which type of evidence-based therapy for posttraumatic stress disorder (PTSD) focuses on correcting faulty attributions from the trauma, such as viewing the world as a dangerous place?

A. Cognitive processing therapy (CPT)
B. Eye movement desensitization and reprocessing therapy (EMDR)
C. Present-centered therapy (PCT)
D. Prolonged exposure therapy (PE)
E. Trauma-focused cognitive behavioral therapy (TFCBT)

10.7. Of the factors listed, which of the following is the most important risk factor for developing posttraumatic stress disorder (PTSD)?

A. Being single or divorced
B. Being very young or very old
C. Having good financial means, being labeled in a high socioeconomic class
D. Participating in the Vietnam war
E. Severity of or proximity to the trauma

ANSWERS

10.1. B. Adjustment disorder
Adjustment disorders are in response to a stressful life event, such as a medical diagnosis, financial difficulties, relationship problems, etc. It can occur within 3 months of the stressor and can result in depressive symptoms and/or anxiety, resulting in a disturbance in functioning and possibly a disturbance in conduct. A PTSD would be more likely to occur with traumatic events such as assault, crimes, physical or sexual abuse, war, etc. The patient would experience nightmares or flashbacks and avoidance symptoms. An acute stress disorder differs from PTSD in that the symptoms occur within 1 day to 1 month of the trauma. A major depressive disorder would likely include other symptoms such as changes in appetite, sleeping, energy, suicidal thoughts, etc. (429)

10.2. A. Arousal alterations
In addition to a history of exposure to trauma, a PTSD diagnosis requires one symptom of intrusion (i.e., reenactment, nightmares, dissociative responses, etc.), one of avoidance (i.e., avoiding memories or external reminders of the trauma), two symptoms of negative mood/cognition (i.e., negative perceptions of self, cognitive distortions, excessive guilt, decreased interest in activities, etc.), and two in arousal alterations (i.e., irritability, anger, hypervigilance, risk taking, sleep disturbances, etc.). (431)

10.3. E. The stressor and severity descriptions
One of the challenges in diagnosing an adjustment disorder is that there are no clear criteria that define the stressors that are required to make this diagnosis and specific affective, cognitive, and autonomic descriptions are not specified. Another challenge is that the symptoms can be of any severity. It is defined that the symptoms need to occur within 3 months of the stressor. The disorder can occur at any age. Specific criteria are included for avoidance and hyperarousal symptoms for a posttraumatic stress disorder (PTSD) diagnosis. The symptoms for both PTSD and an adjustment disorder should result in some impairment in functioning. (433)

10.4. E. Persistent symptoms exist for at least 1 month
Many people experience PTSD symptoms including shock, nightmares, and flashbacks after a traumatic event. However, most resolve on their own and some will meet criteria for an acute stress disorder. A diagnosis of PTSD can only be made if the symptoms persist for at least 1 month. It is normal for symptoms to fluctuate with various degrees of intensity over time. PTSD may or may not be associated with comorbid anxiety or depression. Two negative mood/cognition and two arousal alteration symptoms are required to make a diagnosis of PTSD though only one symptom of intrusion and one of avoidance are required. A rapid presentation of symptoms is not required. There is a modifier criterion for delayed expression with symptoms not presenting until at least 6 months after the trauma. (431, 434)

10.5. B. Paroxetine
The patient described has a diagnosis of posttraumatic stress disorder (PTSD). The selective serotonin reuptake inhibitors (SSRIs), particularly sertraline and paroxetine have the most robust evidence for efficacy. There is some supportive evidence that the serotonin and norepinephrine reuptake inhibitors (SNRIs), such as venlafaxine and the atypical antipsychotics, such as risperidone, along with anticonvulsants, such as topiramate could be helpful. Prazosin can help with nightmares found in posttraumatic stress disorder. (434)

10.6. A. Cognitive processing therapy (CPT)
CPT involves correcting faulty attributions as mentioned above such as views of the world being uncontrollable and unpredictable. EMDR involves recalling distressing images of the trauma while receiving sensory inputs. Patient-centered therapy focuses on the current relationship and work challenges and does not directly address the trauma. TFCBT includes prolonged exposure therapy and involves reexperiencing the traumatic event through imaginal and in vivo exposures. (435)

10.7. E. Severity of or proximity to the trauma
While certain factors increase the risk of PTSD such as being a young adult, single, divorced, widowed, socially withdrawn, or of low socioeconomic class, the most important risk factors include the severity, duration, and proximity of a person's exposure to the trauma. While one survey showed approximately 30% of males developed PTSD from the Vietnam war, other trauma aside from war can also lead to the development of PTSD. (435)

11

Dissociative Disorders

11.1. A wife brings her husband to the emergency room (ER) presenting with unusual behavior. She noted that he doesn't remember her or his name, his job, and is acting like a child. Which diagnosis is most likely?

A. Acute stress disorder
B. Dissociative amnesia
C. Dissociative fugue
D. Malingering
E. Transient global amnesia

11.2. Which symptom is more indicative of a seizure disorder rather than a dissociative amnesia?

A. Alterations in consciousness
B. Ongoing depersonalization
C. Persistence of memory impairment
D. Sudden wandering and traveling away from a main residence
E. Quick resolution of bizarre behaviors

11.3. Which of the following DSM-5 criteria for depersonalization/derealization disorder is only present for derealization symptoms and not for depersonalization?

A. Detachment from surroundings
B. Feelings of observing oneself
C. Perceptual distortions
D. Sense of unreality
E. Time distortion

11.4. Which personality traits are most commonly seen with dissociative identity disorder?

A. Avoidant
B. Borderline
C. Obsessive compulsive
D. Narcissistic
E. Schizotypal

11.5. A patient is evaluated in the emergency room after being brought in off the street and was found to be in a trance-like state. The patient is unable to identify their age or address. Upon cognitive testing, the patient replies that 2 + 2 is 5 and hands the doctor a key when asked to hand a pencil. When asked to point to the color green, the patient points to something gray. The patient reports feeling confused due to hearing voices and seeing strange things. These symptoms best fit which of the following diagnoses?

A. Depersonalization disorder
B. Derealization disorder
C. Dissociative identity disorder
D. Ganser syndrome
E. Transient global amnesia

11.6. While often a treatment-refractory group, those with depersonalization and derealization disorders appear to partially benefit from which of the following medication treatments?

A. Atypical antipsychotics
B. Mood stabilizers
C. Serotonin reupdate inhibitors
D. Tricyclic antidepressants
E. Typical antipsychotics

11.7. Which is the first step in psychotherapy in treating a patient with dissociative identity disorder?

A. Establishing safety and symptom stabilization
B. Fusion and integration of all states
C. Improved communication and collaboration with self-states
D. Hypnotherapeutic interventions
E. Processing of traumatic memories and life experiences

11.8. Limitations of dialectical behavioral therapy (DBT) for treatment of dissociative identity disorder include a lack of focus in which of the following areas?

A. Affect regulation
B. Depersonalization/derealization and flashbacks
C. Distress tolerance
D. Safety and wellness
E. Therapy-interfering behaviors

11.9. Which somatic treatment strategy is most useful for patients with dissociative identity disorder?

A. Selective serotonin reuptake inhibitor (SSRI) treatment should be initiated as first-line therapy
B. Stick with smaller doses of alpha-antagonists to best help with nightmares
C. Treat comorbid symptoms present across most personalities
D. Use typical antipsychotics to decrease anxiety and flashbacks
E. Utilize electroconvulsive therapy (ECT) for those with persistent psychotic features

11.10. After depression and anxiety, which of the following is the third most commonly reported psychiatric symptom?

A. Attentional/focusing issues
B. Auditory/visual hallucinations
C. Body checking/restricting
D. Delusions/paranoia
E. Depersonalization/derealization

ANSWERS

11.1. B. Dissociative amnesia
This case presents a classic description of dissociative amenia, including a patient with a history of an acute trauma and physical symptoms including alterations in consciousness, a trance state, age regression, anterograde dissociative amnesia, etc. Dissociative fugue involves a sudden, unexpected travel away from the usual place where the person resides, along with the amnesia and identity confusion. While there is no absolute way to differentiate dissociative amnesia from a factitious disorder or malingering, often there is a history of the individual trying to escape legal, financial, or personal difficulties. Often, these patients will confess spontaneously when confronted. While dissociative amnesia can be a part of an acute stress disorder, the other acute stress features are not also present in this case. Transient global amnesia involves a sudden onset of complete anterograde amnesia, along with retrograde amnesia, while there is preservation of personal identity and an anxious awareness of the memory loss. (438)

11.2. E. Quick resolution of bizarre behaviors
While seizures should be part of the differential diagnosis for dissociate amnesia and in some cases, the diagnosis can only be clarified by EEG monitoring, for the most part, the clinical presentation of seizures differs from dissociate amnesia. With seizure, there are clear-cut ictal events and the patient can show wandering, semipurposeful, or bizarre behavior and memory problems but rarely do after postictal event. Changes in consciousness and depersonalization can be seen with dissociative amnesia and a sudden change in residence can be seen with dissociative fugue. (438, 439)

11.3. A. Detachment from surroundings
While feelings that things aren't real can be a part of depersonalization or derealization symptoms, the only other DSM-5 criteria to describe derealization includes feeling detached from one's surroundings. Depersonalization symptoms including feeling detached from oneself and feeling as if observing oneself, along with time and perceptual distortions. (441)

11.4. C. Obsessive compulsive
Obsessive compulsive disorder (OCD) symptoms along with obsessive compulsive personality traits are most commonly seen in dissociative identity disorder. Compulsive checking, handwashing, and counting often occur in those with dissociative phenomena, abuse, and post-traumatic stress disorder (PTSD) symptoms. (444)

11.5. D. Ganser syndrome
Ganser syndrome is characterized by giving approximate answers and often the correct answer is passed over for a related, but incorrect one. It also includes clouding of consciousness or conversion symptoms, along with dissociative symptoms, such as amnesia, along with trance-like behaviors, and in half of the cases, visual and auditory hallucinations are also reported. In dissociative identity disorder, acute forms of amnesia along with a fugue episode can be present. These patients report multiple forms of complex amnesia including recurrent blackouts, and have fluctuations in skills, habits, and knowledge. Depersonalization disorder is the persistent feeling of detachment or estranged from one's self. Derealization involves feelings of unreality or being detached from one's environment. Transient global amnesia includes a sudden onset of complete anterograde amnesia, along with pronounced retrograde amnesia but preservation of memory for personal identity is intact. (445)

11.6. C. Serotonin reuptake inhibitors
Those with depersonalization and derealization disorders might partially respond to medication including serotonin reupdate inhibitors, benzodiazepines, and stimulants. Also, there is some evidence for opioid antagonists and cognitive enhancers in helping with depersonalization and derealization disorders. There is absolutely no empirical evidence to support the use of either typical or atypical antipsychotics and these medications may increase feelings of emotional deadness. (446)

11.7. A. Establishing safety and symptom stabilization
Psychotherapy using a phasic model to treat the complex posttraumatic disorder is mainstay treatment for dissociative identity disorder. Phase 1 consists of stabilization of the dissociative symptoms and comorbid symptoms and establishing safety. Phase 2 involves working on the traumatic memories and making sure the patient is stabilized and aware of the risk of acute worsening of PTSD symptoms. Phase 3 involves fusion, reintegration, and recovery. While hypnotherapy can alleviate some symptoms such as flashbacks and dissociative hallucinations, some controversies exist and it should not be the first step in psychotherapy. (446)

11.8. B. Depersonalization/derealization and flashbacks

DBT was developed for the treatment of borderline personality disorder. Given many patients with borderline personality disorder report trauma histories, it has been thought that DBT might help those with dissociative identity disorder as well. DBT focuses on safety, therapy-interfering behaviors, affect regulation strategies, distress tolerance, and radical acceptance, all of which can be helpful in the treatment of dissociative identity disorder. However, one limitation is that it does not directly focus on the main symptoms of dissociative identity disorder, including depersonalization/derealization and dissociative amnesia, along with flashbacks, and trauma-based symptoms. (447)

11.9. C. Treat comorbid symptoms present across most personalities

Various medications might be useful in the treatment of dissociative identity disorder. Often nightmares are responsive to higher doses of alpha-adrenergic antagonists, such as prazosin, if tolerated. Antidepressant medications including SSRIs, tricyclics, and monoamine oxidase inhibitors (MAOIs) can be helpful in reducing depression and stabilizing mood. Atypical neuroleptics are more effective and better tolerated compared to typical ones for helping with severe anxiety and PTSD symptoms. However, the most effective strategy is to target comorbid symptoms that are present across most or all personalities. Given rapid symptom fluctuations in this disorder, it is important to avoid chasing each symptom with a new medication or change in dose. (448)

11.10. E. Depersonalization/derealization

Transient experiences of depersonalization/derealization can be prevalent in both normal and clinical populations and are the third most commonly reported psychiatric symptom following depression and anxiety. A lifetime prevalence is estimated to be anywhere from 26% to 74%. (449)

12

Somatic Symptom and Related Disorders

12.1. Which of the following DSM-5 criteria are no longer required for a diagnosis of a somatic disorder?

A. Abnormal labs and medical findings
B. Anxiety and depressive symptoms
C. Impairment daily
D. Persistent belief of an undetected disease
E. Symptoms that cannot be medically explained

12.2. Which feature differentiates illness anxiety from somatic symptom disorder?

A. Addiction to internet searches about the feared illness
B. Daily social or occupational impairment
C. Lack of medical evidence to explain the symptoms
D. Need for excessive reassurance from medical doctors
E. No significant physical symptoms

12.3. A patient is in the hospital for being unable to walk and having fainting spells after being in a car accident. The patient was driving his car when getting in the accident and witnessed his friend being killed. Multiple medical workups have not found any medical explanation for these neurologic symptoms. Which psychiatric diagnosis is most likely?

A. Conversion disorder
B. Dissociative disorder
C. Factitious disorder
D. Illness anxiety disorder
E. Somatic symptom disorder

12.4. International Classification of Diseases, Tenth Revision (ICD-10) criteria for somatization disorder differs from DSM-5 criteria for somatic symptom disorder in which of the following ways?

A. More than one pain symptom is required
B. No exclusion of a medical cause of the symptoms is required
C. Social or interpersonal impairment is not necessary
D. The duration of the symptoms lasts for a much longer time frame
E. The patient must be anxious about the symptoms

12.5. Which of the following test findings is more consistent with a conversion disorder rather than an underlying neurologic issue?

A. A patient reporting arm paralysis hits his hand on his face when his hand is dropped
B. A patient reporting blindness can touch his index fingers together
C. No flinching is noted when sudden bright lights are flashed in the eyes of a patient complaining of complete blindness
D. Sensory loss conforming to a specific pattern of distribution is found in a patient endorsing anesthesia
E. There is an absence of relative afferent pupillary defect in a patient complaining of blindness in one eye

12.6. An inpatient with many past psychiatric hospitalizations at various places reports severe depression and hallucinations after years of no response to various antidepressant treatments and electroconvulsive therapy (ECT). The patient reported the depression happened after witnessing a child being run over and killed. The patient won't sign consent to contact any relatives for collateral and reports worsening of symptoms the day before discharge, with no clear triggers. The patient is requesting further stay so that more in-depth medical and psychological testing can be done. This history is most consistent with which of the following psychiatric disorders?

A. Conversion disorder
B. Factitious disorder
C. La belle indifference
D. Major depressive disorder
E. Malingering

12.7. Which of the following history elements should trigger suspicion of a factitious disorder? Choose four correct answers.

A. Deterioration early in the hospital stay
B. Fixed fear of having a specific disease
C. History of opiate prescriptions without cause
D. History of working in the health care field
E. Lack of concern about symptoms
F. Resistance to a psychiatric assessment required for surgical clearance
G. Request for disability papers to be filled out
H. Request for invasive medical treatment

12.8. Which is a physical examination or test finding that can be indicative of a factious disorder?

A. A fever of 40 °C with diaphoresis
B. Anemia with blood found in the stool
C. Dermatitis on the back
D. Electrocardiogram (EKG) changes along with changes in creatine kinase levels
E. Healing of chronic wounds when casted

12.9. Somatic symptom disorder can be distinguished from factitious disorder, or malingering, in which of the following ways?

A. La belle indifference is present
B. No simulations of the reported symptoms are shown
C. Siblings also show unexplained illnesses
D. Symptoms are transient and lack focus on a specific disease
E. The patient insists on invasive medical procedures

12.10. What percentage of those with conversion disorder is later diagnosed with a neurologic or nonpsychiatric medical disorder explaining the symptoms?

A. 0 to 15
B. 25 to 50
C. 50 to 75
D. 75 to 90
E. 85 to 95

12.11. Somatic symptom disorder is most often comorbid with which of the following psychiatric disorders?

A. Eating
B. Depressive
C. Posttraumatic
D. Psychotic
E. Substance

12.12. Which antidepressants seem to be more effective for treatment of pain related to somatic symptom disorders?

A. Dopamine reupdate inhibitors
B. Serotonin antagonist and reuptake inhibitors
C. Serotonin-norepinephrine reuptake inhibitor
D. Selective serotonin reuptake inhibitors
E. Tricyclics

12.13. Which is a crucial first step in treating a child once the diagnosis of a factitious disorder imposed on them by a parent has been made?

A. Calling child welfare services
B. Discharging the patient from the hospital
C. Educating the parent of the dangers of their actions
D. Notifying the police
E. Performing further medical procedures to confirm the diagnosis

12.14. A higher prevalence of conversion disorder exists among which of the following populations?

A. Adults over 35 years old
B. Children under 6 years old
C. Males of all ages
D. People with no prior outpatient psychiatric treatment
E. Surgical referral to a psychiatry consultation service

ANSWERS

12.1. E. Symptoms that cannot be medically explained

An older perspective for somatic disorders involved only including symptoms that could not be medically explained. We now know that patients with medically established diagnoses can have a disproportionate amount of anxiety or physical symptoms from their medical disorder. Thus, in DSM-5, it is no longer required for symptoms to be medically unexplained. Patients with somatic symptom disorder believe they have an undetected disease, and the symptoms are typically impairing their lives on a day-to-day basis. Anxiety and depression are common comorbid symptoms, in addition to the somatic symptoms with this disorder. (451)

12.2. E. No significant physical symptoms

Similarities between illness anxiety disorder and somatic symptom disorder include a strong belief that the person has a serious undiagnosed medical illness despite evidence to the contrary. Significant impairment in day-to-day functioning remains. These patients are often addicted to searches about their feared illness and often seek excessive reassurance from medical providers. Unlike those with somatic symptom disorder, patients with illness anxiety disorder do not have significant physical symptoms. (451)

12.3. A. Conversion disorder

Patients with conversion disorders, also known as functional neurologic symptom disorder, often appear to have a neurologic condition such as a sensory or motor problem, which are found to be incompatible with true neurologic conditions The symptoms are not intentionally produced and often follow a trauma or other stressor. Paralysis, dysphasia, seizures, blindness, or deafness are common symptoms seen, along with disturbances in consciousness. (451)

12.4. D. The duration of the symptoms lasts for a much longer time frame

While perhaps the major difference between ICD-10 somatization disorder versus DSM-5 somatic symptom disorder is that the DSM-5 omitted the criteria requiring evidence that there is no underlying medical cause of the disorder, another difference is that the symptoms for somatic symptom disorder are only required to last a relatively short amount of time, more than 6 months, whereas the ICD-10 criteria for somatization disorder require the symptoms must last for more than 2 years. Other minor differences include that for somatic symptom disorder, anxiety about the symptoms is a necessary criterion. (452)

12.5. E. There is an absence of relative afferent pupillary defect in a patient complaining of blindness in one eye

In testing for true monocular blindness, the Marcus Gunn, or swinging flashlight test can be done. If no relative afferent pupillary defect is noted, it is consistent with a conversion disorder, rather than actual blindness. Even patients that are fully blind should be able to touch their index fingers together by proprioception, but often those with conversion disorder cannot when complaining of blindness. When bright lights are shown into the eyes of someone with conversion disorder who is complaining of blindness, typically flinching is noted. The Hoover test, dropping someone's hand onto the face, can test for conversion disorder if the patient's hand falls next to, instead of on the face. If the anesthesia is due to conversion disorder rather than an actual organic problem, typically the sensory loss does not conform to a specific nerve pattern. (455)

12.6. B. Factitious disorder

Factitious disorder can be imposed on oneself or others. It involves a patient feigning to have a medical or psychiatric illness to achieve the sick role. Unlike with malingering, in factitious disorder, no clear secondary gain can be found. Elements of the history that can suggest a factitious disorder include a history of bereavement involving a violent or bloody death, often in a child. Symptoms of depression, hallucinations, conversion symptoms, and memory issues are commonly found. Often, these patients take psychoactive substances to produce the symptoms. A history of multiple treatments at various hospitals, along with requests for more tests to be performed, are common features of a factitious disorder. Another feature is that the illness does not follow the typical pattern of remission or show some response to treatment. A flare-up of symptoms before discharge can also commonly be found. (456)

12.7. C. History of opiate prescriptions without cause, D. History of working in the health care field, F. Resistance to a psychiatric assessment required for surgical clearance, and H. Request for invasive medical treatment

Common signs of factitious disorder include the above answers, along with a patient seeking treatment at various hospitals, inconsistent information being given, a history of many medical tests and consultations being performed, findings consistent with self-manipulation, and at least one health care worker considering the diagnoses of factious disorder. (457)

12.8. E. Healing of chronic wounds when casted

A suggestive sign of a factious disorder can include a nonhealing wound that finally heals when casted. Dermatitis with lesions distributed in reachable areas (i.e., not on the back) could be a sign of factitious disorder. High fevers of more than 41 °C with no diaphoresis or other signs of viral infection are typical for a factious disorder. Factitious disorder is often indicated by a history of anemia, but no clear site of bleeding can be found. In a person feigning an infarction and trying to elevate the creatine kinase levels by beating themselves, and EKG would not show changes typical of an infarction. (458–460)

12.9. B. No simulations of the reported symptoms are shown

Somatic symptom disorder is distinguished from factitious disorder and malingering in that those with somatic symptom disorder do not simulate the symptoms they report. La belle indifference can be a sign of conversion disorder, though is an unreliable one. Siblings showing unexplained illness can be common in factitious disorders by proxy. Symptoms of conversion disorder are transient and do not focus on a particular disease. Seeking invasive or painful procedures can be a sign of a factitious disorder. (462, 463)

12.10. B. 25 to 50

It is important to note that an estimated 25% to 50% of those classified with a conversion disorder later receive a neurologic or nonpsychiatric medical diagnosis accounting for their symptoms. This should serve as a reminder that in all cases of conversion disorder, a thorough medical and neurologic workup should always be performed. (463)

12.11. B. Depressive

Depressive and anxiety disorders are highly comorbid with somatic symptoms disorder. Comorbid medical illnesses can also exist. (464)

12.12. E. Tricyclics

While CBT has been found to be most effective for the treatment of somatic symptom disorders, when psychopharmacology is required, the antidepressants seem to work, with data favoring the older antidepressants, such as the tricyclics, over the newer ones, such as the serotonin reuptake inhibitors. (465)

12.13. A. Calling child welfare services

In cases of factitious disorder imposed on another, often legal interventions need to be made. In cases in which the child is being harmed, notifying child welfare or child protective services is the first step. The child should not be discharged home, as they might require placement in another family for safety. The first step is to always make sure the child is safe. Often an inpatient admission is needed for safety and to institute a plan. (466)

12.14. E. Surgical referral to a psychiatry consultation service

Though rare in the general population, around less than 1%, conversion disorder is found in higher rate (5% to 14%) in medical or surgical referrals to a psychiatrist consultation liaison service, and in those receiving outpatient treatment in psychiatric clinics (5% to 25%). Those with conversion disorder tend to be females under the age of 35 years and children as young as 7 years old have been reported to have conversion disorder. (467)

13

Feeding and Eating Disorders

13.1. A 14-year-old female reports not eating during the day because she feels too anxious to eat at school and doesn't like the school lunch. Her parents report she refuses snacks when coming home from school and exercises for 2 hours daily. Parents report she then eats a big dinner and snacks constantly until 7 PM, and then won't eat anything further. She denied any body image concerns though her parents reported she is going to the bathroom more frequently and has reported nausea and vomiting. Her periods stopped and she lost weight and she is now at 105 lb at a height of 5′5″. She reported wanting to gain weight. Which of the following disorders are most likely?

A. Anorexia nervosa, binge/purge subtype
B. Bulimia nervosa
C. Night eating syndrome
D. Other specified feeding or eating disorder
E. Purging disorder

13.2. A 13-year-old female presents with increased isolation and is skipping meals. Her parents report concern of weight loss though noted it is difficult to tell since she wears baggy clothing and is refusing to be weighed. They reported she is exercising multiple times daily and when they see her eat, she cuts her food up until little pieces. Medical evaluation would most likely show which of the following findings (choose three).

A. Bradycardia
B. Hypercholesterolemia
C. Hyperthermia
D. Hypertension
E. Increased gastric emptying
F. Lanugo
G. Leukocytosis

13.3. Which of the following endocrine findings can be seen in patients with anorexia nervosa?

A. Decreased cortisol
B. Decreased reverse triiodothyronine
C. Elevated growth hormone
D. Increased thyroxine
E. Lower levels of prolactin

13.4. Which feature is unique to anorexia versus bulimia nervosa?

A. Absence of menses
B. Body image concerns
C. Excessive exercising
D. Severely low weight
E. Vomiting

13.5. Which of the symptoms below would be more indicative of a binge rather than overeating?

A. Compensatory exercising after the episode
B. Consuming more than 1,000 kcals during the episode
C. Eating excessively after hunger from restricting
D. Eating an excessive amount of food in under 2 hours
E. Excessive eating episodes occurring twice a month

13.6. In general, which symptom is more consistent with a depressive disorder compared to anorexia nervosa?

A. Low energy
B. Difficulty focusing
C. Reports of decreased appetite
D. Ritualistic hyperactivity
E. Weight loss

13.7. A 16-year-old female has a long history of depressive symptoms and suicidality, along with a preoccupation with her weight and will skip breakfast and lunch most days and then eat thousands of calories at night and feeling out of control, will vomit after. She engages in this pattern a few times per week and has also started taking diet pills daily. Her weight has remained stable around 130 lb at a height of 5'6". Which personality disorder is most commonly comorbid with this eating disorder?

A. Avoidant
B. Borderline
C. Obsessive–compulsive
D. Narcissistic
E. Schizotypal

13.8. Which of the following symptoms can distinguish night eating syndrome from bulimia nervosa?

A. Being overweight
B. Consumption of thousands of calories during an episode
C. Eating nonfood items
D. Lack of concern about body image and weight
E. Skipping meals during the day and only eating at night

13.9. Anorexia nervosa is associated with which of the following comorbid psychiatric disorders in approximately half of the patients?

A. Depression
B. Obsessive–compulsive disorder
C. Panic disorder
D. Social phobia
E. Substance use

13.10. The prevalence of posttraumatic stress disorder (PTSD) is most often found to be comorbid with which of the following eating disorders?

A. Anorexia nervosa
B. Avoidant restrictive food intake disorder
C. Binge eating disorder
D. Bulimia nervosa
E. Night eating syndrome

13.11. Which factor is most predictive of a better prognosis for patients with anorexia nervosa?

A. Childhood onset
B. Full weight restoration
C. Lack of purging features
D. Having never lost periods
E. Onset later in life

13.12. Which psychotherapeutic approach is most helpful for treating adolescents with anorexia nervosa?

A. Challenge core beliefs about body image concerns
B. Have parents prepare, plate, and supervise meals
C. Focus on improving interpersonal relationships
D. Motivation to get the patients to change their eating behavior
E. Teach patients to measure their own food and use an exchange system

13.13. Data on the use of atypical antipsychotics for the treatment of anorexia nervosa in adolescents support which of the following findings?

A. Aripiprazole is tolerated better than the other atypicals
B. Eating disorder thoughts are improved when used as an adjunct to selective serotonin reuptake inhibitor (SSRI)
C. Meta-analyses have not supported their use
D. Olanzapine is associated with the most weight gain
E. Risperidone did not show added cardiac risks

13.14. A 15-year-old female has been struggling with skipping meals and has been vomiting and/or using laxatives three to five times a week for the past year. Her weight is 110 lb and her height is 5'3". Which of the following treatments is first line for this eating disorder?

A. Cognitive behavioral therapy (CBT)
B. Family-based treatment (FBT)
C. Fluoxetine
D. Olanzapine
E. Topiramate

13.15. Which treatment type has been proven to have the best results for the treatment of binge eating disorder?

A. Cognitive behavioral therapy (CBT) combined with SSRIs
B. Dialectical behavioral therapy
C. Family-based treatment combined with topiramate
D. Interpersonal psychotherapy (IPT) combined with SSRIs
E. Stimulants

13.16. Which psychological factor is unique to the development of anorexia nervosa, compared to bulimia nervosa?

A. Elevated harm avoidance
B. Elevated negative emotionality
C. Engagement in self-harm
D. High ability to delay rewards
E. Increased impulsivity levels

ANSWERS

13.1. A. Anorexia nervosa, binge/purge subtype

Though reporting wanting to gain weight, the girl described in the vignette above has behaviors consistent with restricting and she lost a large amount of weight and is currently underweight, and has lost her periods. The increased frequency of going to the bathroom and excessively eating large quantities of food after the restricting is suspicious for a binge/purge subtype of anorexia nervosa. With the other disorders listed (bulimia nervosa, night eating syndromes, and purging disorder) the weight would be stable. Purging and night eating disorders do not include restricting and binging. Other specific feeding or eating disorders (OSFEDs) can include night eating and purging disorder, along with atypical anorexia nervosa, which would have similar features to anorexia nervosa, including weight loss, but the weight would appear normal or overweight even after the weight loss. (469)

13.2. A. Bradycardia, B. Hypercholesterolemia, and F. Lanugo

The patient described meets criteria for classic anorexia nervosa, restricting subtype. Common medical complications include bradycardia, hypotension, and arrhythmias and these patients are at increased risk of death, mainly from cardiac complications. Hypothermia, decreased gastric emptying, and leukopenia are other associated findings with malnutrition. Despite decreased cholesterol intake, due to liver damage from the malnutrition, cholesterol is typically increased. (470, 471)

13.3. C. Elevated growth hormone

Often patients with anorexia nervosa lose their menses due to low levels of luteinizing hormone, follicle-stimulating hormone, and low estrogen. Testosterone is suppressed in males with anorexia. Growth hormone increases to help the body compensate. Cortisol, a marker of stress, is also increased. Elevated prolactin is also found. Thyroid hormone changes include low, or a normal thyroxine level, and low triiodothyronine, along with increased reverse triiodothyronine. (471)

13.4. D. Severely low weight

In both anorexia and bulimia nervosa, body image concerns are present, and the binge/purge subtype of anorexia can look like bulimia nervosa except for that those with anorexia nervosa are of a severely low weight, whereas typically those with bulimia nervosa are of normal weight (though some may be under- or overweight). Excessive exercising is considered a type of compensatory behavior that would go under purging. The absence of menses is a nonspecific sign and was eliminated in changing from the DSM-IV to DSM-5 criteria for anorexia nervosa. (471, 472)

13.5. D. Eating an excessive amount of food in under 2 hours

Often, patients with anorexia will report subjective binges of overeating after periods of restriction and feeling out of control though calorie wise and timing wise, these episodes do not necessarily count as actual binges. A true binge per DSM-5 is defined as eating a large quantity of food (i.e., more than 2,000 kcals) in under 2 hours and a feeling of a loss of control during these episodes, along with at least three of the following criteria: eating quicker than normal, eating until uncomfortably full, eating in spite of not feeling hungry, eating alone to avoid embarrassment, and feeling guilty or disgusted afterward. These episodes need to occur at least once a week for 3 months in order to meet criteria. (473)

13.6. C. Reports of decreased appetite

While those with depression could potentially have increased appetite, often decreased appetite is commonly reported and it can help distinguish between depression versus anorexia nervosa since in anorexia nervosa, a normal appetite or hunger are commonly reported. With anorexia nervosa, behaviors to curb the hunger are noted, along with a preoccupation with food, recipes, cooking, etc. Psychomotor retardation or hyperactivity can be seen in both depression and anorexia, though in anorexia, the hyperactivity is typically planned and ritualistic and the focus is on weight loss and there is an intense fear of weight gain and body image disturbance. With both malnutrition and depression, focusing issues can be seen. (474)

13.7. B. Borderline

The patient described above has bulimia nervosa, characterized by binging and purging at least once a week for 3 months, along with a focus on body/shape/weight concerns and unlike anorexia nervosa, binge/purge subtype, for bulimia, the weight is typically normal. Patients with bulimia often engage in impulsive behaviors other than purging including substance use, compulsive shopping, self-harm, etc. They often meet criteria for borderline personality disorder and at times can also meet criteria for bipolar II disorder. (474)

13.8. D. Lack of concern about body image and weight

With many eating disorders, such as anorexia and bulimia nervosa, body image, along with weight and shape concerns are a key feature. While eating large quantities of food can occur in both bulimia and night eating syndrome, those with night eating syndrome do not have body image concerns or a fear of weight gain. Another distinguishing feature is that the binges in bulimia typically involve a higher number of calories consumed compared to night eating syndrome. Timing differs in that for night eating syndrome, these involuntary episodes typically occur after the patient has gone to sleep, and the eating can occur even when asleep or unconscious. Eating nonfood items can happen in night eating syndrome as well as other eating disorders. (474)

13.9. A. Depression

Anorexia nervosa is highly comorbid with other psychiatric disorders, with depression being the most common at 50%. Social phobia is also commonly comorbid at around 22% and comorbidity with obsessive–compulsive disorder is around 35%. (473)

13.10. D. Bulimia nervosa

Patients with bulimia nervosa have higher histories of sexual abuse and PTSD. It is thought that over 26% of those with bulimia have a comorbid PTSD, compared to over 8% for anorexia, and over 13% for binge eating disorder. (475)

13.11. B. Full weight restoration

Overall, patients with anorexia nervosa have recovery rates of 30% to 50%. Mortality rates for individuals with anorexia are six times higher than the general population. Adolescents with a shorter duration of illness tend to have the best prognosis. Individuals who are fully weight-restored on an inpatient unit, along with weight maintenance for a month after discharge are positive signs of a good prognosis, along with those who can have a large variety in their diet and consume high-kcal items. A lower body mass index (BMI) and weight loss after discharge are factors associated with a poor long-term outcome. (476)

13.12. B. Have parents prepare, plate, and supervise meals

Cognitive and behavioral principles can be helpful in treating anorexia nervosa, such as monitoring thoughts, feelings, and emotions and monitoring interpersonal relations, and working on cognitive restructuring for core beliefs. However, in adolescents under 18 years old with anorexia nervosa, a family-based treatment approach (FBT) has been shown to be most helpful. Phase 1 of treatment involves a focus on restoration of the patient's physical health, with the parents making the decisions regarding what the patient should eat. Psychodynamic therapy might involve building an alliance with the patient and empathizing with the patient's point of view rather than directly trying to get them to change their eating behavior. (477)

13.13. C. Meta-analyses have not supported their use

No pharmacologic treatment has been shown to lead to definitive improvement for the treatment of anorexia nervosa. Some studies have looked at atypical antipsychotics, mainly olanzapine, for weight gain, though meta-analyses and large studies have not supported its use. Added cardiac and metabolic complications can be found when using the atypical antipsychotics in this already medically compromised population. (477)

13.14. A. Cognitive behavioral therapy (CBT)

The patient described above has bulimia nervosa, given the presentation of binging, purging, and being of a normal weight. CBT is first-line treatment for bulimia nervosa. FBT and dialectical behavioral therapy (DBT) might also be effective for bulimia, though are not as well studied. While fluoxetine is U.S. Food and Drug Administration (FDA) approved for the treatment of bulimia and topiramate might have some efficacy in reducing binging episodes, CBT should be initiated first. (477, 478)

13.15. A. Cognitive behavioral therapy (CBT) combined with SSRIs

CBT is the most effective treatment for binge eating disorder and should be considered first-line treatment. When combined with SSRIs and other medications, studies have shown better results than CBT alone. Stimulants, such as lisdexamfetamine can help with weight loss and decrease binging.

Anticonvulsants, such as topiramate, can help improve binge eating disorder and lead to more weight loss. Interpersonal psychotherapy and dialectical behavioral therapy might also be effective in helping to treat binge eating disorder, though CBT with the addition of an SSRI is thought to be the most effective. (478)

13.16. D. High ability to delay rewards
While those with anorexia or bulimia nervosa can both engage in self-harm and have elevated harm avoidance, along with increased negative emotionality, typically an increased ability to delay rewards is a unique phycologic predisposing factor to anorexia nervosa. (479)

14

Elimination Disorders

14.1. The diagnosis of encopresis in the DSM-5 includes which of the following symptoms as a specifier?

A. Abnormal sphincter tone
B. Anger
C. Anxiety
D. Constipation
E. Laxative responsive

14.2. Which of the following children would meet DSM-5 criteria for encopresis?

A. An 8-year-old child who soils himself when he has major school examinations
B. A 5-year-old child with constipation, diarrhea, and soiling himself for 3 months
C. A 7-year-old child who soiled his pants once after going to the bathroom
D. A 10-year-old child who soils himself each time after having caffeinated tea at lunch
E. A 3-year-old child who smears feces on his carpet weekly

14.3. Which treatment should be the initial step in treating a child with encopresis without evidence of constipation?

A. Family-based treatment
B. Fluoxetine
C. Polyethylene glycol (PEG)
D. Surgical disimpaction
E. Timed, regular toileting intervals

14.4. Which of the following causes of encopresis is most common?

A. Behavioral and conduct problems
B. Hirschsprung disease
C. Sexual abuse
D. Specific toilet phobia
E. Withholding feces via sphincter tightening due to pain

14.5. A 5-year-old child has been bed-wetting most nights of the week for the past year. Which of the following psychiatric disorders are they at increased risk of getting compared to the general population?

A. Attention deficit hyperactivity
B. Anxiety
C. Depressive
D. Eating
E. Oppositional defiant

14.6. Which of the following outcomes is the most typical course for a child with enuresis?

A. Development of an oppositional defiant disorder
B. Occurrence after 1 year of dryness
C. Progression to a chronic cystitis
D. Relapse in adulthood
E. Spontaneous remission

14.7. What is the minimum age a child can respond to use of a bed-wetting alarm for enuresis?

A. 2
B. 4
C. 6
D. 8
E. 10

14.8. Use of the bell and pad alarm for the treatment of bed-wetting is a form of which type of behavioral therapy?

A. Classical conditioning
B. Operant conditioning
C. Positive reinforcement
D. Punishment
E. Negative reinforcement

14.9. Though rare, which is the most severe side effect documented with the use of desmopressin in the treatment of enuresis?

A. A cardiac arrest
B. Agranulocytosis
C. A hyponatremic seizure
D. Liver failure
E. Renal failure

14.10. Which neurotransmitter reuptake inhibitor is thought to be a safer alternative to imipramine for the treatment of enuresis?

A. Desipramine
B. Duloxetine
C. Reboxetine
D. Strattera
E. Tranylcypromine

14.11. Which type of enuresis is most commonly diagnosed?

A. Adolescent onset
B. Combination (diurnal and nocturnal)
C. Diurnal
D. Nocturnal
E. Structural/anatomical defect

ANSWERS

14.1. D. Constipation
Either constipation or overflow incontinence are specifiers that should be used in the DSM-5 when making a diagnosis of encopresis. Patients without abnormalities in sphincter tone are more likely to respond to laxatives, though it is not included as a specifier. Anger and anxiety can be emotional factors that contribute to encopresis, though are not included as specifiers in the DSM. (481)

14.2. B. A 5-year-old child with constipation, diarrhea, and soiling himself for 3 months
For a diagnosis of encopresis to be made, eliminating feces on the clothes or floor, whether voluntary or unintentional, must occur in someone who is greater than or equal to 4 years old and the episodes have to occur at least once a month for a period of 3 or more months. (482)

14.3. E. Timed, regular toileting intervals
For encopresis with constipation, often daily laxatives, such as PEG are utilized and in severe cases, surgical disimpaction under general anesthesia is initiated prior to the laxative use. When encopresis without constipation is noted, the typical first step is a cognitive behavioral intervention to help institute regular, timed intervals on the toilet. This can also be helpful in cases of encopresis with constipation. Supportive psychotherapy can be helpful in children with comorbid anxiety and self-esteem issue. Family interventions can help when children are smearing feces. (482)

14.4. E. Withholding feces via sphincter tightening due to pain
In 90% of cases of childhood encopresis, children will withhold feces by contracting their gluteal muscles, holding their legs, and then tightening their external anal sphincter, typically as a response to previously painful bowel movements due to constipation. A specific phobia of using the toilet is a less common cause of encopresis. In only about 5% to 10% of cases are medical conditions, such as Hirschsprung disease and spinal cord damage, contributing factors. One study found sexual abuse is higher in a sample of children with encopresis compared to healthy controls, though this disorder is by no means a specific indicator of sexual abuse. (483)

14.5. A. Attention deficit hyperactivity
The patient described above has enuresis, which is defined in DSM-5 as episodes of urinating onto the bed or clothing, either voluntarily or unintentionally for at least 2 weeks for 3 or more months in children 5 years or older. Nocturnal, diurnal, or both should be indicated as specifiers. Children with enuresis are at a higher risk of attention-deficit/hyperactivity disorder (ADHD) compared to the general population. (483)

14.6. E. Spontaneous remission
Medical causes of enuresis should be ruled out including urinary tract infections, bladder dysfunction, spina bifida, cystitis, etc. However, most sophisticated radiographic medical tests are deferred unless there are signs of repeat infections. The most common scenario is that enuresis is self-limited and spontaneous remission is seen. Enuresis most commonly occurs in those without ever having a period of dryness first (80%). The age of onset is older (i.e., 5 to 8) in those in which a year period of dryness occurred first. Relapses can occur. The course is often complicated in those with comorbid ADHD. (484)

14.7. C. 6
A bed alarm has been the mainstay of treatment for enuresis. It alerts a child when they start to void during sleep. The device is attached to the child's underwear and then sounds a loud noise to awaken the child to go to the toilet. At the age of 6 or 7 years, it is thought that the child is old enough to respond optimally to the alarm. (484)

14.8. A. Classical conditioning
Classical conditioning in this case involves associating the involuntary response of nocturnal enuresis with the unconditioned stimulus, the alarm, training the child to get up and go to the bathroom (unconditioned response). It is the mainstay treatment for nocturnal enuresis and typically more effective than bladder training (i.e., delayed urinating for increased times during the day). (484)

14.9. C. A hyponatremic seizure
Desmopressin, a nasal spray that acts as an antidiuretic compound, is used to treat enuresis when it is causing significant social or functional impairment for the child. The most common side effects of desmopressin are headaches, nasal congestion, epistaxis, and stomachaches. A rare complication of a hyponatremic seizure has been documented with use of desmopressin for enuresis treatment. (484)

14.10. C. Reboxetine
Antidepressants with anticholinergic side effects, such as imipramine, were initially used for the

treatment of enuresis. However, due to its considerable side effect profile, such as cardiotoxicity, it has fallen out of favor. Reboxetine, though not currently available in the United States, is a norepinephrine reuptake inhibitor that is a safer alternative to imipramine for the treatment of enuresis, without the potential for cardiac toxicity. (484)

14.11. D. Nocturnal
The three main types of enuresis are diurnal, nocturnal, and a combination of diurnal and nocturnal. In general, enuresis is most commonly present in 5-year-olds (i.e., 5% to 10%). Among the types, nocturnal enuresis accounts for about 80% of children with enuresis. Adolescent onset is rare around 1%. Structural abnormalities, such as genitourinary pathology, are less common and typically present with both diurnal and nocturnal enuresis. (484)

15

Sleep–Wake Disorders

15.1. A 30-year-old woman presents to the outpatient clinic with a chief complaint of, "I'm always so tired." She states that she has always needed more sleep than everyone else "for as long as I can remember," and that she would sleep for 12 hours a day if she could. During the week, she gets in bed around 8 pm, falls asleep in 10 to 15 minutes, and wakes at 6 am to get ready for work at a city government office. She manages to stay awake at work and complete her tasks, though she is drowsy and has some difficulty sustaining attention. On the weekends she goes to bed at the same time but does not wake until 10 am or later the next day. She states that she has tried caffeinated drinks, vitamins, and light therapy, and admits to taking some of a friend's methylphenidate to see if it would help, but she remains drowsy. She laments that she is not able to spend much time with friends because she has to be in bed so early "or I can't function the next day." She denies snoring. Body mass index (BMI) is 18.5. Vital signs are within normal limits. Mental status examination reveals a well-nourished, though slender female in no acute distress. Mood is "tired," with congruent affect. She denies auditory or visual hallucinations. What is the most likely diagnosis?

A. Insomnia disorder
B. Hypersomnolence disorder
C. Narcolepsy
D. Sleep apnea
E. Circadian rhythm sleep disorder

15.2. What brain structure is responsible for maintaining circadian rhythm and a regular sleep–wake cycle?

A. Arcuate nucleus
B. Nucleus accumbens
C. Caudate nucleus
D. Suprachiasmatic nucleus
E. Nucleus basalis

15.3. A 20-year-old male college student reports a 6-month history of excessive daytime sleepiness to his primary care physician. He states that he can fall asleep "instantly" at any time, and that he has nodded off for a few seconds to a few minutes while driving, while at work, and in class on many occasions. Despite those brief periods of sleep, he can sometimes recall "full-on dreams." He notes that when he first gets up in the morning, he is sometimes unable to move for about minute, during which he will "see things from my dreams, but I'm fully awake." He states that he gets about 7 to 8 hours of sleep a night, "but even when I sleep for 12 hours on the weekend, I still just suddenly fall asleep during the day." He reports that he has three to four beers on weekend nights with his friends and denies drug use. He is on no medications and has no medical illnesses. He states that he does not snore. BMI is 20. What hormone is most likely to be deficient in this patient?

A. Leptin
B. Orexin
C. Ghrelin
D. Growth hormone
E. Thyroid-stimulating hormone

15.4. A 5-year-old child is brought to the pediatrician by his parents who report three instances over the past month of the child getting up during the night and wandering around in the house. He does not respond when they call his name and does not appear to do anything purposeful as he walks around. He is easily redirected to his bed and sleeps without incident for the rest of the night. He has no memory of the episode the next day. What is the most likely course of these episodes?

A. They will spontaneously remit after adolescence
B. They will sharply decrease in frequency prior to puberty
C. They will slowly decrease in frequency during young adulthood
D. They will persist throughout his life
E. They will increase until puberty, then sharply drop off

15.5. Chronic alcohol use can lead to insomnia through what mechanism?

A. Decreased proportion of time in non-rapid eye movement (NREM) sleep
B. Central nervous system suppression of breathing
C. Arousal-induced sleep cycle fragmentation
D. Increased anxiety prior to sleep
E. Increased sleep latency

15.6. The multiple sleep latency test (MSLT) is essential in the diagnosis of what sleep–wake disorder?

A. Obstructive sleep apnea
B. Central sleep apnea
C. Narcolepsy
D. Circadian rhythm sleep disorder
E. Rapid eye movement (REM) sleep behavior disorder

15.7. A 40-year-old woman reports a 10-year history of difficulty falling asleep. She believes that the problem began when she worked a highly stressful job during which she "went to sleep worried about getting yelled at by my boss the next day." Even after she changed jobs, the anxiety about not being able to sleep remained. She states that she is now at the point where she gets in bed frustrated because she knows she will be awake for hours. She used to watch the clock, but stopped doing that a month ago, as it was making her more upset at night. However, it has not improved the insomnia. She tried melatonin, which she felt was initially helpful, but she no longer derives benefit even after increasing the dose. She has also tried over-the-counter diphenhydramine, but felt that she was getting addicted to it. She denies symptoms of depression. What should be the next step in her treatment?

A. Eszopiclone therapy
B. Sleep hygiene
C. Relaxation therapy
D. Suvorexant therapy
E. Cognitive behavioral therapy for insomnia (CBTi)

15.8. Treatment of cataplexy involves medications with what physiologic effect as the mechanism of action?

A. Inhibition of muscle atony
B. Suppression of REM sleep
C. Central nervous system (CNS) stimulation
D. Suppression of sleep-related hormones
E. Muscle relaxation

15.9. A 50-year-old woman complains of difficulty sleeping for the last 6 months. She states that when she gets in bed, she tosses and turns because she feels that "I just need to move." She also reports that she sometimes feels like bugs are crawling on her skin, particularly her legs, which is alleviated by getting out of bed and walking around. She then gets back in bed, but the sensations return in about 30 minutes. She ends up staying awake almost all night two to three times a week. She notes that she is falling asleep at work because she is so tired. After further history and a physical examination, what lab test should be ordered?

A. Complete blood count with differential
B. Liver function tests
C. Urine drug screen
D. Ferritin level
E. Triglyceride level

15.10. The narcolepsy medication pitolisant works through what pharmacologic mechanism?

A. Norepinephrine–dopamine reuptake inhibition
B. Dopamine reuptake inhibition
C. H3 receptor antagonism/inverse agonism
D. D2 receptor partial agonism
E. 5HT3 antagonism

ANSWERS

15.1. B. Hypersomnolence disorder
The patient in this case easily falls asleep and reports no difficulty staying asleep or having early morning awakening, thus ruling out insomnia disorder. She does not report sudden periods of sleep during the day or drop attacks of cataplexy. Though her BMI and lack of snoring do not eliminate sleep apnea as a possibility, they make the diagnosis less likely. She is sleeping at night as she desires, and though the lack of improvement with light therapy does not preclude a diagnosis of circadian rhythm sleep disorder, it makes it much less likely. Her symptoms fit best with hypersomnolence disorder, as she reports reduced attention and excessive daytime sleepiness and time spent asleep. (486)

15.2. D. Suprachiasmatic nucleus
The nucleus accumbens mediates motivational and emotional processes and is considered the neural interface between motivation and action. The caudate nucleus is a part of the basal ganglia that is involved in working memory and executive functioning. The nucleus basalis is involved in cortical activation and memory function. The arcuate and suprachiasmatic nuclei are both located in the hypothalamus. The function of the arcuate nucleus is control of the anterior pituitary and feeding, while the function of the suprachiasmatic nucleus is regulation of biologic rhythms, such as the circadian rhythm. (486)

15.3. B. Orexin
Orexin is a hypocretin that was discovered in 1998 and is associated with narcolepsy to the extent that the disorder is now considered to be caused by hypocretin/orexin deficiency. Ghrelin and leptin are hormones that help mediate energy balance and satiety. Though growth hormone surges during sleep, it is not associated with narcolepsy. A low amount of thyroid-stimulating hormone can lead to fatigue, but not narcolepsy. (491)

15.4. A. They will spontaneously remit after adolescence
Sleepwalking most commonly affects children ages 4 to 8 years. Episodes do not usually require treatment, aside from making sure the environment is safe (locking doors and windows, keeping dangerous objects out of reach, not letting the child sleep in a bunk bed, etc.). For most children, sleepwalking spontaneously remits after puberty. (497)

15.5. C. Arousal-induced sleep cycle fragmentation
Alcohol is believed to lead to insomnia due to arousals during the sleep cycle, which lead to a decreased proportion of time spent in REM sleep. Alcohol can exacerbate obstructive sleep apnea, but a strong correlation between alcohol and central sleep apnea has not been shown. Alcohol usually decreases sleep latency and anxiety in the short term, which can fool people into thinking that it is helpful for insomnia. (491)

15.6. C. Narcolepsy
A polysomnogram can be used in the evaluation of sleep apnea, REM sleep behavior disorder, narcolepsy, and other causes of daytime sleepiness. If after assessing sleep quality and quantity during the polysomnogram narcolepsy is still suspected, an MSLT will be performed. The MSLT involves five, 20-minute opportunities for a patient to nap. If the patient falls asleep and REM sleep waves are detected on two occasions (or one occasion if the previous polysomnogram revealed REM sleep within 15 minutes of sleep onset), the diagnosis of narcolepsy is made. (503)

15.7. E. Cognitive behavioral therapy for insomnia (CBTi)
CBTi has repeatedly shown sustained improvement, up to at least 36 months in some studies, in insomnia. While it does not work as quickly as pharmacologic means, there is no apparent rebound effect from discontinuation, thus making pharmacologic treatments less effective long term, even those approved for long-term use such as eszopiclone. Sleep hygiene is a component of CBTi, and by itself is not as effective. Relaxation therapy can be helpful for those who experience tension prior to bedtime, and is often paired with other insomnia treatments such as sleep hygiene. (510–512)

15.8. B. Suppression of REM sleep
Medications such as tricyclic antidepressants and selective serotonin reuptake inhibitors (SSRIs) are used in the treatment of cataplexy for their ability to suppress REM sleep, not sleep hormones. Inhibition of muscle atony occurs in REM sleep behavior disorder. CNS stimulation, which occurs with psychostimulants, can be helpful for narcolepsy, though not cataplexy. CNS depressants such as sodium oxybate can be helpful for cataplexy. There have been case reports of muscle relaxants used for cataplexy, but this is not first line and should be avoided when sodium oxybate is used. (513)

15.9. D. Ferritin level
About 15% of patients with restless leg syndrome have an iron deficiency, with a serum ferritin level of <50 mcg/L. In these patients, in addition to first-line, dopaminergic agonists such as pramipexole, rotigotine, and ropinirole, iron supplementation can be helpful. (501)

15.10. C. H3 receptor antagonism/inverse agonism
Pitolisant, an U.S. Food and Drug Administration (FDA)-approved treatment for narcolepsy, is a selective H3 receptor agonist/inverse agonist. Another FDA-approved medication for narcolepsy, solriamfetol, acts through norepinephrine–dopamine reuptake inhibition, as do stimulants, which are often used. Modafinil and armodafinil block dopamine reuptake. (512–513)

16
Human Sexuality and Sexual Dysfunctions

16.1. A 23-year-old man presents to a primary care clinic as a new patient. During the sexual history, he states that he has never had sexual fantasies or a desire for sexual activity. He notes that he was teased for this in high school, "but I don't care. Sex just isn't something I'm interested in." He states that he has a strong group of friends and enjoys his job as a department store assistant manager. He has had a girlfriend for the past year, "and she's not interested in sex, either." He reports that he tried masturbating a few times when he was a teenager, and that each time he ejaculated quickly. He stopped masturbating "because it didn't do anything for me." He states that he rarely gets erections. He has no medical illnesses and is on no medications. Vitals are within normal limits. Physical examination reveals a well-developed, well-nourished male in no acute distress. Sexual maturity rating is 5. What is the most likely diagnosis?

A. Male erectile disorder
B. Male hypoactive sexual desire disorder
C. No diagnosis
D. Premature ejaculation

16.2. A woman can be diagnosed with female sexual interest/arousal disorder despite the presence of which of the following circumstances?

A. Vaginal lubrication and congestion
B. Medications which can cause decreased libido
C. Relationship problems with the sexual partner
D. A medical condition which can interfere with arousal
E. A psychiatric condition that can lead to reduced sexual interest

16.3. A 22-year-old male presents to the outpatient clinic with a complaint of, "It takes me over a half hour to orgasm." He states that he first had intercourse at the age of 19, and that he is sexually active exclusively with women. He has had two previous sexual partners with whom he had the same difficulty. His girlfriend of 2 months recently told him that she loved him, which "freaked me out." He is on no medications and has no chronic medical illnesses. Vital signs are within normal limits, and physical examination is noncontributory. The patient is most likely to experience a more average time to ejaculation under what circumstance?

A. Anal sex
B. Masturbation
C. Use of sildenafil
D. Sex with a different partner
E. Use of selective serotonin reuptake inhibitor (SSRI)

16.4. What is the maximum length of time from penetration to ejaculation in which the diagnosis of premature (early) ejaculation can be made?

A. 15 seconds
B. 30 seconds
C. 1 minute
D. 2 minutes
E. 5 minutes

16.5. In addition to effects on serotonin, tricyclic antidepressant medications can lead to erectile and ejaculatory dysfunction due to effects on what neurotransmitter?

A. Norepinephrine
B. Dopamine
C. Acetylcholine
D. Gamma-aminobutyric acid (GABA)

16.6. A 50-year-old man presents to the outpatient clinic for follow-up of hypercholesterolemia, hyperlipidemia, and borderline hypertension. He is on simvastatin, and was told at his last visit 6 months ago that he would benefit from weight loss. He reports that he has had three episodes of "squeezing" chest pain, nausea, shortness of breath, and sweating over the last 2 months. The episodes last around 5 minutes. He takes over-the-counter sildenafil for erectile dysfunction. He is 5'8" and 113 kg (250 lb), body mass index (BMI) is 38. Vitals are within normal limits except for blood pressure, which is 140/95. Physical examination is unremarkable. An ECG shows no chronic ischemia. What medication is contraindicated in the management of this patient's symptoms?

A. Metoprolol
B. Nitroglycerin
C. Ranolazine
D. Amlodipine
E. Aspirin

16.7. Sildenafil has what sexual effect on women?

A. Increased arousal
B. Vaginal lubrication
C. Increased orgasm intensity
D. Loosening of pelvic floor muscles
E. Decreased pelvic pain

16.8. A 35-year-old woman presents to her OB/GYN physician with a complaint of low sexual desire for the last 2 years. She states that she has been in therapy for the last 8 months to address possible relationship factors, and though the communication with her husband has improved, libido remains low. She denies vaginal pain or dryness. She has no chronic medical or mental illnesses and is on no medications. Vital signs are within normal limits. Physical examination is noncontributory. What evidence-based pharmacologic agent could be effective for this patient?

A. Sildenafil
B. Yohimbine
C. Desvenlafaxine
D. Fluoxetine
E. Flibanserin

16.9. What is the sexual side effect a woman is likely to experience from estrogen replacement therapy used to relieve symptoms of menopause?

A. Decreased libido
B. Vaginal dryness
C. Vaginal mucous membrane thinning
D. Dyspareunia

16.10. A 25-year-old woman presents to a sex therapist for help with "my fear of intimacy and sex." She reports that she was sexually assaulted when she was 21 years old, and since then has been on dates but has had no sexual contact, including kissing. "When he leans in to kiss me, I freeze up and start sweating." She has been in therapy for post-traumatic stress disorder (PTSD), which she feels is helpful for working through the trauma, and is now ready to "become physical in a relationship again." She wants to overcome anxiety from holding hands, and eventually progress to intercourse. What type of therapy is most likely to help her achieve her goal?

A. Dual-sex therapy
B. Mindfulness
C. Group therapy
D. Behavior therapy
E. Analytically oriented sex therapy

16.11. In addition to significant distress from or acting on sexual fantasies or impulses, what is required to diagnose an individual with a paraphilic disorder?

A. Intense sexual arousal from the fantasy or impulse
B. Involvement of a nonconsenting person in the fantasy or impulse
C. Acting on the fantasy or impulse would be a criminal offense
D. Lack of sexual response to typical erotic stimuli
E. Having a sexual fantasy or impulse outside of typical erotic stimuli

16.12. What ages of the child and patient and age difference between them are required for a diagnosis of pedophilia?

	Child	Patient	Age difference
A.	<10 years	≥16 years	≥3 years
B.	<14 years	≥18 years	≥3 years
C.	<10 years	≥18 years	N/A
D.	<14 years	≥16 years	≥5 years
E.	<10 years	≥16 years	N/A
F.	<14 years	≥18 years	≥5 years

16.13. A 24-year-old man tells a psychiatrist that he has engaged in acts of exposing his penis to unsuspecting women for the last 5 years. He states that he has done this about 30 times, has never been caught, and that he does it for a "sexual rush," usually when he has been drinking. He also states that he saw his neighbor having sex through her window when he was 10 years old. Since then, he has sought out opportunities, often when drunk, to watch unsuspecting people engage in sexual activity or in states of undress, and masturbates during or soon afterward. He states that he has had a girlfriend for the last year with whom he is sexually active, and wants to stop the voyeuristic and exposing behaviors before she finds out. What factor most predicts that he will be successful in treatment?

A. Alcohol use prior to the behaviors
B. Having more than one paraphilia
C. Being in a sexual relationship
D. The age of his first voyeuristic act

16.14. A 31-year-old single man presents to an outpatient primary care clinic to establish care. During the sexual history, he states that he has had around 30 sexual partners a year for the past 10 years. He describes a "need" to have intercourse resulting in orgasm. He notes that he has had a few girlfriends over the years, but they have broken up with him "because I can't stop cheating." He has tried several times to decrease the behavior, but relapses within a few weeks each time. He was fired once because he would not stop using a dating app while at work. What is the most likely comorbid disorder in this patient?

A. Bipolar disorder
B. Major depressive disorder
C. Substance use disorder
D. Obsessive compulsive disorder
E. Narcissistic personality disorder

16.15. Gender identity is developed in most children by what age?

A. 2 to 3 years
B. 3 to 4 years
C. 4 to 5 years
D. 5 to 6 years
E. 6 to 7 years

16.16. What part of the nervous system is ultimately the epicenter of both male and female orgasms?

A. Orbitofrontal cortex
B. Limbic system
C. Anterior cingulate cortex
D. Caudate nucleus
E. Spinal cord

16.17. Children begin normal genital self-stimulation around what age?

A. 1.5 years
B. 3 years
C. 5 years
D. 7.5 years
E. 10 years

ANSWERS

16.1. C. No diagnosis
The patient meets all of the criteria for lifelong male hypoactive sexual desire disorder except for the lack of psychosocial impact of marked distress, which is a requirement of all sexual dysfunction diagnoses. He is satisfied with his relationships and expresses no desire for sexual activity. Therefore, no diagnosis would be given. (519, 520)

16.2. A. Vaginal lubrication and congestion
Vaginal lubrication is not necessarily caused by arousal, and can be present in women with or without female sexual interest/arousal disorder. Relationship problems, substances or medications, and medical or psychiatric conditions that can lead to the decreased desire must be excluded before making the diagnosis. (520)

16.3. B. Masturbation
The patient is describing symptoms of delayed ejaculation. This rarely occurs during masturbation, and most often occurs during coitus, which would include anal sex. Sildenafil could be useful for treatment of erectile dysfunction. Use of an SSRI is often a cause, not a cure, of delayed ejaculation. Though his girlfriend's profession of love for him may create additional anxiety, the problem has been present with all his partners, so neither his current anxiety nor a change of partners will likely make a difference. (522)

16.4. C. 1 minute
The diagnosis of premature (early) ejaculation can be given if the time from penetration until ejaculation is 1 minute or less. Severity is considered mild if ejaculation occurs between 30 and 60 seconds, moderate when between 15 and 30 seconds, and severe when less than 15 seconds. (524)

16.5. C. Acetylcholine
Anticholinergic effects of antidepressants such as tricyclics can lead to problems with erections and delayed ejaculation. Enhanced dopaminergic activity and increased norepinephrine production by some antidepressants such as bupropion may increase sex drive. GABA enhancement, such as in novel antidepressants under development and in benzodiazepines, can lead to less anxiety and sometimes improved sexual function. (528, 529)

16.6. B. Nitroglycerin
The patient is experiencing episodes of angina, for which antianginals such as aspirin, nitrates, beta-blockers, statins, calcium channel blockers, and ranolazine can be used. In patients on sildenafil, nitrates are contraindicated, as the combination can cause a dangerous, and sometimes fatal, drop in blood pressure. (529)

16.7. B. Vaginal lubrication
Sildenafil can result in vaginal lubrication, but not increased arousal or orgasm. Pelvic pain from vaginismus is caused by involuntary pelvic floor muscle tightening, which sildenafil does not affect. (529)

16.8. E. Flibanserin
Flibanserin is U.S. Food and Drug Administration (FDA) approved for generalized hypoactive sexual desire disorder. Pharmacotherapy can be used by itself or along with psychotherapy such as insight-oriented or behavioral sex therapy. Sildenafil does not help with desire. Acute depression can contribute to decreased libido, for which antidepressants such as desvenlafaxine and fluoxetine could be helpful. Yohimbine has been used as an aphrodisiac, but has not been shown in studies to be effective. (530)

16.9. A. Decreased libido
Estrogen therapy, regardless of purpose of use, can lead to decreased libido, and is sometimes used to treat compulsive sexual behavior in men. However, it prevents vaginal mucous membrane thinning and facilitates lubrication, the latter of which can be a cause of dyspareunia. Androgens, such as testosterone, can help with the decreased libido caused by estrogen. (530, 531)

16.10. D. Behavior therapy
Much like with the treatment of phobias, behavior therapy can be helpful for patients who fear sexual interaction. The patient will first learn relaxation techniques to decrease anxiety, then progress to exposure and response prevention. Dual-sex therapy focuses on communication between partners who are both in a sexually distressing situation. Group therapy provides support for patients who share similar sexual problems, and sometimes uses behavioral techniques within the groups for treatment of sexual problems. Mindfulness is a cognitive technique used to center on sensations that lead

to arousal or orgasm. Analytically oriented sex therapy helps patients learn or relearn sexual satisfaction, and is sometimes combined with behavioral treatments to treat sexual dysfunctions. (532, 533)

16.11. A. Intense sexual arousal from the fantasy or impulse
All paraphilic disorders require at least 6 months of "recurrent and intense sexual arousal" from the sexual fantasy or impulse. They do not all involve a nonconsenting person (such as with fetishistic disorder or sexual masochism disorder) or result in a criminal offense if acted upon (such as with fetishistic disorder or transvestic disorder). Simply having a sexual fantasy or impulse outside of typical erotic stimuli (a paraphilia) is necessary but not sufficient for a diagnosis of a paraphilic disorder. A person with a paraphilic disorder often has a lack of a sexual response to normophilic sexual interests, but this is not a criterion for the diagnosis. (533)

16.12. D. <14 years ≥16 years ≥5 years
To make a diagnosis of pedophilia, the child must be under 14 years old, the patient must be at least 16 years old, and there must be at least a 5-year age difference. These age requirements can be different than those for statutory rape, which can vary from state to state. (535)

16.13. C. Being in a sexual relationship
Though paraphilic disorders are challenging to treat, some factors, such as engaging in regular sexual activity, having a single paraphilia, and self-referral, are good treatment predictors. Poor prognostic indicators include the presence of substance abuse and early age of onset. (538)

16.14. C. Substance use disorder
Sex addiction has many of the same signs as an addiction due to a substance use disorder, which is the most common comorbidity. Treatment can also follow a similar course by way of 12-step groups such as Sexaholics Anonymous, Love Addicts Anonymous, and Sex Addicts Anonymous. (540)

16.15. A. 2 to 3 years
By 2 to 3 years of age, most children who have an unambiguous sexual identity have developed a secure identification of being male or female. (542)

16.16. E. Spinal cord
Both sexual arousal and orgasm are organized at the spinal level, though many parts of the nervous system are involved in sexual behavior. The orbitofrontal cortex is involved in the emotion of sexual behavior. Caudate nucleus activity is a factor in whether sexual activity follows arousal. The left anterior cingulate cortex is involved in hormone control and sexual arousal. Structures of the limbic system that are activated by emotions such as fear and anxiety are hypoactive during orgasms in women. (543)

16.17. A. 1.5 years
Children discover the pleasurable feelings from self-stimulation between 15 and 19 months old. They also begin to develop a normal, healthy curiosity about the genitals of others around that time. (543)

17

Gender Dysphoria, Gender Identity, and Related Conditions

17.1. A 13-year-old born as a female has insisted since he was 3 years old that he is really a boy. He has always preferred to play sports with boys, as opposed to engaging in traditional gender-role activities for girls. He wears boys' clothing at all times and has never worn a dress. Since the beginning of puberty, he has worn a binder around his torso to flatten out his breasts. He has told his parents, friends, and teachers to use the "he" pronoun since he was 9 years old. He eventually wants to transition physically to being a male. He is sexually attracted to females. His karyotype is 23, XX. What term best describes the sexual identity of this individual?

A. Transexual
B. Transgender
C. Homosexual
D. Genderqueer
E. Cross-dresser

17.2. The parents of a 4-year-old boy present to the outpatient clinic concerned about their son, who they state tells everyone that he is a girl. They say that he has always played with "girl toys" such as dolls, and that they have caught him several times putting on his 6-year-old sister's dresses. His karyotype is 23, XY. What is the most likely outcome for the child regarding his gender identity/expression in adulthood?

A. He will identify as a gender-dysphoric male
B. He will transition surgically to a female
C. He will identify as a male
D. He will identify as a gender-dysphoric female

17.3. A 23-year-old transgender man decides to begin hormone treatment for phenotypical masculinization. In addition to liver function tests, which of the following labs should be routinely monitored?

A. Thyroid stimulating hormone (TSH)/T3/T4
B. Blood urea nitrogen (BUN)/creatinine
C. Na^+/K^+
D. Hemoglobin/hematocrit
E. Follicle stimulating hormone (FSH)/Leutenizing hormone (LH)

17.4. What is the default sex of a human embryo, and what causes it to develop into the opposite sex?

A. Default female—becomes male from Y chromosome–induced androgens
B. Default male—becomes female from lack of Y chromosome–induced androgens
C. Default female—becomes male from Y chromosome estrogen suppression
D. Default male—becomes female from a double dose of X chromosome estrogen

ANSWERS

17.1. A. Transexual
The individual can be described as transgender, the term referring to someone who identifies with a gender different than their assigned gender. However, the term transexual is a better fit, as he wants to have the body of a male. Genderqueer refers to someone who feels that they are between genders, are both genders, or are neither gender. Cross-dressing is wearing the clothes typically associated with a different gender than the one assigned at birth, but maintaining the identity of the assigned gender. Given that he identifies as a male and is attracted to females, his sexual orientation is heterosexual, not homosexual. (547)

17.2. C. He will identify as a male
Several studies have shown that a majority of children with gender dysphoria identify with their birth-assigned gender as adults. Most who continue to identify as a different gender do not have gender reassignment surgery. (549)

17.3. D. Hemoglobin/hematocrit
Testosterone supplementation can lead to an increase in red blood cell counts which can lead to stroke, so hemoglobin and hematocrit should be monitored routinely. Liver function tests should also be monitored because testosterone is metabolized by the liver. Glucose and lipids should be monitored as well, as testosterone can increase the chance of lipid abnormalities and diabetes. (550)

17.4. A. Default female—becomes male from Y chromosome–induced androgens
The default state of mammalian embryos is female. Androgens produced by the presence of the Y chromosome convert the tissue into male. (551)

18
Disruptive, Impulse Control, and Conduct Disorders

18.1. What is the common feature in the diagnosis of pyromania, intermittent explosive disorder (IED), and kleptomania?

A. Guilt following the incident
B. Incidents result in legal trouble
C. Increasing tension prior to the incident
D. A personal benefit from the incident
E. A desire to cause harm by the incident

18.2. What is the age requirement for a diagnosis of intermittent explosive disorder?

A. The patient must be at least 3 years old
B. The patient must be at least 6 years old
C. The patient must be under 12 years old
D. The patient must be under 18 years old
E. The patient must be at least 18 years old

18.3. Parents bring their 16-year-old son to the outpatient clinic because of "his emotional outbursts over the last year. We're walking on eggshells around him. We never know what will set him off." He agrees with his parents and adds that he cannot control himself. He states that some situations get him "so mad that I start breaking things and punching holes in the wall." During the most recent episode, he was playing a video game with friends until his team started to lose. He started cursing loudly and threw the controller at the TV and broke the screen. "The anger just rose up in me until I couldn't control it." His parents note that he often cries and will "beat himself up with guilt afterward," but that in between episodes, "he's fine." He denies feeling depressed or manic, and denies auditory or visual hallucinations or suicidal ideation. He has no chronic illnesses and is on no medications. Vitals are within normal limits and there are no abnormal findings on physical examination. What should be the next step in the management of this patient?

A. Refer him for cognitive behavioral therapy
B. Begin a trial of carbamazepine
C. Perform a medical workup
D. Admit him to the hospital
E. Begin a trial of valproate

18.4. A 25-year-old man who was arrested and jailed 2 days ago on a charge of petit larceny tells the judge that he could not resist stealing a plastic vase from a department store, even though he had no use for it. He is shown video from three other stores which captured him stealing other relatively valueless objects over the past 2 weeks. He states that he does not plan to steal, "but I get this urge that I can't resist and I have to do it." Afterward, he feels a sense of relief. He has never confronted someone to take their possessions. He admits to stealing since he was 18 years old. What is the most likely course of his stealing behavior over the next 10 years?

A. It will wax and wane
B. It will become more frequent
C. It will stay constant
D. It will slowly decrease
E. It will remit completely

18.5. Parents present with their 22-year-old son to the outpatient clinic because of the son's aggressive behavior. They state that he seems to "get angry over nothing," and will fly into a rage consisting of screaming, slamming doors, and verbally abusing them. He states that he cannot control himself and that he has lost several jobs because of his outbursts. Afterward, he always apologizes "and I promise not to do it again. I really mean it, but then the rage just builds up sometimes and I have to let it out." He has tried meditation, deep breathing, and anger management classes, but they have not been effective. His parents state that he is a joy to be around outside of the outbursts, but those times are overshadowed by the behaviors. He lives at home, and they are worried that he will never keep a job long enough to be able to move out. He has no chronic illnesses and is on no medications. What treatment is most likely to be effective?

A. Family therapy and an antipsychotic medication
B. Cognitive behavioral therapy and an anticonvulsant medication
C. Family therapy and selective serotonin reuptake inhibitor (SSRI)
D. Cognitive behavioral therapy and an antipsychotic medication
E. Contingency management and an SSRI
F. Contingency management and an anticonvulsant medication

ANSWERS

18.1. C. Increasing tension prior to the incident
The disruptive, impulse-control disorders of IED, kleptomania, and pyromania are all similar in that there is a sense of rising tension prior to the incident, followed by a decrease in tension afterward. Guilt usually occurs in IED, may occur in kleptomania, and often does not occur in pyromania. The incidents do not necessarily result in legal trouble. The object stolen in kleptomania may have little to no value to the person, just as in pyromania there is no personal benefit, financial or otherwise, from the fire. The acts are not caused by a desire to harm, but to relieve the tension that builds up. (553, 554)

18.2. B. The patient must be at least 6 years old
Intermittent explosive disorder is one of the few disruptive, impulse-control disorders with an age requirement. A diagnosis cannot be made in an individual until they are at least 6 years old. (554)

18.3. C. Perform a medical workup
The patient and his parents are reporting symptoms of intermittent explosive disorder (IED). Since IED is a diagnosis of exclusion, medical causes of his symptoms, such as substance use, brain tumors, endocrine disorders, etc. should first be ruled out, so a full medical workup should be performed. There is no current indication for hospital admission. Recommending or starting treatment would be premature before the other diagnoses are ruled out. (555)

18.4. A. It will wax and wane
Kleptomania tends to be a chronic disorder, with the frequency of stealing ranging from less than one to several episodes a month. The course waxes and wanes over time. (557)

18.5. C. Family therapy and an SSRI
The treatment most likely to be successful for intermittent explosive disorder is a combination of psychotherapy and medication. For a young adult living at home, family therapy is particularly useful, though cognitive behavioral therapy and contingency management may also be effective. SSRIs are helpful in reducing impulsivity and aggression. Antipsychotics and anticonvulsants both have mixed results. (557)

Personality Disorders

19.1. Which personality disorder is associated with traits of chronic social withdrawal and isolation, along with discomfort with interacting with others and a constricted affect?

A. Antisocial
B. Avoidant
C. Paranoid
D. Schizoid
E. Schizotypal

19.2. Criticism of the DSM-5 personality disorder diagnoses include which of the following concerns?

A. A categorical approach is used
B. An approach based on temperament is utilized
C. Comorbid substance use and other medical illnesses are not accounted for
D. Impairment is limited to only a focus on dysfunctional relationships
E. The focus is on a dimensional approach

19.3. On mental status examination, a patient has thought content significant for projection, themes of jealousy, and ideas of reference. The patient's speech is goal-directed and logical, with no signs of psychosis, and motor is significant for tension. Which of the following personality disorders best fits this description?

A. Avoidant
B. Dependent
C. Obsessive compulsive
D. Paranoid
E. Schizotypal

19.4. Which personality disorder is classified under a psychotic disorder, rather than personality disorder in the international classification of diseases, Tenth revision (ICD-10)?

A. Antisocial
B. Borderline
C. Paranoid
D. Schizoid
E. Schizotypal

19.5. A patient presents as having lifelong stormy relationship and is always in a state of crisis. The patient has struggled with self-harm and feelings of anger, alternating with numbness and emptiness. This patient is most likely to use which of the following defense mechanisms?

A. Intellectualization
B. Isolation
C. Projective identification
D. Rationalization
E. Reaction formation

19.6. A patient presents as attention-seeking and as emotionally labile and hypersexual or flirtatious at times. Which of the following defense mechanics is most likely to be utilized by this patient?

A. Dissociation
B. Intellectualization
C. Projection
D. Reaction formation
E. Sublimation

19.7. Which personality disorder is only included in DSM-5 and in ICD-10 is listed under an "other specific personality disorder"?

A. Borderline
B. Dependent
C. Histrionic
D. Narcissistic
E. Paranoid

19.8. Which personality disorder in ICD-10 is defined by excessive attention to detail and checking behaviors, along with rigidity and self-doubt?

A. Anankastic
B. Avoidant
C. Borderline
D. Dependent
E. Not otherwise specified

19.9. Which of the following symptoms is a distinguishing factor between schizophrenia versus paranoid personality disorder?

A. Hallucinations
B. Hostile or threatening demeanor
C. Ideas of reference
D. Jealousness
E. Suspiciousness

19.10. Which of the following symptoms are more commonly found in borderline personality disorder, as compared to histrionic personality disorder?

A. Egocentrism
B. Exaggerated speech and emotions
C. Flirtations and being sexually provocative
D. Identity diffusion
E. Somatic symptoms

19.11. A patient with chronic self-esteem issues and a fear of loneliness and abandonment calls her one friend daily and will only go out with her. She needs to call her to ask her opinion of trivial things daily and struggles with making any decisions on her own. The friend describes her as kindhearted and has not had any recent arguments with her. Which is the most likely personality disorder this patient has?

A. Dependent
B. Borderline
C. Histrionic
D. Obsessive compulsive
E. Schizoid

19.12. A patient presents with chronic fears of being disliked by others and avoids relationships due to fears of shame, rejection, and criticism by others. Which of the following personality disorders is most commonly comorbid with this one?

A. Antisocial
B. Histrionic
C. Narcissistic
D. Obsessive compulsive
E. Schizoid

19.13. Which is the most likely course of borderline personality disorder?

A. Completed suicide in the fifth decade of life
B. Development of a comorbid psychotic disorder by one's fifth decade
C. Functional improvement is noted by the second decade in life
D. History of multiple arrests by the time one reaches their 20s
E. Greater relationship stability is achieved in one's 40s and 50s

19.14. Which type of psychotherapy is best suited toward patients with antisocial personality disorder?

A. Contingency management
B. Dialectical behavioral therapy
C. Group therapy
D. Psychodynamic psychotherapy
E. Social skills training

19.15. Which is an important component of dialectical behavioral therapy in treating patients with borderline personality disorder?

A. Contingency management
B. Mentalization training
C. Phone consultation
D. Reliance on clarification
E. Use of confrontation

19.16. Evidence suggests that which medication might be most helpful in treating those with obsessive compulsive personality disorder with depressive symptoms?

A. Amitriptyline
B. Carbamazepine
C. Fluvoxamine
D. Citalopram
E. Quetiapine

19.17. Which personality disorder is more commonly found in women compared to men and in younger patients?

A. Avoidant
B. Borderline
C. Histrionic
D. Obsessive compulsive
E. Paranoid

19.18. A biologic inheritance is suggested by studies showing saccadic eye movements during smooth pursuit tests in which of the following personality disorders?

A. Antisocial
B. Avoidant
C. Borderline
D. Histrionic
E. Schizotypal

19.19. Fantasy is a defense mechanism most utilized in which of the following personality disorders?

A. Borderline
B. Histrionic
C. Obsessive compulsive
D. Paranoid
E. Schizoid

19.20. Persons showing decreased harm avoidance have been found to have been given drugs that affect which of the following neurotransmitters?

A. Acetylcholine
B. Dopamine
C. Glutamate
D. Norepinephrine
E. Serotonin

19.21. Plasma levels of oxytocin are positively correlated with differences in which of the following personality dimensions?

A. Harm avoidance
B. Novelty seeking
C. Persistence
D. Reward dependence
E. Slow to warm up

ANSWERS

19.1. D. Schizoid
Schizoid personality disorder is characterized by lifelong social withdrawal, and they are often described as eccentric. They have discomfort with interacting with others and a bland, constricted affect is noted on mental status examination. In contrast, those with avoidant personality disorder are also socially withdrawn but they are not asocial and show a great desire for companionship and are very sensitive to rejection. Antisocial personality disorder is characterized by lack of ability to conform to social norms and can include criminal acts. Those with paranoid personality disorder are often mistrustful, hostile, and irritable. Those with schizotypal personality disorder often have magical thinking and ideas of reference and derealization. (560)

19.2. A. A categorical approach is used
The categorical approach to personality disorders in DSM-5 is thought to be problematic to describe complex personality disorders in a few symptoms. A dimensional approach is better supported by research, incorporating temperament and functional impairment. (561)

19.3. D. Paranoid
Those with paranoid personality disorder present as formal and tense on mental status examination and often have a humorless mannerism. Speech is often goal-directed and logical though thought content shows evidence or projection and often ideas of reference. A patient with schizotypal personality disorder often presents as inappropriate with psychotic symptoms. Avoidant personality disorder presents as an anxious patient with a tense manner, along with vulnerability to the interviewer's comments, feeling criticized at times. A patient with dependent personality disorder often presents as complaint and often looks for guidance. Obsessive compulsive personality disorder is notable for a stiff demeanor, constricted affect with a serious mood, and defense mechanism of rationalization, isolation, intellectualization, and undoing are utilized. (562–566)

19.4. E. Schizotypal
Schizotypal personality disorder is characterized by pervasive discomfort with an inability to maintain close relationships. It presents with eccentric behavior, and oddities in thinking and appearance. These patients may have peculiar speech and express superstitious thoughts, thinking they possess special powers and can present as having brief psychotic symptoms at times. In ICD-10 schizotypal personality disorder is classified under psychotic disorders, rather than personality disorder. (563)

19.5. C. Projective identification
The patient described above most likely has borderline personality disorder. Patients with this disorder can present as argumentative and have episodes of psychosis and depression with unpredictable, self-destructive behavior, including self-harm. Feelings of anger, numbness, loneliness, and emptiness are characteristic of this disorder. Projective identification, in which the patient projects their own intolerable aspects of themselves onto others, is a classic defense mechanism for this disorder. (564)

19.6. A. Dissociation
The patient described above has histrionic personality disorder. Traits include attention-seeking behavior along with seductive behavior. They can present as suggestible and emotionally labile. The major defenses these patients utilize are dissociation and repression. (564, 565)

19.7. D. Narcissistic
In DSM-5, narcissistic personality disorder is defined as those persons with a grandiose sense of self-importance, characterized by strained relationships, often exploiting others, lacking empathy, jealousy, and having a fragile self-esteem. In the ICD-10, it is not included as a separate personality disorder, rather it is listed under an "other specified personality disorder." (565)

19.8. A. Anankastic
Anankastic personality disorder is the ICD-10 term for obsessive compulsive personality disorder. Features include those mentioned about included self-doubt, perfectionism, checking, attention to detail, stubbornness, being overly cautious, and having unwanted thoughts of impulses. (566)

19.9. A. Hallucinations
Paranoid personality disorder differs from schizophrenia in that no hallucinations or formal thought disorders are noted. All of the other features mentioned above can be symptoms of either schizophrenia or a paranoid personality disorder. (567)

19.10. D. Identify diffusion
Though features of borderline and histrionic personality disorders overlap, identity diffusion, suicide attempts, and brief psychotic episodes are more common in borderline personality disorder. (568)

19.11. A. Dependent
Dependent traits can occur in many psychiatric disorders, including both histrionic and borderline personality disorders, as well as dependent personality disorder. With dependent personality disorder, the person usually has a long relationship with one person. In contrast, with borderline and histrionic personality disorders, a series of tumultuous relationships are seen. (568)

19.12. A. Schizoid
The patient described above has avoidant personality disorder. Paranoid, schizotypal, schizoid, dependent, and borderline are the most commonly co-occurring personality disorder with avoidant personality disorder. (569)

19.13. E. Greater relationship stability is achieved in one's 40s and 50s
Functional improvement in borderline personality disorder is often not noted until the fourth and fifth decades of life. While brief psychotic episodes can be a component of borderline personality disorder, comorbid psychotic disorders are rare. While death from suicide is a risk of this disorder, the suicide and self-harm risks are highest in the young adult years and wane as time goes on. A history of multiple arrests is more common with antisocial personality disorder. (570)

19.14. A. Contingency management
Those with antisocial personality disorder are thought to have a limited response to therapy. A limited evidence base supports that these patients repose better to contingency management and rewards-based interventions, compared to cognitive behavioral therapy. (571)

19.15. B. Phone consultation
Dialectical behavioral therapy has the most empirical support for treating borderline personality disorder. It involves utilizing four modalities: group skill training, individual therapy, phone consultation, and a consultation team. Contingency management is useful for treating antisocial personality disorder. Mentalization-based therapy (MBT) is another type of therapy used to treat borderline personality disorder, as is transference-focused psychotherapy (TFP), in which the therapy relies on the use of clarification and confrontation in working with the patient using a psychodynamic approach. (573)

19.16. D. Citalopram
Limited evidence for medication management in treating obsessive compulsive personality disorder suggests that citalopram may be helpful in treating those with comorbid depression. In one study comparing citalopram and sertraline, which both reduced symptoms, citalopram performed better than sertraline. Some studies have suggested benefits from fluvoxamine and carbamazepine as well, though citalopram has specifically been shown to target depression in this population. (574)

19.17. B. Borderline
Borderline personality disorder is more common in women than in men and is typically seen in younger compared to older patients, as there is natural tendency toward remission as one ages. Histrionic personality disorder used to be thought to occur more frequently in women, but data suggest it might occur equally among men and women Avoidance, obsessive compulsive, and paranoid personality disorders are all more commonly found in men. (574)

19.18. E. Schizotypal
Biologic factors have been examined in personality disorders often to help examine inheritance or best guide treatment. Smooth pursuit eye movements are found to be saccadic, or jumpy, in those with introversion, withdrawal, and schizotypal personality disorder. Low platelet monoamine oxidase (MAO) levels have also been found in some patients with schizotypal personality disorder. (575)

19.19. E. Schizoid
Common defense mechanisms to each personality disorder can be found, helping the patient to resolve inner conflicts. Awareness of these defense mechanisms can help the psychiatrist in treating the patient. Those with schizoid personality disorder utilize fantasy and retreat to imaginary lives to help with feelings of loneliness and fear. Those with borderline often use dissociation. Isolation is common in those with obsessive compulsive personality disorder. Those with paranoid personality disorder utilize projection, while those with histrionic personality disorder often utilize dissociation. (376)

19.20. E. Serotonin
Temperament, biases in the modulation of conditioned behavioral response to physical stimuli, plays a role in personality formation. Four temperaments of harm avoidance, novelty seeking, reward dependence, and persistence have been studied. The anterior serotonergic cells in the dorsal raphe nucleus and the dopaminergic cells of the ventral tegmental area innervate the same structures and provide opposing influences to modulate approach and avoidance behaviors. When given serotonin drugs, harm avoidance behavior is decreased. (578)

19.21. D. Reward dependence
Reward dependence reflects behavior in response to social rewards. Noradrenergic and serotonergic projections likely modulate reward conditions. Plasma levels of oxytocin are thought to positively correlate with reward dependence. (578)

20

Other Conditions that May Be a Focus of Clinical Attention

20.1. In what section is the diagnosis of malingering categorized in the DSM-5?

A. Disruptive behavior disorders
B. Other conditions that may be a focus of clinical attention
C. Personality disorders
D. Psychotic disorder
E. Somatic symptom and related disorders

20.2. Common potential causes of feigning symptoms as a part of malingering include which of the following scenarios? (Choose three correct answers)

A. Enjoyment of being in the sick role
B. Gaining free room and board at a hospital*
C. Getting worker's compensation
D. Having severe depression
E. Inflicting pain upon minors by subjecting them to medical tests
F. Obtaining drugs for abuse

20.3. Patients with conversion disorder as opposed to malingering are more likely to display which of the following symptoms?

A. Avoidance of diagnostic evaluations
B. Behave as clingy and dependent
C. Possess a suspicious demeanor
D. Provide extremely detailed description of events leading to their illness
E. Refuse opportunities for employment

20.4. Which symptom is more typical of a major depressive disorder rather than normal grief?

A. Difficulty carrying out daily activities for a few weeks
B. Guilt about not seeing the loved one enough
C. Hearing the voice of the loved one
D. Irritability and insomnia
E. Significant psychomotor retardation

20.5. Which neurologic abnormality is found in half of aggressive criminals?

A. Abnormal EEGs
B. Brain tumors
C. Cerebral atrophy
D. Loss of grey matter in the brain
E. Migraines

20.6. Which is one of the most common symptoms noted in adult antisocial behavior?

A. Drug abuse
B. Pathologic lying
C. Somatic complaints
D. Suicide attempts
E. Work problems

20.7. Though antisocial behavior often continues through a person's life, some evidence exists that which of the following treatments might be helpful?

A. Acceptance and commitment therapy
B. Dialectical behavior therapy and phone coaching
C. Cognitive behavioral therapy
D. Group therapy and therapeutic communities
E. Interpersonal psychotherapy

20.8. Which group of people appears to be more vulnerable to negative experiences in dealing with phases of life problems?

A. Men
B. Minorities
C. People who utilize sublimation
D. Those of a higher socioeconomic status
E. Younger people

20.9. Which parenting style is most likely to be associated with children who are more aggressive, impulsive, and struggle with achieving?

A. Attachment
B. Authoritarian
C. Authoritative
D. Helicopter
E. Permissive

20.10. Studies support which of the following findings for physician marriages compared to other occupational groups?

A. Conflicts and separation are less likely to occur
B. Psychiatrists have the highest rate of divorce
C. Surgeons are most likely to get married
D. They occur later in life, on average in their 30s
E. They have higher satisfaction rates

ANSWERS

20.1. B. Other conditions that may be a focus of clinical attention
Malingering, a deliberate falsifying of physical or psychological symptoms to achieve a secondary gain (i.e., avoiding work, obtaining financial compensation, avoiding criminal prosecution, etc.) is not considered a mental health disorder, rather is listed in a section in the DSM-5 called "Other conditions that may be a focus of clinical attention." (580)

20.2. B. Gaining free room and board at a hospital, C. Getting worker's compensation, and F. Obtaining drugs for abuse
Malingering involves faking psychological or physical symptoms or secondary gain. Common causes of faking symptoms include to obtain drugs for abuse, or faking psychiatric symptoms to get free room and board in a hospital if homeless. Other cause of malingering includes faking injury to get money, or to get out of testifying in court. When there is no clear secondary gain and enjoyment of the sick role is noted, factitious disorder should be considered. Munchausen disorder by proxy should be considered if the adult is inflicting medical tests on a child and lying about their medical symptoms. (580, 581)

20.3. B. Behave as clingy and dependent
Malingering should be differentiated between conversion disorder with both, objective signs cannot account for their subjective experience. Those with conversion disorder are often dependent, clingy, friendly, and cooperative, compared to those with malingering who are suspicious and aloof. While those with conversion disorder want an answer and search for evaluations, those with malingering avoid them. Malingerers often avoid employment opportunities as well to circumvent their disability. Those with conversion disorder often have vague descriptions of their illness and inaccuracies and gaps in their history but those with malingering often provide excessively detailed accounts of events leading to their disability. (582)

20.4. E. Significant psychomotor retardation
Signs of normal bereavement can include sadness, irritability, insomnia, tearfulness, and difficulty carrying out daily activities, though if prolonged marked functional impairment, it is more consistent with a major depressive disorder. Excessive guilt about things (other than actions taken around the time of the loved one's death), along with thoughts of dying (other than wanting to be with the loved one) are symptoms consistent with a major depressive disorder. Significant psychomotor retardation and worthlessness, along with hallucinations that don't just involve the lost loved one, can also point toward a diagnosis of a major depressive disorder, rather than just grief. (582)

20.5. A. Abnormal EEGs
Neurologic conditions are often associated with adult antisocial behavior. Abnormal EEGs are commonly found in violent offenders, with studies estimating around 50% of aggressive criminals have abnormal EEG findings. Complex partial seizures should be ruled out in those with antisocial behavior. In cases of epilepsy or encephalitis, careful examination should be done to examine the extent those disorders are contributing to the behavior. (584)

20.6. E. Work problems
Though all the symptoms noted above can be features of antisocial behavior in adults, work problems are thought to be the most prominent symptoms (around 85%) followed by marital, financial dependency, and arrests, along with alcohol abuse. Less common symptoms include somatic complaints (11%), drug abuse (15%), suicide attempts (11%), and pathologic lying (16%). (585)

20.7. D. Group therapy and therapeutic communities
Though often outcomes for treating adult antisocial behavior are poor, in general, it is thought that behavior seems to decrease after 40 years old. Psychological therapy and medication treatment are typically not very effective, though for incarcerated criminals in institutional settings, some forms of group therapy have been shown to help and therapeutic communities are also thought to be helpful. (585)

20.8. B. Minorities
Phases of life problems can occur at any age. Common problems include divorce of parents, illness, having children, etc. Men appear to handle these phases of life problems better externally, whereas women, those of lower socioeconomic status, and minorities appear most vulnerable to the negative experiences, resulting in anxiety and depression. Positive attitudes, family relationships, mature

defense mechanisms, with use of sublimation, creativity, and flexibility appear to be protective factors against depression and anxiety from these phases of life problems. (587)

20.9. E. Permissive
Permissive parenting, which can be described as minimally restrictive and accepting, is associated with kids who are more aggressive, impulsive, and tend to be low achievers. Authoritarian parents can be described as cold and restrictive, and these children tend to be withdrawn or conflicted. Parents should aim for an authoritarian approach involving restriction as needed in a warm and accepting way. These children are thought to be the most socially well-adjusted and do better cognitively and are the highest achievers. (588)

20.10. B. Psychiatrists have the highest rate of divorce
Physicians have the highest risk of divorce compared to other occupation groups, with psychiatrists having the highest rates (50%), followed by surgeons (33%), internist pediatricians, and pathologists. Stress of work, including dealing with life–death situations, long hours, malpractice risks, and increased risk of depression and substance use are likely factors that contribute to the high divorce rate. (589)

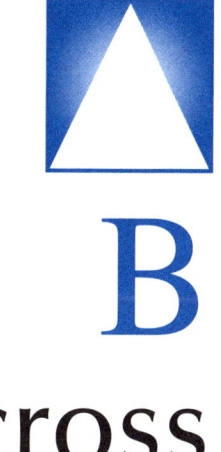

B
Treatment Across the Lifespan

21

Psychopharmacology

21.1. An 80-year-old woman in an assisted care facility was started 2 weeks ago on nightly doses of quetiapine due to episodes of drowsiness, confusion, and ataxia. The symptoms largely resolved after two doses. However, she now has had muscle stiffness and drooling for the last 3 days, and the ataxia has been replaced by a shuffling gait. She is also on memantine and hydrochlorothiazide. Vital signs on evening nursing rounds are T 98.8 F, BP 130/85, pulse 80, and respirations 16. Mental status examination reveals a well-nourished female in no acute distress. She is pleasant and cooperative. Her mood is "7 out of 10" with congruent affect. She denies suicidal ideation or auditory or visual hallucinations. She is oriented to person, place, time, and situation. What is the most appropriate treatment to address this patient's current symptoms?

A. Begin propranolol
B. Begin bromocriptine
C. Discontinue quetiapine
D. Begin tetrabenazine
E. Begin benztropine

21.2. What neuroleptic-induced movement disorder is more likely to occur in men than women?

A. Neuroleptic-induced parkinsonism
B. Neuroleptic malignant syndrome (NMS)
C. Acute dystonia
D. Acute akathisia
E. Tardive dyskinesia (TD)

21.3. A 27-year-old man presents to the outpatient clinic for medication management of his 9-year diagnosis of schizophrenia. He is currently on risperidone, which has kept him stable and out of the hospital for the past year. He has been on haloperidol, fluphenazine, quetiapine, and ziprasidone. Though each was initially helpful, he was eventually hospitalized because "they just stopped working." He remarks that this has been his longest period without hospitalization since he was first diagnosed, and does not want to make medication changes. However, he complains that he "can't keep my tongue in my mouth. It's embarrassing." He notes that he also cannot stop clenching and unclenching his fists. Abnormal involuntary movement scale (AIMS) test reveals a severity rating of 3, incapacitation rating of 2, and awareness rating of 3. What is the best step to relieve this patient's movement symptoms?

A. Decrease risperidone dose
B. Change risperidone to clozapine
C. Begin benztropine
D. Begin valbenazine
E. Change risperidone to aripiprazole

21.4. Which serotonin–dopamine antagonist is most likely to cause akathisia?

A. Aripiprazole
B. Olanzapine
C. Clozapine
D. Quetiapine
E. Ziprasidone

21.5. Which serotonin–dopamine antagonist is most likely to cause extrapyramidal symptoms?

A. Aripiprazole
B. Risperidone
C. Olanzapine
D. Quetiapine
E. Ziprasidone

21.6. A 37-year-old man with bipolar disorder presents to the urgent care clinic with complaints of painful sores on his chest and in his mouth. He states that, 3 days ago, he developed a cough, body aches, and felt "sick." He believed he had the flu, so he stayed home and hydrated. Yesterday, he noticed a purplish rash on his chest. When he woke this morning, part of the rash had blistered and peeled, and had become painful. He also noticed an ulcer in his mouth. His medications are valproic acid and lamotrigine. Vitals are temperature 99.8, pulse 90, and respirations 20. BP taken on the lower left arm is 160/90. Examination reveals a purplish rash on his chest and upper part of his arms, with intermittent peeling and blistering. Four blisters are present on the oral mucosa. What is the next most appropriate step in treatment?

A. Give a dose of oral diphenhydramine and a prescription to take twice a day until the rash resolves
B. Send him to the emergency department
C. Administer IV diphenhydramine in the office and observe the rash
D. Prescribe bromocriptine and advise him to go to the emergency department if symptoms do not resolve by the next day
E. Advise he discontinue his medications and follow up the next day with the prescribing physicians

21.7. A 78-year-old man is brought to the emergency department by nursing home staff following 2 weeks of increasing agitation and confusion. He has diagnoses of hypertension, bipolar disorder, and diabetes mellitus, for which he is on hydrochlorothiazide (HCTZ), aripiprazole, metformin, and oxcarbazepine. The nursing home staff reports that his vitals have been normal over the past week, and he has had no physical complaints except for being more tired than usual. Symptoms do not correlate with a specific time of day. A month ago, his speech started getting pressured and he had difficulty getting to sleep, so oxcarbazepine was increased. At that time, HgB A1c was 5.4, cholesterol was 180, and triglycerides were 150. Currently, vital signs are within normal limits. On examination, he is lethargic, and is alert and oriented to person, but not place and time. What lab result is most likely to be abnormal?

A. Glucose
B. Potassium
C. Sodium
D. Hemoglobin
E. White blood cell count

21.8. A 27-year-old woman is brought by emergency medical services (EMS) on a hotter-than-usual summer day to the emergency department due to an abrupt onset of difficulty standing, hand tremors, and confusion. She had just completed a citywide marathon 30 minutes ago when she was noticed by other runners to stumble and fall to the ground. She was not able to give her name, and said at the time that she was in her house in a different city. She has a diagnosis of bipolar disorder and has been stable on extended-release lithium and lamotrigine for the last 10 years. The electronic medical record shows that her lithium level was 1.0 at her last outpatient psychiatry appointment a week ago. Current vitals are T 99.7 F, BP 100/60, pulse 60, and respirations 14. Lithium level is 2.0. Physical examination reveals coarse hand tremors, ataxia, and horizontal nystagmus. What is the next best step in treatment?

A. Intravenous saline
B. Gastric lavage
C. Administration of activated charcoal
D. Hemodialysis
E. Whole bowel irrigation

21.9. A 36-year-old male is discovered by his mother on the floor of his bathroom after she returned home from work. EMS is called, and he is found to be dead at the scene. On the floor is an empty bottle of her amitriptyline and an empty bottle of his lamotrigine, both of which had been filled the day before. She states that he had no medical illnesses besides bipolar disorder and did not use drugs. A suicide note is found at the scene. What is the most likely mechanism of his death?

A. Inhibition of sodium current into myocardial cells
B. Acute hypothalamic dopamine blockade
C. Stimulation of postsynaptic 5-HT1A and 5-HT2A receptors
D. Acute norepinephrine release secondary to tyramine ingestion
E. Delayed type IV hypersensitivity reaction

21.10. In addition to alcohol and benzodiazepines, withdrawal from what class of psychoactive medications can be fatal?

A. Stimulants (cocaine, methamphetamine, etc.)
B. Monoamine oxidase inhibitors (MAOIs)
C. Barbiturates
D. Tricyclic antidepressants
E. Opioids

21.11. In addition to lithium, what psychotropic medication carries an U.S. Food and Drug Administration (FDA) warning for pregnant women due to an increased risk of cardiac malformation?

A. Carbamazepine
B. Valproic acid
C. Lamotrigine
D. Citalopram
E. Paroxetine

21.12. A 9-year-old boy diagnosed with autism spectrum disorder at age 2 is brought to the outpatient clinic due to worsening aggression and irritability over the last 2 months. He was started on sertraline for depression 6 months ago. At that time, in addition to irritability, he displayed decreased appetite, loss of interest in playing video games, lethargy, and poor concentration at school, resulting in his grades dropping from Bs to Ds. Since treatment, only the irritability has remained. He now occasionally bites himself and shows aggression toward his parents, teachers, and behavioral therapist. He has not physically attacked anyone, but his parents are worried that may soon occur. New therapeutic techniques have been marginally ineffective. The parents note that he has always displayed these behaviors, but that they have increased in frequency and intensity. He has no chronic medical illnesses and is on no other medications. Vital signs are within normal limits and physical examination is noncontributory. He is begrudgingly cooperative, but calm. What is the next best step in treatment for this child?

A. Increase sertraline
B. Obtain a head CT
C. Begin aripiprazole
D. Admit the child to the hospital
E. Change therapists

21.13. What atypical antipsychotic is most likely to lead to weight gain?

A. Risperidone
B. Quetiapine
C. Olanzapine
D. Paliperidone
E. Aripiprazole

21.14. An 18-year-old man is admitted to the hospital for first-break psychosis after locking himself in his college dorm room for 2 days because he felt that was the only way "to keep the demons away from me." Medical workup in the emergency department found no etiology for the psychotic symptoms. He was first started on haloperidol, which led to a stiff neck, which was mostly relieved with benztropine. A trial of fluphenazine caused his eyes to fix in an upward deviation. Risperidone led to the same effects. He is on no other medications and has no chronic medical illnesses. Body mass index (BMI) is 17. What medication should be tried next to manage his symptoms?

A. Aripiprazole
B. Quetiapine
C. Clozapine
D. Chlorpromazine
E. Asenapine

21.15. In addition to lurasidone, what serotonin–dopamine antagonist must be taken with food to achieve maximum effect?

A. Aripiprazole
B. Iloperidone
C. Lurasidone
D. Quetiapine
E. Ziprasidone

21.16. A 24-year-old man presents to the outpatient clinic for follow-up of schizophrenia. He was diagnosed 6 months ago, and symptoms have been adequately controlled with risperidone. He is greatly distressed by breast enlargement, and states that he stopped taking the medication a week ago after he noticed milk discharge from his chest. He is willing to try another medication, but refuses to take anything that can cause the same symptoms. He has a current BMI of 23. BMI prior to starting medication was 21. He is also on amiodarone for congenital heart disease. He has no known drug allergies. Which of the following medications should be considered for this patient?

A. Aripiprazole
B. Asenapine
C. Iloperidone
D. Quetiapine
E. Ziprasidone

21.17. The parents of a 26-year-old man who is diagnosed with schizophrenia called the office to say that they were not able to get him to the lab yesterday for his weekly complete blood count (CBC) for clozapine. When they went to the pharmacy, they were denied the patient's dose of medication. They note that the patient has not missed a lab appointment in 4 months, and state that they can get his blood drawn the next morning. They request assistance with getting him the clozapine. How should the physician respond?

A. Send in a prescription for one dose of medication
B. Call the pharmacy to authorize an override
C. Send a prescription to a different pharmacy
D. Affirm that the medication cannot be dispensed
E. Call the lab and explain the situation

21.18. Iloperidone must be titrated slowly to avoid what side effect?

A. Sedation
B. Tachycardia
C. Orthostatic hypotension
D. QTc prolongation
E. Akathisia

21.19. A 19-year-old man presents to the outpatient psychiatry clinic for follow-up management of his diagnosis of schizophrenia 8 weeks ago. At the time of initial presentation, he had had a 6-month history of auditory hallucinations and paranoia, which were preceded by an 8-month history of withdrawing from family and friends and staying in his room so that he would not "be subject to the influence of the emperor." After an extensive workup, he was started on aripiprazole, and he and the family were provided with psychoeducation on the illness. He was on a low dose for 2 weeks, then a medium dose for 2 weeks, then the maximum recommended dose for 4 weeks. Today, his parents report that his behavior is unchanged. They attest that they watch him take and swallow his medication every morning, which he does with no hesitation. What should be the next step in treatment?

A. Augment with a first-generation antipsychotic
B. Continue aripiprazole for another 4 weeks
C. Change to clozapine
D. Change to a different, nonclozapine, serotonin–dopamine antagonist
E. Change to the long-acting injectable form of aripiprazole

21.20. A 30-year-old woman on a telepsych appointment with a psychiatrist complains of "being so depressed for the last month that I can't get out of bed. That's why I couldn't come in." She states that she was diagnosed with major depressive disorder (MDD) 10 years ago, and has had six such episodes in that time, which also included increased appetite, decreased concentration, withdrawal from friends and family, and poor energy. She reports that the symptoms usually resolve in about 2 months, and that she will "ride it out" because she does not like to take medication. She notes that her husband is very understanding during these periods and does extra work around the house while she recovers. She is concerned this time because she has started to hear voices over the last 3 days telling her that she should kill herself. "This is the most depressed I have ever been, and these voices are scaring me. I don't know what to do!" She is diagnosed with hypothyroidism, which has been well controlled with synthetic thyroid hormone. Thyroid function tests done 3 months ago were in the normal range. She has no other medical illnesses and is on no other medications. Mental status examination reveals an anxious affect. She is tearful at times. She states that she is willing to "do whatever it takes" to get better. What should be the treatment for this patient?

A. An antidepressant medication only
B. An antipsychotic medication only
C. An antidepressant and an antipsychotic medication
D. Electroconvulsive therapy (ECT) only
E. ECT and an antidepressant medication

21.21. What is the usual mechanism of orthostatic hypotension from first-generation antipsychotics?

A. Beta-2 receptor agonism
B. D2 receptor antagonism
C. Alpha-1 receptor blockade
D. Acetylcholine receptor antagonism
E. H1 receptor blockade

21.22. Increased secretion of prolactin caused by antipsychotic medication dopamine receptor blockade occurs via what neuroanatomical tract?

A. Mesocortical
B. Mesolimbic
C. Nigrostriatal
D. Tuberoinfundibular

21.23. A 25-year-old man is hospitalized for the third time in 6 years for acute psychosis after attacking his girlfriend "to make her less attractive to the men on the TV." During the first hospitalization, he was diagnosed with schizophrenia after an extensive medical workup and started on ziprasidone. Per the electronic medical record, he stopped going to the outpatient psychiatrist 6 months later and received no more refills. He was prescribed risperidone during his last hospitalization 3 years ago, which markedly decreased auditory and visual hallucinations. He then followed up monthly at the outpatient clinic and was moderately compliant with his medications. Over the last year, his visits became infrequent and he reported taking his medication only one to two times a week at his last visit 3 months ago. Vital signs are within normal limits and urine drug screen is negative. He is stabilized on paliperidone in the hospital and discharged on paliperidone palmitate. After discharge, he asks the outpatient psychiatrist how long he needs to stay on the medication. What is the most appropriate response?

A. 3 to 6 months
B. 1 year
C. 2 to 3 years
D. 4 to 5 years
E. Indefinitely

21.24. A 55-year-old woman who was diagnosed with obsessive-compulsive disorder (OCD) 2 months ago returns to the outpatient clinic for a follow-up appointment. At the time of diagnosis, she reported that she was greatly distressed by her ritual of checking the house several times to make sure that she left no electrical appliances on prior to leaving the house and going to bed which has made her late for work and shortened her sleep time. The Yale-Brown Obsessive-Compulsive Scale (Y-BOCS) showed symptoms in the severe range. She was started on sertraline at that time and quickly titrated up to a medium dose. At her follow-up appointment 4 weeks later, she reported that she no longer is late for work, but has been close to being so several times. Y-BOCS at that time was in the high-moderate range, and sertraline was titrated to the maximum dose. Today, she states that she has had some more improvement, and is comfortably on time for work due to checking a fewer number of times, but she still checks. Y-BOCS is in the low-moderate range. She is also diagnosed with diabetes, for which she is on metformin. Vitals are within normal limits. Physical examination is noncontributory. Mental status examination reveals a mood of "better, but not great," with congruent affect. Which is the most appropriate next step in treatment?

A. Prescribe a supratherapeutic dose of sertraline
B. Augment with risperidone
C. Continue current dose
D. Change to a different selective serotonin reuptake inhibitor (SSRI)
E. Change to serotonin norepinephrine reuptake inhibitor (SNRI)

21.25. What is the most common long-term side effect of SSRIs?

A. Nausea
B. Headache
C. Sedation
D. Sexual dysfunction
E. Anxiety

21.26. A 30-year-old woman presents to the outpatient clinic with complaints of anxiety "all the time over every little thing." She states that she has always been "the family worrywart," and that others tell her that she is making life more stressful than it has to be, "but I just can't help it. I always think of the worst possible scenario for everything." She endorses difficulty getting to sleep due to "thinking about all the things I have to get done the next day." She also complains of headaches, poor concentration, and feeling "edgy." Though this has been a lifelong problem, she came today because "I'm just tired of feeling this way." She reports that she has had a "heart rhythm issue" since birth, but is on no medications. She reports a family history of anxiety and breast cancer. Vitals are within normal limits and physical examination is noncontributory. What SSRI is relatively contraindicated in this patient?

   A. Citalopram
   B. Escitalopram
   C. Fluoxetine
   D. Fluvoxamine
   E. Sertraline

21.27. A 40-year-old woman who has a 15-year history of bipolar disorder, which has been well controlled with lithium, calls the clinic to report symptoms of diarrhea, headache, and restlessness since taking her new dose of escitalopram 6 hours ago. Four weeks ago, she reported difficulty sleeping, poor concentration and appetite, lethargy, and anhedonia. She had not had a manic episode in 10 years, and agreed to begin escitalopram. At her clinic appointment yesterday, she reported that symptoms of depression had improved, but she still had some depressed mood and anhedonia, so the dose of escitalopram was increased. Lithium level was 0.9. What is the most likely cause of the patient's current symptoms?

   A. Emergence of a co-occurring anxiety disorder
   B. The beginning of a manic episode
   C. A sharp increase in plasma serotonin
   D. An acute increase in plasma lithium concentration
   E. Atypical symptoms of depression

21.28. The likelihood of SSRI discontinuation syndrome is most closely associated with what property of the medication?

   A. Half-life
   B. Protein binding
   C. CYP 450 metabolism
   D. Potency
   E. Bioavailability

21.29. A 54-year-old man who has been on a moderate dose of venlafaxine for generalized anxiety disorder for 20 years tells his physician that he feels the medication is beginning to lose effectiveness. He is noticing that he is starting to worry about "anything and everything," which is disrupting his sleep, and would "like to get a handle on this before it gets out of control." He has been happy with his medication so far, and wants to increase it. He is also diagnosed with hypercholesterolemia, type I diabetes, and has smoked a pack a day for the last 35 years. He has an insulin pump and is on simvastatin. Vital signs are T 98.8 F, BP 130/85, pulse 90, and respirations 18. The venlafaxine is increased to the highest dose. Which of the following physiologic measurements should now be monitored more closely?

   A. Blood glucose
   B. BMI
   C. Blood pressure
   D. Serum lipids
   E. Oxygen level

21.30. The low level of sexual dysfunction from bupropion is thought to be attributed to what pharmacologic property of the medication?

   A. Downstream stimulation of dopamine reward pathways
   B. Short half-life of 12 hours
   C. Decreased evening plasma levels
   D. Lack of serotonin reuptake inhibition
   E. Downstream stimulation of norepinephrine receptors

21.31. Bupropion is contraindicated in individuals with what medical condition?

A. Hepatitis
B. Epilepsy
C. Congenital QT prolongation
D. Hypertension
E. Renal disease.

21.32. In addition to blockade of postsynaptic serotonin 5HT2 and 5HT3 receptors, mirtazapine's antidepressant effects are mediated through what pharmacologic mechanism?

A. Inhibition of serotonin and norepinephrine reuptake
B. Inhibition of norepinephrine and dopamine reuptake
C. Antagonism of presynaptic alpha-2 receptors
D. Activation of serotonin 5HT1A receptors
E. Serotonin–dopamine antagonism

21.33. An 86-year-old female resident at a senior living facility complains of difficulty remembering the names of others in the facility over the last 3 weeks. Her adult children report that she has been calling them over the last 3 weeks and crying about how she was a horrible mother. They note no pattern in the time of day of her calls. She has been waking up in the morning 2 to 3 hours earlier than usual, with difficulty returning to sleep. Appetite has decreased to the point that she picks at her meals or skips them altogether. She has not gone to the community bingo games in the past week, and makes little effort to get out of the bed. On mental status examination, she is alert and oriented to person, but responds with "I don't know" when asked about place and time, as well as on several measures of cognition, such as serial 7s. She gives minimal effort on the clock-drawing test. Her mood is, "I just don't feel good," with congruent, dysphoric affect. Vital signs are within normal limits. Which of the following medications should be used in the treatment of this patient?

A. Mirtazapine
B. Memantine
C. Risperidone
D. Trimethoprim-sulfamethoxazole
E. Hydroxyzine

21.34. A 60-year-old man presents to an outpatient psychiatrist to establish care after moving to a new city. He states that he was diagnosed with major depressive disorder 35 years ago and has been on nefazodone since then and does not want to discontinue it. Prior to continuing the prescription, the psychiatrist should order what lab test?

A. Liver function
B. Serum glucose
C. Thyroid stimulating hormone (TSH)
D. Creatinine
E. Complete blood count

21.35. Trazodone can cause what physiologic medical emergency?

A. Status epilepticus
B. Priapism
C. Ventricular fibrillation
D. Acute renal failure
E. Ketoacidosis

21.36. Tricyclic antidepressants (TCAs) exert their therapeutic effect by what primary pharmacologic mechanism?

A. Alpha-1 and alpha-2 receptor antagonism
B. Serotonin and norepinephrine reuptake inhibition
C. Cholinergic muscarinic receptor antagonism
D. Norepinephrine and dopamine reuptake inhibition
E. Serotonin, norepinephrine, and dopamine reuptake inhibition

21.37. A 43-year-old female with a diagnosis of obsessive-compulsive disorder (OCD) returns to the outpatient clinic due to continued symptoms despite being on sertraline for the last 3 months. She states that the medication has been no more effective than the fluoxetine and paroxetine she has been on, each for 12 weeks at the highest dose. She has no other illnesses and is on no other medications. What medication should be tried next?

A. Bupropion
B. Fluvoxamine
C. Clomipramine
D. Amitriptyline
E. Selegiline

21.38. A 76-year-old man presents to the outpatient clinic with a complaint of, "I'm depressed and I can't go on." He states that since his spouse died 4 weeks ago, "I can't sleep, I can't eat, and there is no reason to live. We were together for 50 years!" He has stopped socializing with friends and stays in his house, crying on and off throughout the day out of grief and because "I'm too exhausted to do anything else." He has lost 10 pounds in the last month. He denies suicidal ideation, but states that "even though I would never kill myself, I want to die." He is on metformin for diabetes and pilocarpine and acetazolamide for narrow-angle glaucoma. Which of the following medications for his symptoms is relatively contraindicated?

A. Vortioxetine
B. Paroxetine
C. Venlafaxine
D. Amitriptyline
E. Selegiline

21.39. A tricyclic should be used as the antidepressant of last resort in individuals with which health condition?

A. Heart disease
B. Pregnancy
C. Liver disease
D. Epilepsy
E. Renal disease

21.40. The 2-week washout period needed before starting another antidepressant after the last dose of an irreversible monoamine oxidase inhibitor (MAOI) is to give time for what physiologic mechanism to occur?

A. The drug to detach from monoamine presynaptic transporters
B. The drug to detach from postsynaptic monoamine receptors
C. The body to synthesize new monoamine oxidase
D. Decrease in plasma concentration after five half-lives of time
E. Hepatic metabolism and excretion of both the parent drug and active metabolite

21.41. A 55-year-old man presents to his primary care physician with feelings of "not having any get up and go" for the last month. He states that for nearly all of his life he has enjoyed fishing every weekend, but now "I just don't feel like doing it." He is surprised that he often feels run down, even though he is in the bed for 10 to 12 hours some weekends, which is an increase from his prior 7 to 8. He reports gaining 10 pounds in the last 6 months, even though his appetite has been decreased for the last month. He denies current or past suicidal ideation. He occasionally takes colchicine for flares of gout, but otherwise has no history of medical problems and is on no other medications. Vital signs are within normal limits and physical examination is noncontributory. Mental status examination reveals a "down" mood with congruent affect. There is no suicidal ideation. Cognition is intact. What lab tests should the physician order as part of the workup for the patient's current symptoms?

A. Uric acid
B. Complete blood count (CBC)
C. Urinalysis
D. Thyroid function
E. Plasma colchicine level

21.42. Ketamine acts with what pharmacodynamic effect on N-methyl-D-aspartate (NMDA) receptors?

A. Allosteric modulator
B. Antagonist
C. Agonist
D. Partial agonist
E. Inverse agonist

21.43. A 28-year-old man returns to the outpatient clinic after being diagnosed with bipolar I disorder, most recent episode manic, and starting on lithium 4 weeks ago. He states that he feels "stable, not so up and down," and that he has been able to sleep for 7 hours a night again, which is a sharp increase from the previous 1 to 2 hours. He feels that the medication has been helpful, but he complains of his hands shaking, most notably when he writes with a pen or engages in some other fine-motor task. He is on no other medications and has no other illnesses. He last took the medication 8 hours ago. On examination, a fine tremor is present, most notably in his fingers when he holds his arms out. Neurologic examination reveals a normal gait and reflexes. Extraocular muscles are intact with no nystagmus. What is the most likely cause of the patient's tremor?

A. Gradual lithium toxicity
B. Lithium-induced hyperthyroidism
C. Normal lithium side effect
D. Lithium withdrawal
E. Acute lithium overdose

21.44. Lithium use during the first trimester of pregnancy is associated with which congenital birth defect?

A. Tetralogy of Fallot
B. Spina bifida
C. Neural tube defects
D. Ebstein anomaly
E. Anencephaly

21.45. In a person who takes immediate-release lithium twice a day, when should the lithium level be drawn?

A. At any time
B. As soon as possible after taking a dose
C. Around 12 hours after taking a dose
D. Around 6 hours after taking a dose
E. Between 1 and 6 hours after taking a dose

21.46. A 27-year-old female, who was diagnosed with bipolar I disorder 7 years ago, comes to the outpatient clinic for a routine follow-up appointment. Her illness has been well-controlled with valproate for the past 5 years. During the 2 years since her diagnosis, she has been hospitalized six times due to acute manic episodes and suicidal ideation. She was initially prescribed lithium but stopped it because, "It took away my creativity and dulled me out." She has also been on paliperidone, olanzapine, aripiprazole, risperidone, lamotrigine, and carbamazepine, all of which were discontinued either due to side effects or lack of efficacy. She does not want to take a long-acting injection. She reports that her current medication "keeps me stable. Without it, I would be back in the hospital." She reports that she and her husband now want to have a child, and are concerned about the effects of valproate on the fetus, but states, "I can't get sick and go back into the hospital. I finally have my life together." What should the physician recommend regarding the patient's concerns?

A. Discontinuing valproate until after the first trimester
B. Beginning folic acid supplementation
C. Changing to a different antiepileptic medication
D. Changing to a different antipsychotic medication
E. Lowering the dose of valproate until it reaches below 50 μg/mL

21.47. In addition to a complete blood count (CBC), what laboratory test should be routinely ordered in patients taking valproate?

A. Blood urea nitrogen (BUN)/creatinine
B. Liver function
C. Thyroid function
D. Lipid panel
E. Glucose

21.48. A 36-year-old man diagnosed with bipolar I disorder with rapid cycling was started on olanzapine 3 weeks ago when he was hospitalized during his first manic episode. One week after that, while still hospitalized, he was started on lamotrigine and discharged a week later. He has been titrating as directed, and would be on day 21 today. He calls the outpatient clinic this morning to report that he left the lamotrigine at home while the family was on a weeklong trip, and asks how he should proceed with taking it. He is on no other medications besides olanzapine. What should be recommended to the patient?

A. Restart the titration from the beginning (day 1)
B. Restart the titration time from the most recent increase (day 14)
C. Resume the titration from where he left off (day 16)
D. Continue with the scheduled titration (day 21)

21.49. A 35-year-old woman was started on carbamazepine and diagnosed with bipolar I disorder while hospitalized due to acute mania 4 months ago. She has been on the same dose for the last 2 months. She presents to the outpatient clinic today for a routine follow-up. Though she complains of occasional nausea from the medication, she has found that it is tolerable if she takes it with food, "and a little nausea is much better than being in the hospital, so I still take it every day." She notes that she started thyroid hormone replacement therapy a month ago due to hypothyroidism. She worries that she is becoming manic because she is only needing to sleep 6 hours instead of her usual 8, and because "I think my concentration isn't as good." She denies other symptoms of mania, suicidal ideation, or impairment at her job. What is the most likely cause of the patient's current symptoms?

A. Decreased efficacy over time ("poop out")
B. Noncompliance due to side effects
C. Increase in carbamazepine metabolism
D. Drug interaction with thyroid hormone
E. Induction of mania from thyroid hormone

21.50. A 24-year-old man with a diagnosis of bipolar disorder presents to the outpatient clinic for a routine follow-up. He has been on quetiapine for the past 4 months, resulting in a "stable" mood. He is pleased with the treatment except for an increase in weight of 10 pounds over the past 2 months, leading to an increase in BMI from 23 to 24.4, despite exercising four times a week and eating a 1,800 cal/day diet. He takes no other medications. Vital signs are normal, and physical examination is unremarkable. Glucose and lipid profile prior to the start of the treatment were within normal limits. Besides metformin, what medication could be most helpful in mitigating this patient's weight gain?

A. Aripiprazole
B. Methylphenidate
C. Topiramate
D. Oxcarbazepine
E. Mixed amphetamine salts

21.51. What is the most common side effect of benzodiazepine use?

A. Ataxia
B. Dizziness
C. Mild cognitive impairment
D. Drowsiness
E. Drug rash

21.52. Flumazenil can reverse the adverse effects of what drug?

A. Alcohol
B. Barbiturates
C. Opioids
D. Benzodiazepines
E. Tricyclics

21.53. A 21-year-old man is brought to the emergency department after his friends called EMS due to him passing out and not being able to be aroused 2 hours later. His friends told the emergency medical technicians (EMTs) that they had all been drinking more heavily than usual, and that he had consumed seven drinks in 3 hours. In the emergency department, the EMR from the outpatient clinic reveals that he is diagnosed with type I diabetes mellitus (DM) and panic disorder, and that he has an insulin pump and was started on sertraline and clonazepam a week ago. What vital sign is most likely to be abnormal?

A. Blood pressure
B. Heart rate
C. Respirations
D. Temperature

21.54. Buspirone has been shown to be effective as a primary treatment of what disorder?

A. Obsessive-compulsive disorder (OCD)
B. Major depressive disorder
C. Generalized anxiety disorder
D. Panic disorder
E. Social phobia

21.55. A 45-year-old woman presents to the outpatient clinic with a complaint of, "I have performance anxiety." She states that she has been a concert pianist for the last 15 years, and that she started becoming anxious before she had to perform after she made a mistake 6 months ago during a concert, "and probably no one noticed, but I did. Since then, I've been terrified that I'll mess up again." She denies anxiety in other situations, and continues to perform, "but it's getting harder every time. If this keeps up, I'm going to have to stop playing." She is diagnosed with type II diabetes mellitus, for which she is on metformin. She also takes fish oil and vitamin C "to keep myself healthy." Vital signs are within normal limits. Physical examination is unremarkable. Which of the following medications often used in the treatment of her symptoms is relatively contraindicated in this patient?

A. Clonazepam
B. Propranolol
C. Sertraline
D. Desvenlafaxine
E. Hydroxyzine

21.56. A 30-year-old woman is brought to the emergency department (ED) by EMS after her husband called due to her being confused, calling him by her father's name and lapsing in out of consciousness. At the ED, he reports that she told him before bed she had mistakenly mixed up her thyroid medicine, of which she takes three pills a night, with her sleeping medicine, of which she only takes one a night. He adds that she told him she had acquired the sleeping medicine "from a friend." He does not know the names of the medications. Temperature is 98.8 F, blood pressure is 140/95, pulse 90, and respirations 10. Neurologic examination reveals ataxia, hyporeflexia, and lateral nystagmus. On mental status examination, she is confused and oriented to person, but not place or time. What is the likely causal agent of her current symptoms?

A. Temazepam
B. Trazodone
C. Amobarbital
D. Hydroxyzine
E. Doxepin

21.57. What medication used for sleep can cause amnesia and automatic behaviors, such as nighttime eating and driving as side effects?

A. Melatonin
B. Ramelteon
C. Eszopiclone
D. Zolpidem
E. Prazosin

21.58. A 28-year-old man presents to the VA outpatient department 3 months after returning from overseas, where he served in the armed forces as a combat medic. He states that he has had problems sleeping for the last 10 weeks because "every time I close my eyes at night, I have vivid dreams of limbs blown off and dead soldiers littering the field." He states that he saw a fellow soldier "die in my arms before we could get him to a medical field station." He adds that he gets startled and is triggered by sudden loud noises, which "take me right back to the battlefield." During a recent holiday in which neighbors shot off fireworks, he had to stay in a rural hotel "because the flashbacks were so bad." He has never been on medication. He states that the lack of a full night's sleep is what bothers him the most, and that "I can handle the other stuff by myself if it weren't for these dreams every night." Vitals are within normal limits. Physical examination is noncontributory. What is the most common side effect of the medication used to treat this patient's chief complaint?

A. Priapism
B. Amnesia
C. Weight gain
D. Dizziness
E. Automatic behaviors

21.59. A 9-year-old boy who was diagnosed 4 weeks ago with attention-deficit/hyperactivity disorder (ADHD), hyperactive-impulsive type, returns to the outpatient clinic for follow-up after starting methylphenidate. His mother reports that she started him on 5 mg twice a day, and increased the medication by 5 mg/week up to 20 mg twice a day with minimal effect except for a decrease in appetite. He is still getting notes from school about his unruly behavior. What is the next step in the medication management of this child?

A. Increase the methylphenidate to a maximum of 30 mg twice a day
B. Change the medication to atomoxetine
C. Augment the medication with clonidine
D. Change the medication to mixed amphetamine salts
E. Augment the medication with bupropion

21.60. A 10-year-old girl is brought to the outpatient clinic by her parents after a referral from school due to the child "staring off into space" for the last 4 months. Her teacher reported that she has forgotten to turn in her homework several times and that her desk is disorganized. At home, she takes 30 minutes to do a 10-minute school assignment, which is then littered with careless mistakes. "She is making C's when we know she has the ability to make A's." Her parents also report that she "sometimes doesn't seem to be listening when we talk to her. She's not ignoring us, her mind is just somewhere else." She was diagnosed with persistent motor tic disorder 3 years ago, and though she displays symptoms, she says she is not bothered by them. She is on no medications. Vital signs are within normal limits. Physical examination is noncontributory. What is the first-line pharmacologic treatment for this child?

A. Atomoxetine
B. Methylphenidate
C. Clonidine
D. Bupropion
E. Guanfacine

21.61. A 7-year-old boy who has been on lisdexamfetamine for the last 6 months is brought by his parents to the outpatient clinic for a 2-month follow-up on his progress at school. He is seen by the nurse, who takes his height, weight, and vitals. What measurement is most likely to have decreased since he began the medication?

A. Heart rate
B. Respirations
C. Weight
D. Height
E. Blood pressure

21.62. What is atomoxetine's mechanism of action?

A. Alpha-2 agonism
B. Dopamine reuptake inhibition
C. Increased dopamine release
D. Norepinephrine reuptake inhibition
E. GABA inhibition

21.63. Place buprenorphine, methadone, and naltrexone in order of effect on the μ-opioid receptor from agonist to antagonist.

A. Methadone > naltrexone > buprenorphine
B. Naltrexone > methadone > buprenorphine
C. Buprenorphine > methadone > naltrexone
D. Naltrexone > buprenorphine > methadone
E. Methadone > buprenorphine > naltrexone
F. Buprenorphine > naltrexone > methadone

21.64. A 45-year-old man on methadone maintenance therapy for the last 5 years presents to the emergency department with complaints of headache, anxiety, nausea, and jitteriness. He states that the symptoms began 4 days ago when he stopped going to the methadone clinic and have gotten progressively worse. He states that he wants to "be done with all this addiction stuff, so I figured I'd go cold turkey." He now feels he underestimated the withdrawal symptoms, but still wants to "push through." What medication would be most appropriate for the patient at this time?

A. Methadone
B. Buprenorphine
C. Clonidine
D. Naltrexone
E. Tramadol

21.65. A 55-year-old woman is being discharged from the hospital after her sixth day of detoxification from alcohol. During the admission, she had been on a protocol to monitor for alcohol withdrawal and was given chlordiazepoxide on two occasions. Today, she states that she is ready to stop drinking, but the craving for alcohol is what perpetually leads to relapse. She is on sertraline for depression. Vital signs are within normal limits. What pharmacologic agent would be most helpful to decrease the chance of relapse?

A. Diazepam
B. Disulfiram
C. Clonidine
D. Acamprosate
E. Naltrexone

21.66. Disulfiram works by what mechanism?

A. Glutamate transmission reduction
B. Aldehyde dehydrogenase inhibition
C. Opioid receptor antagonism
D. GABA transmission enhancement
E. Displacement of ethanol from GABA receptors

21.67. A 10-year-old boy is brought to the urgent care by his grandmother, who reports that the child became sweaty and shaky 2 hours ago. She states that he did not eat breakfast or lunch today "because he said his stomach hurt." The child states that his head hurts and that he could not sleep well last night. His grandmother reports that she picked him up from his parents' house after school 2 days ago to keep him over the weekend. She adds that he usually takes medication for ADHD every day, "but I don't think he really needs it, so I didn't give it to him. If they want to give it to him again tonight when I take him home, they can." He is on no other medications and has no other illnesses. Vitals are T 98.8 F, BP 140/85, pulse 90, respirations 22. Physical examination is significant for bilateral hand tremors. What is the most likely medication the child is prescribed?

A. Atomoxetine
B. Amphetamine salts
C. Methylphenidate
D. Clonidine
E. Lisdexamphetamine

21.68. A 78-year-old woman is brought by her son to the outpatient clinic who states, "I'm ready for medicine for my mother now." He recounts how his mother was diagnosed with Alzheimer dementia 5 years ago. At that time, the physician suggested that his mother starts on a cognitive enhancement medication, but he did not want her on another medication in addition to the atorvastatin, lisinopril, and metformin she was already taking for hypercholesterolemia, hypertension, and diabetes. He states that her dementia has progressed to the point that neither he nor his two siblings can safely care for her anymore at any of their homes. She has wandered out of the house during the night, frequently forgets who they are, and has left the stove and oven on, nearly burning down the house on more than one occasion. They are actively looking for a secure living facility. Vitals are normal, and physical examination reveals an agitated woman who looks older than her stated age, with no acute examination findings. Which of the following cognitive enhancement medications is most appropriate?

A. Donepezil
B. Tacrine
C. Galantamine
D. Rivastigmine
E. Memantine

21.69. An 18-year-old man presents to the outpatient primary care clinic for a yearly physical examination. He has no chronic medical illnesses and is on no medications. During the sexual history, he states that he has never had sexual intercourse, "and the guys at school are giving me a hard time about being a virgin." He has been dating the same girl for a month, and admits that he has no romantic feelings for her. He has tried to have vaginal sex with her "so that everyone will stop making fun of me," but found that he could not maintain an erection. He admits to trying sildenafil, "but it didn't work. I still couldn't get hard." He denies drug use, states that he gets morning erections, and has no difficulty with masturbation. What is the most likely cause of the lack of response to the medication?

A. He has a fast nitric oxide metabolizer
B. The dose he is taking is too low for his age
C. He is not sexually attracted to his girlfriend
D. He did not take the medication with a high-fat meal
E. Nitric oxide depletion due to frequent masturbation

21.70. A 22-year-old man with a diagnosis of schizoaffective disorder, who has been hospitalized for 2 days due to acute psychosis, was noted by staff yesterday to have been "quieter than usual." He walked around the unit looking confused, though when questioned, was oriented to person, place, and situation. The next morning, he did not report to the day area for breakfast. The unit nurse found him in bed with his pillow soaked with sweat. He did not respond to questions. When the nurse attempted to take his blood pressure, she had difficulty bending his arm to get it out from under the sheet. Vitals are T 39 C (102.2 F), BP 150/95, pulse 110, and respirations 20. He was started on haloperidol 3 days ago upon admission. He is also on escitalopram. What is the most likely cause of this patient's current condition?

A. Serotonin syndrome
B. Malignant hypothermia
C. Neuroleptic malignant syndrome (NMS)
D. Malignant catatonia
E. Extrapyramidal side effects (EPS)

ANSWERS

21.1. E. Begin benztropine
The patient is displaying symptoms of neuroleptic-induced parkinsonism, for which the treatment of choice is an anticholinergic agent such as benztropine, amantadine or diphenhydramine. Neuroleptic malignant syndrome, for which dantrolene or bromocriptine would be used, would present with autonomic instability such as hyperthermia and increased pulse and blood pressure. As she has shown marked improvement in the original symptoms with the quetiapine, it would be best to try to treat the side effect as opposed to starting a new medication which may or may not be effective, and which can lead to the same side effect. Propranolol would be used for akathisia, which would present with hyperkinesis as opposed to bradykinesis, while tetrabenazine would be used for tardive dyskinesia, which likely would not appear this quickly, and would involve choreoathetoid movements. Antihistamines such as diphenhydramine can also be used as an alternative to anticholinergics. (594, 703)

21.2. C. Acute dystonia
Of all of the common neuroleptic-induced mood disorders, medication-induced acute dystonia is more likely to occur in men, particularly those under age 30 years. Neuroleptic-induced parkinsonism is more likely to affect older women, NMS is more likely to affect younger women, and acute akathisia and TD are most likely to affect middle-aged women. (594–597)

21.3. D. Begin valbenazine
The patient has a moderate level of tardive dyskinesia (TD) which is causing him a moderate amount of distress. The first approach considered should be to lower the dose of the offending agent. However, given the patient's history of hospitalizations and his stated preference not to adjust his current regimen, neither a decrease in dose nor a change to another agent would be the best choice. If the risperidone becomes ineffective in the future, clozapine would be a strong consideration, as it is unlikely to cause TD and can even decrease it. Benztropine is not helpful for TD. A VMAT2 inhibitor such as valbenazine would be first-line treatment. (598)

21.4. A. Aripiprazole
Aripiprazole is the most likely of the serotonin–dopamine antagonists to cause akathisia due to its high potency (high D2 blockade). Olanzapine and clozapine have low levels of D2 blockade, while quetiapine and ziprasidone have low to medium levels of D2 blockade. (595, 597, 613)

21.5. B. Risperidone
Risperidone is most likely of the serotonin–dopamine antagonists to cause extrapyramidal symptoms, and resembles haloperidol, in terms of side effects, at higher doses. Aripiprazole is most likely to cause akathisia. (598, 610)

21.6. B. Send him to the emergency department
The patient is showing classic signs and symptoms of Stevens–Johnson syndrome. Though it can be caused by any medication, it is linked to lamotrigine and can manifest at any time the medication is used, not just during titration. The presence of valproic acid raises the blood level of lamotrigine, so if the two are used simultaneously, the lamotrigine either should be reduced, or titrated very slowly. As Stevens–Johnson is a potentially life-threatening condition, those who show symptoms should go to the emergency department immediately. He will need to permanently stop the lamotrigine. (600)

21.7. C. Sodium
Symptoms of confusion, agitation, and lethargy can be caused by hyponatremia, which can occur in individuals taking oxcarbazepine, especially the elderly. Acute hyperglycemia can cause confusion and lethargy, but his A1c would be expected to have been higher a month ago if he were having several repeated episodes of glucose spikes. Infection could cause similar symptoms, but a fever would be expected. Fatigue can be a symptom of both low hemoglobin and low potassium (from HCTZ), but confusion and agitation are usually not. (600)

21.8. D. Hemodialysis
The patient is experiencing acute lithium toxicity caused by increased blood levels secondary to dehydration. This can occur when someone perspires more than usual and does not properly rehydrate. The first-line treatment for acute lithium intoxication is hemodialysis, though gastric lavage could be considered in the case of regular-release preparations, and whole-bowel irrigation for sustained-release preparations. Lithium does not adhere well to activated charcoal. The lithium needs to be removed, not just diluted by IV saline, as lithium toxicity can be fatal. (601)

21.9. A. Inhibition of sodium current into myocardial cells

Tricyclic antidepressants (TCAs) have largely been replaced by SSRIs due to the safety profile of the latter. A concern with TCAs is suicide by overdose, with death being caused by cardiac toxicity. The overall mechanism of death is hypotension caused by a reduction in peripheral resistance and QRS complex prolongation due to an inhibition of sodium into myocardial cells. Acute hypothalamic dopamine blockade is the mechanism behind neuroleptic malignant syndrome. Stimulation of postsynaptic 5-HT1A and 5-HT2A receptors is the mechanism behind serotonin syndrome. Acute norepinephrine release following tyramine ingestion is the mechanism of a hypertensive crisis caused by some monoamine oxidase inhibitors (MAOIs). A delayed type IV hypersensitivity reaction is a theoretical mechanism of Stevens–Johnson syndrome. https://emj.bmj.com/content/18/4/236 (600)

21.10. C. Barbiturates

Though the muscle aches, abdominal cramping, agitation, GI upset, and other unpleasant symptoms of opioid withdrawal can make people wish they were dead, the process is not life-threatening. Stimulant withdrawal can lead to fatigue, vivid dreams, sleep disturbances, hyperphagia, and psychomotor changes, but is not deadly. Stopping tricyclics and MAOIs can lead to a nonfatal discontinuation syndrome consisting of flu-like symptoms, insomnia, nausea, imbalance, sensory disturbances, and hyperarousal. Barbiturate withdrawal includes anxiety, restlessness, tremor, dizziness, psychosis, and seizures. If left untreated, withdrawal can lead to hyperthermia, circulatory failure, and death. (604)

21.11. E. Paroxetine

Carbamazepine and valproic acid both can lead to neural tube defects. Lamotrigine may cause oral clefts. Citalopram can cause QT interval prolongation and ventral tachycardia at high doses in the person taking the medication, but is not known to be associated with birth defects. In 2005, the FDA issued an alert that paroxetine increases the risk of heart defects when taken during the first trimester. (606, 626)

21.12. C. Begin aripiprazole

Irritability can be a core symptom of depression in children. However, given that he no longer displays any of the other symptoms of depression, his current behaviors are likely not a relapse or exacerbation, so increasing sertraline would be of little benefit. There are currently no indications for a head CT. He is not at present a danger to himself or others, so hospitalization is not indicated. Aripiprazole, as is risperidone, is indicated for irritability in children and adolescents with autism spectrum disorder. Given that they have tried many other measures, and behaviors are intensifying, a medication intervention is warranted. A decrease in irritability and aggression may help him engage more in therapy. Given that his current symptoms are not limited to just the therapist, and that his therapist is trying new techniques, changing to a different therapist would likely be of little benefit. (612)

21.13. C. Olanzapine

Though all atypicals can cause weight gain, olanzapine consistently leads to more weight gain more frequently. The weight gain is not dose related and continues over time. Clozapine is also consistent in leading to weight gain. (611)

21.14. B. Quetiapine

The patient has had extrapyramidal side effects (EPS) with two first-generation antipsychotics and a serotonin–dopamine antagonist (albeit risperidone, which behaves most like a first-generation medication in regards to EPS), which shows how sensitive he is to this particular side effect. Quetiapine would be the next best option given that it is the serotonin–dopamine antagonist least likely to lead to EPS. Though chlorpromazine is a low potency, highly anticholinergic medication, first-generation antipsychotics lead to more EPS in general, so it should be avoided as well. (611)

21.15. E. Ziprasidone

Bioavailability of ziprasidone doubles when taken with food of at least 500 calories. Though it was originally believed that the calories had to be high in fat, that was not supported in studies. https://pubmed.ncbi.nlm.nih.gov/18007569/ (612)

21.16. A. Aripiprazole

Though any serotonin–dopamine antagonist antipsychotic can elevate prolactin levels, asenapine, like risperidone, can cause galactorrhea and gynecomastia. It also, like quetiapine, iloperidone, and ziprasidone, can increase QTc interval and should be avoided in patients on antiarrhythmics, such as amiodarone, that prolong QTc. Even if he were not on an antiarrhythmic, a diagnosis of congenital heart disease should give pause to the prescription of a medication that is known to prolong QTc interval. Aripiprazole does not cause significant QTc interval changes and does not usually cause significant weight gain or prolactin elevation. (612–614)

21.17. D. Affirm that the medication cannot be dispensed
Clozapine absolutely cannot be dispensed without current lab results sent to the pharmacy, so sending a prescription to another pharmacy, or writing a prescription for one dose, would be of no use. As this rule in inviolable, explaining the situation to the pharmacy or the lab will also prove fruitless. The parents will need to be told that the medication cannot be dispensed. Missing a blood draw also means that he has to restart the 6 months of weekly blood draws before he can move to biweekly draws. (614)

21.18. C. Orthostatic hypotension
While sedation and tachycardia are common side effects of iloperidone, the medication must be titrated slowly in order to avoid orthostatic hypotension. Titration speed does not affect the QTc prolongation that may occur at doses of 12 mg bid. The rate of akathisia is similar to that of placebo. (614)

21.19. D. Change to a different, nonclozapine, serotonin–dopamine antagonist
The patient appears to have gotten no therapeutic benefit from 8 weeks of aripiprazole, with 4 of them being at the maximum dosage. At this point, aripiprazole can be considered a treatment failure, and would likely be no more effective with additional time on the medication. Had he shown any improvement, continuing the current dose for another 4 weeks, or augmentation with a first-generation antipsychotic would have been reasonable. Clozapine is used once a person has been shown to be refractory to several antipsychotic medications. The treatment of choice at this time would be to change to a different serotonin–dopamine antagonist. (615)

21.20. C. An antidepressant and an antipsychotic medication
The patient is experiencing MDD with psychotic features, as the psychosis emerged during the most severe of her depressive episodes. Had she had steady psychotic symptoms with intermittent episodes of depression, the diagnosis would be schizoaffective disorder, depressive type. First-line treatment for MDD with psychotic features consists of treating both the depression with an antidepressant and the psychosis with an antipsychotic. Though treatment with only an antidepressant should eventually lead to resolution of the psychosis once the depression remits, this would likely take weeks, and she is having command hallucinations of suicide, which warrants aggressive treatment. ECT is also effective for this diagnosis, but given that she is medication naïve and not in imminent danger of self-harm, medication should be tried first. (617)

21.21. C. Alpha-1 receptor blockade
Orthostatic hypotension is a result of alpha-1 receptor blockade. H1 receptor blockade leads to sedation. D2 receptor antagonism is the mechanism that leads to symptom relief in psychotic disorders, as well as Parkinsonian and prolactin side effects. Acetylcholine antagonism, which is stronger in low-potency, first-generation antipsychotics, includes side effects such as dry mouth, blurred vision, constipation, and urinary retention. Beta-2 receptor agonism can lead to trembling, increased heart rate, nervousness, and headache. (619, 620)

21.22. D. Tuberoinfundibular
Prolactin secretion is usually kept in check via dopamine release. Once that dopamine release is blocked by antipsychotics, prolactin increases. Dopamine blockade in the mesocortical pathway leads to a blockade of reward and pleasure, as well as an increase in negative symptoms. Dopamine blockade in the nigrostriatal pathway can lead to Parkinsonian symptoms. Blockade in the mesolimbic system leads to the desired reduction in positive symptoms. (620)

21.23. E. Indefinitely
After one psychotic episode, a patient should be maintained on an antipsychotic for about 1 to 2 years, and after the second episode, about 5 years. After the third episode, medication should be maintained indefinitely, with possible attempts to decrease the dosage every 6 to 12 months, depending on the patient's history. (622)

21.24. C. Continue current dose
OCD typically takes a higher dose of an SSRI for a longer amount of time than when treating depression. Whereas maximum effect at a certain dose for depression may be reached around 6 weeks,

maximum effect for OCD may not be achieved for several months. The patient continues to improve at every 4-week visit, and the medication is at the highest dose. Therefore, the medication should be continued at the current dose. Though there is some evidence for supratherapeutic dosing in some individuals, that is not considered best practice. This also would speak against adding risperidone, as would her current diagnosis of diabetes, and also speaks against changing to a new medication when the one she is on is effective. (627)

21.25. D. Sexual dysfunction
Nausea is a common side effect of SSRIs due to activation of 5HT3 gut receptors. However, this usually resolves in a few weeks. SSRIs are often used for headache, especially migraine prophylaxis, and result in an incidence of headaches of about 20%, similar to that of placebo. Some SSRIs can lead to initial anxiety or worsening of anxiety, which can be often mitigated by starting at a lower dose and titrating slowly, and usually resolves in a few weeks. About 25% of people taking an SSRI report sleep difficulty such as insomnia or somnolence. Between 50% and 80% of people who take SSRIs report sexual side effects such as anorgasmia, delayed orgasm, and premature ejaculation. Sexual dysfunction tends not to remit with time, and may lead to changing to a non-SSRI such as bupropion or mirtazapine. (628, 629)

21.26. A. Citalopram
Citalopram has been shown to lengthen the QT interval, more so when taken with an antipsychotic. It is not recommended for anyone with congenital long QT syndrome. Thought this patient is not exactly sure what her heart rhythm issue is, given the chance that it could be long QT syndrome, and the multiple other SSRIs available, it would be prudent to avoid using citalopram. (629)

21.27. C. A sharp increase in plasma serotonin
Addition of an SSRI to lithium can lead to serotonin syndrome, which can occur when the SSRI is first added or when the dose is increased. Symptoms usually begin hours after taking the medication and start with diarrhea, restlessness, and agitation, and can progress to symptoms including autonomic instability, hyperthermia, delirium, coma, and death if left untreated. The first order of treatment is to immediately stop taking the SSRI. If symptoms progress, she should go to the nearest emergency department. Diarrhea is not a symptom of anxiety disorders, atypical depression, or mania. Co-administration of SSRIs does not raise the lithium level, as lithium is not metabolized by the liver. (630)

21.28. A. Half-life
The likelihood of developing SSRI discontinuation syndrome is based on the half-life of the medication. For this reason paroxetine, with a half-life of 21 hours, is most likely to lead to discontinuation syndrome, while fluoxetine, with a half-life of 4 to 6 days of the parent drug and 9.3 days of the active metabolite, is least likely. Therefore, one strategy to mitigate withdrawal effects caused by the termination of other SSRIs is to change the person's medication to fluoxetine, then taper off of that. (630)

21.29. C. Blood pressure
Venlafaxine, most notably the instant release formulation, can lead to a dose-related sustained increase in blood pressure. Unlike serotonin–dopamine antagonists, venlafaxine is not known to lead to changes in weight, blood glucose, or serum lipids. Impaired oxygenation could result from the smoking history, not venlafaxine. (633)

21.30. D. Lack of serotonin reuptake inhibition
Sexual side effects of antidepressants are mostly mediated by serotonin, though the exact mechanism is still unknown. Bupropion does not act on serotonin, which is thought to be the reason that it leads to low sexual dysfunction. Bupropion both ultimately stimulates dopamine reward pathways and norepinephrine receptors, as the medication inhibits the reuptake of both neurotransmitters. Those actions do not correlate with sexual dysfunction, though increased reward pathway stimulation could lead to *increased* libido. Bupropion is usually administered in the morning, leading to decreased evening plasma levels, but this is unrelated to sexual dysfunction, as is the half-life of the medication. (635)

21.31. B. Epilepsy
Bupropion confers a dose-dependent risk of seizures of 0.05% at 300 mg/day and 0.1% at 400 mg/day, and is contraindicated for persons with epilepsy. Hypertension may occur in some patients, so it should be used with caution in those with that condition. Likewise, it should be used with caution in individuals with severe cirrhosis or hepatic impairment, or renal impairment, but is not

contraindicated. Bupropion is not known to affect QTc interval. (636)

21.32. C. Antagonism of presynaptic alpha-2 receptors

Mirtazapine is unique in that it increases the amount of serotonin and norepinephrine via antagonism of presynaptic alpha-2 adrenergic receptors, which inhibit release of those two neurotransmitters. Inhibition of serotonin and norepinephrine reuptake is the mechanism of action of SNRIs such as venlafaxine and duloxetine. Inhibition of serotonin and dopamine reuptake is the mechanism of action of bupropion. Stimulation of serotonin 5HT1A receptors is one of the mechanisms of vilazodone and buspirone. Serotonin–dopamine antagonism is the mechanism of action of "atypical" antipsychotics such as risperidone, ziprasidone, and olanzapine. (637)

21.33. A. Mirtazapine

The patient is showing symptoms of depression and depression-related cognitive dysfunction (also known as pseudodementia). As opposed to primary dementia, the progression of memory loss was rapid, she is distressed by the memory loss, and she does not try hard on the mental status examination, as opposed to trying and getting answers wrong. Also, her symptoms do not follow a pattern of worsening in the evening, which would be suggestive of sundowning, a delirium that is sometimes present in those with dementia. In this patient, the cognitive symptoms are in addition to the regular symptoms of major depressive disorder, so she should be treated with an antidepressant. Mirtazapine would be an especially good choice due to its side effects of appetite stimulation and somnolence. Memantine would be given for a true dementia. Risperidone could be given if she were sundowning. An antibiotic could be given if she were shown to have a UTI or other infection which could lead to delirium. Though hydroxyzine can be helpful for sleep, it would not help with the primary problem of depression, and should be used with caution, as should any anticholinergic medication in the elderly. (237, 637)

21.34. A. Liver function

Brand-name nefazodone (Serzone) has been discontinued in the United States since 2004. However, generic formulations are still available. The medication can cause severe elevation of hepatic enzymes, which in rare cases has led to death. Patients on the medication should have serial hepatic function tests. (638)

21.35. B. Priapism

Though rare at a rate of about one in 10,000, trazodone can lead to priapism, usually within the first 4 weeks of treatment. This is a medical emergency that can require an injection of an alpha-1 agonist agent into the cavernosum of the penis. In some cases, surgery is required. (640)

21.36. B. Serotonin and norepinephrine reuptake inhibition

TCAs work by blocking reuptake of serotonin and norepinephrine in a similar manner to medications such as venlafaxine and duloxetine. However, TCAs have greater anticholinergic and antihistaminergic side effects due to their antagonism of cholinergic muscarinic receptors. They also antagonize H1 receptors, which leads to sedation. In addition, they block alpha-1 receptors, which leads to orthostatic hypotension, the most common cardiovascular autonomic side effect. Serotonin, norepinephrine, and dopamine reuptake inhibition are part of the mechanism of monoamine oxidase inhibitors (MAOIs). (641, 642)

21.37. C. Clomipramine

Clomipramine is uniquely effective for the treatment of OCD, with some symptom relief observed in as little as 2 to 4 weeks, and improvement sometimes continuing for 4 to 5 months. Other tricyclic antidepressants (TCAs) do not show the same efficacy. Monoamine oxidase inhibitors (MAOIs) such as selegiline have not been shown to be especially helpful for OCD. Though SSRIs are first line for OCD, trying a fourth SSRI would likely not be of much benefit after failing three. Bupropion is not effective for OCD, as it has no action on serotonin. Though fluvoxamine is approved and known for treatment of OCD, it has not been shown to be any more or less effective than any other SSRI. (641)

21.38. D. Amitriptyline

Though all of the medications are possible treatments for depression, tricyclic antidepressants (TCAs) should be avoided in patients with narrow-angle glaucoma, as their anticholinergic effects can exacerbate the condition. (702)

21.39. A. Heart disease

Tricyclic antidepressants (TCAs) can cause a myriad of side effects and can exacerbate problems from preexisting conditions. They can possibly induce seizures in patients with epilepsy, but such persons can still use TCAs with a "start low, go slow" initiation and titration. There is not a definitive link between TCAs and birth defects, though TCAs should be discontinued 1 week before delivery, if possible, as they cross the placenta and neonatal withdrawal can occur. TCAs can cause increases in serum transaminases, and in a small percentage, fulminant acute hepatitis. However, they can still be used in patients with liver disease. There is no contraindication in persons with renal disease, as it is metabolized in the liver with little to no excretion in the urine. TCAs, at usual therapeutic doses, can cause tachycardia, flattened T waves, prolonged QT intervals, and depressed ST segments, and should be used in persons with any heart disease only after SSRIs and other antidepressants have been deemed ineffective. They are contraindicated in persons with a QTc greater than 450 ms. (642)

21.40. C. The body to synthesize new monoamine oxidase
Irreversible MAOIs work by permanently inhibiting monoamine oxidase. The body takes about 2 weeks to synthesize new, uninhibited enzyme. (646)

21.41. D. Thyroid function
The patient is describing classic symptoms of depression, for which hypothyroidism can be a cause, and therefore should be a part of a standard depression workup. Colchicine is not known to cause depression either in standard doses or in overdose. Likewise, gout itself, which can lead to an increase in uric acid, is also not known to primarily cause depression, though in some studies people with recurrent attacks of gout were more likely to be depressed compared with the general population. There is no indication in the history for a urinalysis or CBC, which are not typical labs drawn during the workup for depression. (648)

21.42. B. Antagonist
The putative antidepressant mechanism of ketamine and esketamine is the antagonism of NMDA receptors. (648)

21.43. C. Normal lithium side effect
A fine motor tremor is not uncommon at a therapeutic lithium dose. However, a course tremor could indicate lithium toxicity or overdose. Though lithium has been known to cause both hyper and hypothyroidism, the latter of which could cause a tremor, neither would likely develop within 4 weeks. Lithium withdrawal does not cause tremor, and with a half-life of 18 to 24 hours in young adults, he would not be withdrawing after only 7 hours. (651, 652)

21.44. D. Ebstein anomaly
Neural tube defects and anencephaly are associated with valproate use during pregnancy. Spina bifida is associated with carbamazepine and valproate. Ebstein anomaly is associated with lithium. (653, 657)

21.45. C. About 12 hours after taking a dose
Blood levels for lithium, like that for carbamazepine and valproic acid, should be drawn at the trough, right before the next dose. In twice-a-day dosing, that would usually be about 12 hours after a given dose. (654)

21.46. B. Beginning folic acid supplementation
As with any pregnancy and mental illness, the risk of an exacerbation or relapse must be weighed against the risk of harm to the fetus. In this case, given six hospitalizations for acute mania in 2 years despite trying several other medications, the risk of relapse, and possible fetal harm due to actions taken while manic, is high. The patient also states that she does not want to risk relapse. She has already been on numerous other antiepileptic and antipsychotic medications, so the likelihood of another proving to be as effective and without intolerable side effects within the next year is relatively low. Though one should "treat the patient and not the lab results," a valproate level below 50 μg/mL is considered to be subtherapeutic, and would be risky for someone who easily becomes manic. Likewise, discontinuing the medication until she gets pregnant and gets through the first trimester is risky. Daily folic acid supplementation of 1 to 4 mg daily can decrease the risk of valproate-induced neural tube defects. If after preconceptual education about this option she wishes to continue with the plan for pregnancy, this would be the safest course for her. (657)

21.47. B. Liver function
Valproate can lead to thrombocytopenia, so a CBC should be drawn at 1 month and every 6 to 24 months afterward. Valproate can also lead to hepatotoxicity, so liver function tests (LFTs) should be drawn on the same schedule. Thyroid and renal

function tests should be drawn periodically for patients on lithium. Glucose and lipid panels should be drawn periodically for patients on atypical antipsychotics. (658)

21.48. A. Restart the titration from the beginning (day 1)
Due to the possibility of Stevens–Johnson syndrome when lamotrigine is titrated too rapidly, if more than four consecutive doses are missed, titration should be restarted from the beginning. (659)

21.49. C. Increase in carbamazepine metabolism
Carbamazepine induces its own metabolism over time by autoinducing the hepatic enzymes that metabolize it, leading to a decrease in half-life from an average of 26 hours to an average of 12 hours. The enzyme induction reaches its maximum level after 3 to 5 weeks. Four months of therapy is likely too early for "poop out," especially since she has been on the current dose for only 2 months. The patient is not giving indications of noncompliance. Carbamazepine does not interact with thyroid hormone, and its antimanic effects are often augmented by thyroid hormone. Thyroid hormone is not known to induce mania. (660, 661)

21.50. C. Topiramate
Topiramate is sometimes used to mitigate the weight gain caused by some psychotropic medications and can even lead to weight loss. Metformin is used to mitigate changes in blood glucose caused by atypical antipsychotics and can also reduce body weight. While aripiprazole is less likely to lead to significant weight gain than many other atypicals, it is not associated with weight loss. Similarly, oxcarbazepine, while not usually leading to weight gain, does not usually lead to weight loss. While mixed amphetamine salts and methylphenidate could lead to weight loss, they are not used for that purpose, and would not be used in someone with a psychotic disorder, if possible. (664, 709)

21.51. D. Drowsiness
Drowsiness is the most common adverse effect of benzodiazepines, which is sometimes exploited to treat insomnia. Ataxia occurs in fewer than 2%, and dizziness in fewer than 1%. Mild cognitive impairment is infrequent, and allergic reactions to benzodiazepines are rare. (671)

21.52. D. Benzodiazepines
Flumazenil can be used to reverse the adverse psychomotor, amnestic, and sedative effects of benzodiazepines. It does not reverse the effects of ethanol, barbiturates, or opioids, and in patients who have also overdosed on other drugs, such tricyclics, the reversal of benzodiazepine effects on those drugs can lead to their toxic effects, such as seizures and cardiac arrhythmias. (671)

21.53. C. Respirations
The combination of a benzodiazepine and alcohol or other central nervous system (CNS) depressant can lead to severe and possibly fatal respiratory depression. Some stimulants such as cocaine can raise blood pressure and lead to tachycardia, while others such as MDMA can raise body temperature. (672)

21.54. C. Generalized anxiety disorder
Buspirone has only shown effectiveness as a primary agent in the treatment of generalized anxiety disorder. It has also shown some effectiveness in major depressive disorder, but only as an augmenting agent. It has not been shown to be effective in the treatment of panic disorder, OCD, or social phobia. (673)

21.55. B. Propranolol
The patient is describing social anxiety, for which the treatment of choice is an SSRI, though an SNRI could also be used. For more immediate relief, a benzodiazepine or a beta blocker is often used. Hydroxyzine would be less useful for such a situation due to its sedative properties. A beta blocker is relatively contraindicated in someone with diabetes, as it can antagonize the normal physiologic response to hypoglycemia. However, there are times during which the benefit of treatment with a beta blocker can outweigh the risk. (675)

21.56. C. Amobarbital
Signs and symptoms of overdose of barbiturates such as amobarbital include confusion, nystagmus, ataxia, areflexia or hyporeflexia, delirium, and respiratory depression. In decades past, they were commonly prescribed for sleep, but their use has fallen out of favor with the advent of much safer alternatives. (677)

21.57. D. Zolpidem
Zolpidem has been associated with amnesia and automatic behaviors, such as eating and driving, while not conscious. Though eszopiclone is in the same family of medications as zolpidem (nonbenzodiazepine GABA agonists), eszopiclone does not seem to have the same side effect. Melatonin and ramelteon (melatonin receptor agonists) do not have this side effect, nor does prazosin, often used for nightmares associated with posttraumatic stress disorder (PTSD). (681)

21.58. D. Dizziness
Though not FDA approved for treating nightmares, prazosin is often used for that purpose, especially in patients with PTSD. As it is an alpha-2 antagonist that lowers blood pressure in standing and supine positions, dizziness is the most common side effect. Priapism can be caused by trazodone, but that is relatively rare. Amnesia and automatic behaviors can be caused by zolpidem. Some use an atypical antipsychotic for insomnia, which should not routinely be done as the risk of weight gain and metabolic problems is not necessarily dose related. (681)

21.59. D. Change the medication to mixed amphetamine salts
Both methylphenidate and amphetamine preparations of stimulants are effective about 75% of the time. In patients who do not respond to one of the medications, about 70% will respond to the other, which should be tried unless there is a contraindication. Atomoxetine is considered second-line therapy for ADHD, and alpha-2 agonists and bupropion are further down. If there has been a negligible therapeutic effect at 20 mg twice a day, yet the patient is experiencing side effects, increasing the dose further is unlikely to be of much benefit. (682)

21.60. B. Methylphenidate
The first-line pharmacologic treatment for ADHD, inattentive type is a stimulant. It had long been thought that stimulants can exacerbate tics, but current research has shown that this is not an absolute, with some research showing that tics may improve after stimulant treatment. However, some tics may worsen with methylphenidate, but this is not a contraindication to attempting a stimulant. The other treatments may be effective, but they are not first line. (683)

21.61. C. Weight
Stimulant medications can cause the heart rate and blood pressure to increase, not decrease. Though growth suppression is often a concern, studies do not support long-term growth suppression as a side effect. Even if it were to occur, the child would not lose height, just not gain as much as projected. A notorious and common side effect of stimulants is anorexia, which can lead to a measurable weight loss. This can sometimes be mitigated by giving the medication after a meal or by adding caloric supplements during the day. (683, 684)

21.62. D. Norepinephrine reuptake inhibition
Atomoxetine works by inhibiting the presynaptic norepinephrine transporter, thus decreasing norepinephrine reuptake. Clonidine and guanfacine are alpha-agonists used in the treatment of ADHD. Bupropion works by inhibiting norepinephrine and dopamine reuptake. Stimulants increase dopamine and norepinephrine release. Flumazenil is a GABA inhibitor used to reverse the effects of benzodiazepines. (686)

21.63. E. Methadone > buprenorphine > naltrexone
Methadone is a full μ-opioid receptor agonist which is used for short- and long-term opioid detoxification as well as maintenance. Buprenorphine is a partial μ-opioid receptor agonist, and therefore produces a milder withdrawal than a full agonist. Naltrexone is a μ-opioid antagonist that reverses the effects of opioid receptor agonists and precipitates a withdrawal reaction. (687, 689)

21.64. C. Clonidine
The patient is experiencing classic withdrawal from a μ-opioid agonist. Given that he has expressed a desire to come off of such drugs/medications, restarting methadone, or starting buprenorphine or tramadol, would be counter to his wishes. Naloxone could make him feel worse, as it would displace any residual methadone. Clonidine is used to mitigate the adrenergic effects of withdrawal, such as jitteriness and anxiety. However, it will not help the gastrointestinal (GI) symptoms. (689)

21.65. E. Naltrexone
The patient cites alcohol cravings as the main reason for relapse, which opioid receptor antagonists can reduce, especially when paired with an SSRI, according to some studies. Diazepam, like alprazolam and chlordiazepoxide, is often used in protocols such as the Clinical Institute Withdrawal Assessment Alcohol Scale Revised to treat agitation from withdrawal and prevent seizures. Clonidine is used in the treatment of some acute symptoms of opioid withdrawal. The COMBINE study did not show evidence for an increased benefit from acamprosate over naltrexone. Disulfiram does not help with cravings. https://www.ncbi.nlm.nih.gov/pmc/articles/PMC2945872/ (691, 693)

21.66. B. Aldehyde dehydrogenase inhibition
Disulfiram exerts its therapeutic effect of causing adverse physiologic reactions after the consumption of alcohol by inhibiting aldehyde dehydrogenase, which therefore blocks alcohol metabolism.

This subsequently causes an increase in blood acetaldehyde which leads to nausea, headache, vomiting, flushing, and many other unpleasant reactions. Acamprosate theoretically works by increasing GABA transmission and decreasing glutamate transmission. Though opioid receptor antagonists such as naloxone can be used in the treatment of alcohol use disorder, that mechanism is not present in disulfiram. Disulfiram does not compete with ethanol's binding to GABA receptors (in the way that flumazenil works by blocking GABA benzodiazepine receptors). (693)

21.67. D. Clonidine
The child is exhibiting signs and symptoms of clonidine withdrawal, which can begin about 20 hours after the last dose, or if one to two doses have been missed. The child likely took the medication for ADHD at night, and therefore would have last taken it on Thursday night and missed it on Friday and Saturday nights. Discontinuation syndrome consists of anxiety, restlessness, agitation, tremor, abdominal pain, and increased heart rate, blood pressure, and respirations, all of which would be expected with rebound alpha-2 agonist disinhibition. Once he restarts the clonidine, his blood pressure should return to normal. (696)

21.68. E. Memantine
The patient's disease has progressed in severity to the point that she needs constant, supervised care. She is also forgetting some of the most well-known people in her life. Donepezil, rivastigmine, galantamine, and tacrine are all cholinesterase inhibitors that are indicated for mild to moderate Alzheimer disease. Only memantine, an NMDA blocker, is indicated for moderate to severe disease. (697)

21.69. C. He is not sexually attracted to his girlfriend
Sildenafil ultimately works by inhibiting phosphodiesterase (PDE)-5, which regulates the concentration of cyclic guanosine monophosphate (cGMP). cGMP causes smooth muscle relaxation in the corpus cavernosum of the penis, which allows for blood flow, leading to turgidity and tumescence. The whole cascade starts with nitric oxide (NO) increasing cGMP synthesis. NO is only released with sexual stimulation. Therefore, if someone is not sexually stimulated for whatever reason, NO will not be released, and the sildenafil will have no substance upon which it can act. (699)

21.70. C. Neuroleptic malignant syndrome (NMS)
The patient is showing classic signs and symptoms of NMS brought on by haloperidol. Malignant hyperthermia can have a similar presentation, but is precipitated by anesthetic agents and succinylcholine. Malignant catatonia can also present in a similar fashion, but is usually heralded by a prodrome of several weeks of psychosis, agitation, and catatonic excitement. Serotonin syndrome usually includes shivering, ataxia, nausea, and vomiting, which are not present in NMS. EPS does not include the autonomic instability of NMS. https://www.uptodate.com/contents/neuroleptic-malignant-syndrome?search=neuroleptic%20malignant%20syndrome&source=search_result&selectedTitle=1~150&usage_type=default&display_rank=1#H11 (594, 595)

22

Other Somatic Therapies

22.1. What type of seizure activity must be induced to be therapeutically effective in electroconvulsive therapy (ECT)?

A. Absence
B. Partial simple
C. Partial complex
D. Generalized

22.2. A 27-year-old man presents to the mental health center because he has experienced a depressed mood for the last 2 months. He first felt "a little down and just couldn't feel happy, even when I played video games, which I like more than anything." He noticed a week later that he had to force himself to eat. He then started calling out sick to work a couple weeks later because he could not get out of bed. Despite feeling continually "run-down," he found himself waking 2 hours earlier than usual. He spent the next few weeks watching television, even though he could not stay focused on the show. He denies suicidal ideation. He has never experienced these symptoms before and has never been on psychotropic medication. He has no medical illnesses and is on no medications. What is the most effective treatment for his condition?

A. A monoamine oxidase (MAO) inhibitor
B. Cognitive behavioral therapy and selective serotonin reuptake inhibitor (SSRI)
C. Electroconvulsive therapy (ECT)
D. Transcranial magnetic stimulation
E. An SSRI and an atypical medication

22.3. What medication used in the treatment of bipolar disorder is relatively contraindicated for a person who may undergo electroconvulsive therapy (ECT) treatment?

A. Quetiapine XR
B. Olanzapine
C. Quetiapine
D. Aripiprazole
E. Lithium

22.4. What medication is used during electroconvulsive therapy (ECT) to decrease the risk of bone fractures during seizure activity?

A. Atropine
B. Methohexital
C. Succinylcholine
D. Etomidate
E. Glycopyrrolate

22.5. A 64-year-old woman is being treated with electroconvulsive therapy (ECT) for severe depression which began 1 month ago. She has lost 15 lb due to decreased appetite. She is on desvenlafaxine and methamphetamine. She is on no other medications and has no other illnesses. After being anesthetized, the electrical stimulus is delivered, which results in a 50-second duration of a seizure visualized on electroencephalography (EEG). What should be the next step in the treatment session?

A. Repeat the stimulus at a higher power
B. Administer IV diazepam
C. Repeat the stimulus at the current power
D. Conclude the session

22.6. A 43-year-old man with a 20-year history of schizophrenia is on day 35 of hospitalization. He was admitted due to intractable command hallucinations telling him that all foods were radioactive. As a result, he had lost 8 lb in the 2 weeks prior to hospitalization and has lost another 10 since then. The voices have prevented him from getting more than 4 hours of sleep at night. He has been tried on numerous first- and second-generation antipsychotic medications, all with minimal effect. Over the past 3 weeks, he has undergone electroconvulsive therapy (ECT) sessions three times a week with no apparent improvement. Electrodes were placed bilaterally and the dose delivered was up to twice the seizure threshold. He is on no medications that would lower seizure threshold or pose increased risk. What should be the next step in treatment?

A. Retry previous medications
B. Switch to unilateral electrode placement
C. Increase weekly frequency of treatments
D. Retry ECT with an increased dose
E. Continue current treatment for at least 2 more weeks

22.7. What is an absolute contraindication for electroconvulsive therapy (ECT)?

A. Pregnancy
B. A space-occupying central nervous system (CNS) lesion
C. Increased intracerebral pressure
D. A recent myocardial infarction
E. There are no absolute contraindications

22.8. A 53-year-old man has completed his 10th and final electroconvulsive therapy (ECT) treatment for major depressive disorder. He reports the course of ECT as successful, as measured by the resolution of anhedonia and suicidal ideation, resumption of daily activities, and return of appetite, concentration, and energy. However, he continues to complain of problems remembering new information since the treatments began. What is the most likely prognosis regarding his memory over the next 6 months?

A. Memory impairment will remain at its current state
B. Memory will return to baseline
C. Memory impairment will continue to increase
D. Memory impairment will increase over the next 2 months, then slowly improve

22.9. What is a commonality between electroconvulsive therapy (ECT) and transcranial magnetic stimulation (TMS)?

A. The requirement of anesthesia
B. The induction of a seizure
C. An electrical effect on neurons
D. Electrode placement on the scalp
E. Bilateral brain stimulation

22.10. Vagus nerve stimulation is indicated for what mental disorder?

A. Obsessive compulsive disorder
B. Panic disorder
C. Schizophrenia
D. Posttraumatic stress disorder
E. Major depressive disorder

22.11. Neurosurgical ablative treatments are reserved for the most severe major depression and what other mental illness?

A. Schizophrenia
B. Obsessive compulsive disorder (OCD)
C. Generalized anxiety disorder
D. Bipolar disorder
E. Panic disorder

22.12. A 55-year-old woman is brought to the emergency department by EMS after being talked out of jumping off of a local bridge 30 minutes ago. She has been hospitalized dozens of times for suicide attempts and has a 40-year history of major depressive disorder. She states that she has been on "every antidepressant ever made" except for MAOIs, as she is diagnosed with hypertension. She is also diagnosed with borderline personality disorder, and states that she has had three full courses of dialectical behavior therapy (DBT), as well as cognitive behavioral therapy (CBT), and that "I know all the skills." She has had two courses of 14 rounds of electroconvulsive therapy (ECT) with minimal improvement over the last 2 years. She is currently on lisinopril, desvenlafaxine, bupropion, and brexpiprazole. She lives in a boarding home and is treated by a psychiatrist on an assertive community treatment (ACT) team. After telling the physician that she wants to die because "I can't go on living like this anymore," she is involuntarily committed to inpatient treatment. On hospital day 3, she refuses to take any of her medications and tells the treatment team, "I'm done! No more meds, no more therapy, no more nothing! Don't touch me! I want to die in peace!" She does not speak for the next 2 days. The team considers deep brain stimulation. What is an absolute contraindication to the procedure in this patient?

A. The diagnosis of borderline personality disorder
B. The diagnosis of hypertension
C. Not having yet tried monoamine oxidase inhibitors (MAOI)
D. Refusal to give informed consent
E. Living in a boarding home

22.13. Ablative procedures for the treatment of severe mental illness are expected to show results after what period of time at the earliest?

A. Immediately following surgery
B. 4 weeks
C. 3 months
D. 6 months
E. 1 year

ANSWERS

22.1. D. Generalized
The induction of a generalized seizure is necessary to obtain the beneficial effects of ECT. Bilateral seizure activity is necessary, which by definition means it cannot be a partial seizure. Therapeutic efficacy also requires tonic–clonic movements or contractions (without muscle relaxants), which means it cannot be an absence seizure. (730, 734)

22.2. C. Electroconvulsive therapy (ECT)
ECT is the most effective treatment available for major depressive disorder, but due to side effects and stigma, it is rarely used first line. It is now usually used when patients have failed multiple medication trials, are acutely suicidal, have melancholic features, or refuse to eat. (729, 731)

22.3. E. Lithium
ECT should not be used for a patient who is on lithium, as the medication can both lower seizure threshold and predispose the patient to postictal delirium. As an antiepileptic medication, divalproex would raise the seizure threshold, making the induction of a therapeutic seizure more difficult. Aripiprazole, both forms of quetiapine, and olanzapine are fine to use in combination with ECT. (731, 732)

22.4. C. Succinylcholine
The risk of bone fractures during ECT comes from muscle contractions during the seizure. To minimize that risk, muscle relaxants such as succinylcholine are used. Atropine and glycopyrrolate are anticholinergic muscarinic drugs that are sometimes used prior to ECT to minimize oral and respiratory secretions, and to block bradycardia and asystole. Methohexital and etomidate are anesthetics that can be used prior to the procedure. (732, 733)

22.5. D. Conclude the session
A seizure needs to last at least 25 seconds to be effective. If the seizure is too short, up to four more attempts may be tried during the session. If it lasts over 180 seconds, the patient is in status epilepticus, and more of the anesthetic agent or IV diazepam can be given to break the seizure. A seizure length of 50 seconds falls within the therapeutic safe range, so the session should end. (734)

22.6. D. Retry ECT with an increased dose
If a patient has not improved after 6 to 10 sessions of ECT, bilateral placement and treatment at three times the seizure threshold should be tried next before ECT can be deemed a failure. Treatment frequency is usually two to three times a week. More frequent treatments are associated with greater memory impairment, but not necessarily greater efficacy. Previous medications can be retried after ECT has failed, as anecdotally, they may now be helpful after a course of ECT. (734)

22.7. E. There are no absolute contraindications
There are no absolute contraindications, but there are several conditions that can place a patient at higher risk for complications from ECT, which can often be mitigated by closer monitoring. In cases of high-risk pregnancy, fetal monitoring may be necessary. There is a risk for edema and herniation after ECT for someone with a space-occupying CNS lesion, which can be mitigated with dexamethasone pretreatment if the lesion is small. Patients with increased intracerebral pressure are at higher risk due to increased cerebral blood flow during the seizure. This risk can be lessened by controlling the blood pressure during treatment. The risk to a patient with a recent myocardial infarction is greatly diminished 2 weeks after the event, and further diminished 3 months afterward. (734, 735)

22.8. B. Memory will return to baseline
Memory impairment is the most common complaint from patients following ECT. Anterograde amnesia often resolves within a couple months. Within 6 months, the patient is likely to be back at their cognitive baseline. (735)

22.9. C. An electrical effect on neurons
TMS involves the induction of electricity through magnetic stimulation. As such, there are no electrodes to place bilaterally. Instead, the TMS device delivers magnetic pulses via a coil that is held on the scalp. The procedure is noninvasive and does not require anesthesia. Seizures are the most severe side effect of TMS, not a therapeutic requirement. (736, 737)

22.10. E. Major depressive disorder
Vagus nerve stimulation is indicated for long-term adjunctive treatment of chronic or recurrent depression in adults. The depression episode being treated can be due to a unipolar or bipolar disorder. The efficacy in other disorders is unknown. (739)

22.11. B. Obsessive compulsive disorder (OCD)
Surgical intervention is predominantly used only in intractable cases of major depression and OCD. Even then, approval must go through a

multidisciplinary committee. Current techniques can yield improvement in 40% to 70% of cases. (739)

22.12. D. Refusal to give informed consent
There are several relative contraindications to psychiatric neurosurgery for the treatment of mental illness, including cardiopulmonary comorbidities, severe personality disorders, and not having tried a wide variety of previous treatments. A patient must have access to follow-up, postoperative care following the surgery. This patient has been on numerous trials of medication throughout the years, and would have adequate follow-up through the ACT team. Living in a boarding home is not in itself a contraindication if the patient is able to follow up with postop care. Borderline personality disorder and hypertension are relative, not absolute, contraindications. The single absolute contraindication is if informed consent is not given, as psychiatric neurosurgery should never be performed on an unwilling patient. (740)

22.13. D. 6 months
Results from ablative surgeries are not expected to show until at least 6 months, and may take up to 2 years. (742)

23

Psychotherapy

23.1. Which scenario would make a patient a good candidate for psychoanalysis?

A. A diagnosis of a new medical condition
B. An absence of suffering
C. Having a high frustration tolerance
D. Possessing an urgent need for symptom relief
E. Undergoing a high-conflict divorce

23.2. A 30-year-old healthy, bright male who works as an attorney has had a series of few long-term failed romantic relationships over the past few years and has been feeling chronically depressed and anxious due to the loneliness and work stress. He has had increasing struggles with sleeping and focusing due to obsessive thoughts about his failures in life and most recently when dating someone new reported being distressed by sexual dysfunction. He has no history of suicidal thoughts or self-harm. He is willing to make a long-term commitment to treatment this time. He would be a good candidate for which of the following types of psychotherapies?

A. Cognitive therapy
B. Couples therapy
C. Dialectical behavioral therapy
D. Exposure and response prevention
E. Psychoanalysis

23.3. A patient expressing, "cabbages to kings" during a therapy session is a good example of which fundamental technique in psychoanalysis?

A. Free association
B. Psychotic ramblings
C. Reaction formation
D. Suspended attention
E. Working through

23.4. Which is a strategy that is utilized in psychoanalytic psychotherapy more heavily as compared to psychoanalysis?

A. A focus on memory recall
B. A longer treatment time frame
C. Face-to-face sessions
D. Suspended attention
E. Use of free associations

23.5. Expressive psychotherapy is different from psychoanalysis in which of the following ways?

A. A focused understanding of problems is achieved by modifying ego function
B. Deeply hidden and past motives are discovered early in treatment
C. Insight through a genetic level is sought
D. Motives and interactions are traced all the way back through infancy
E. Positive transference and regression are more heavily explored

23.6. A 40-year-old woman was just recently diagnosed with cancer and has minimal time, struggling between being compliant with medical treatments, managing her job, and caring for her kids. She expresses concern about having the time and money for therapy. She feels that her life was great prior to her cancer diagnosis and is hoping the symptoms will pass on their own. Her oncologist is concerned about her missing appointments and that she struggles with getting out of bed and caring for herself. Upon expressing feelings of hopelessness, her oncologist encourages her to start therapy though she remains skeptical. Which therapy is she best suited toward?

A. Cognitive behavioral therapy
B. Expressive psychotherapy
C. Interpersonal psychotherapy
D. Psychodynamic psychotherapy
E. Supportive psychotherapy

23.7. Group therapy would be contraindicated for a patient in which of the following scenarios?

A. A new diagnosis of paranoid schizophrenia with active delusions
B. A patient actively engaged in individual therapy, suffering from depression and suicidal thoughts
C. Bipolar disorder with manic symptoms has been diagnosed, though the patient is stable on medications
D. The patient has antisocial personality disorder and is with others in the group with the same diagnosis
E. The patient is suffering from an acute grief reaction after the death of a spouse

23.8. A family has started therapy together for help in managing one of their children with attention-deficit/hyperactivity disorder (ADHD), oppositional defiant disorder (ODD), and worsening behavior problems. The patient is being bullied in school and the therapist externalizes the problem and helps the family to focus on the outside stressors and diagnoses. Each family member writes a therapeutic letter to another family member in hopes of resolving the conflict within the family and enhancing insight about the story that each member is going through. Which school of family therapy is most likely being employed?

A. Cognitive behavioral
B. Experiential-humanistic
C. Integrative
D. Narrative
E. Psychodynamic

23.9. During a family therapy session, a mother comments that their daughter acts like a monster, screaming, hitting them, and throwing things each morning when trying to get her dressed to go to school. The therapist comments that she acts out due to severe social anxiety and struggles with transitions, and then points out that mother has done a great job at handling her daughter's anxiety in the past when she realizes it is occurring. The therapist also highlights that the child's perseverance helps her to get good grades in school and that her anxious temperament has helped her to be empathic and a good friend to her sibling.

A. Clarification
B. Family management
C. Paradoxical intervention
D. Reframing
E. Unbalancing

23.10. A 20-year-old female has seen multiple therapists over the past few years, noting none of them were helpful and they all offended her. She continues to struggle with depression, poor social relations, lack of ability to maintain a job or relationship, and intermittent self-harm and suicidal thoughts. Which psychosocial treatment has the most empirical support to help her?

A. Acceptance and commitment therapy
B. Cognitive behavioral therapy
C. Dialectical behavior therapy (DBT)
D. Insight-oriented psychotherapy
E. Interpersonal psychotherapy

23.11. Which type of therapy asks patients to direct their attention to specific body area while thinking certain phrases reflecting a relaxed state, progressing through various themes including cardiac regulation and breathing adjustment?

A. Applied tension
B. Autogenic training
C. Biofeedback
D. Progressive muscular relaxation
E. Relaxation therapy

23.12. A patient being treated for anxiety and depression tells the therapist about how embarrassed she was in forgetting the words for her class presentation today and states that she knows she will never make it as a teacher in the future. This is an example of which of the following cognitive distortions?

A. All-or-nothing thinking
B. Labeling
C. Mind reading
D. Overgeneralization
E. Tunnel vision

23.13. Scheduling activities on a daily basis, keeping records, and performing mastery ratings are first steps in which of the following types of treatment for depression?

A. Brief supportive psychotherapy
B. Cognitive behavioral therapy
C. Dialectical behavioral therapy
D. Interpersonal psychotherapy
E. Narrative psychotherapy

23.14. A patient is being treated for a severe phobia of needles. Teaching the patient relaxation strategies, while showing pictures of needles, working toward having them see an actual needle in the office, and then getting a shot at the doctor while experiencing minimal anxiety, is an example of which of the following types of therapies?

A. Aversion therapy
B. Biofeedback
C. Flooding
D. Participant modeling
E. Systematic desensitization

23.15. A therapist is helping to treat agoraphobia in a child by accompanying them to a crowded playground to help them unlearn the fears by observing the therapist having fun at the playground with other children. This is an example of which of the following types of therapies?

A. Applied relaxation
B. Behavioral activation
C. Cognitive therapy
D. Participant modeling
E. Social skills training

23.16. Caution should be used in conducting hypnosis on a patient with which of the following characteristics?

A. Dissociative symptoms
B. Low levels of control
C. Paranoia
D. Suggestibility
E. Trauma

23.17. During the first few initial sessions, a therapist explains the diagnosis of a major depressive disorder to the patient and discusses how the patient is sick and is allowed to not feel well, while emphasizing that they are responsible for their recovery. The therapist starts to explore relationships in the person's life and discusses the role that loss has seemed to play. The therapist is conducting which type of therapy?

A. Acceptance and commitment therapy
B. Insight-oriented psychotherapy
C. Interpersonal psychotherapy (ITP)
D. Psychodynamic psychotherapy
E. Supportive psychotherapy

23.18. A group therapist is helping the patients to foster connections between one another in sharing their goals and continuously encourages the group members to go out into the world and do activities with others and then to come back to the group and share how these experiences have gone. The therapist reflects on the group members' relationship with one another and draws connections between these group relationships and the relationships they have with others outside of the group and their symptoms. This is an example of which of the following phases and types of group therapy?

A. Initial phase of self-help group
B. Intermediate phase of interpersonal psychotherapy (ITP)
C. Middle phase of dialectical behavioral therapy
D. Midtreatment phase of cognitive behavioral therapy
E. Termination phase of social network therapy

23.19. Which of the following is a primary task of narrative psychotherapy?

A. Analyze faulty cognitions and automatic thoughts brought up in the patient's story
B. Be a good listener and connect empathically with the patient's story
C. Determine the validity of the patient's story and help the patient write a new ending
D. Find a problem area in the story and use it to help the patient change social interactions
E. Help the patient write a timeline of their life and decide what area to focus on in treatment

23.20. Which of the following is an alternative, effective treatment to dialectical behavioral therapy for severe borderline personality disorder?

A. Eye movement desensitization and reprocessing
B. Interpersonal psychotherapy
C. Mentalization-based treatment (MBT)
D. Narrative psychotherapy
E. Social skills training

23.21. A psychiatrist discusses with a teen and his parent about the diagnosis and symptoms of the illness, along with strategies to help with medication compliance and reviews signs of worsening illness to look out for. The psychiatrist also reviews how to help the teen and mother to manage a crisis. This intervention is best described as which of the following forms of therapy?

A. Attribution
B. Cognitive behavior
C. Family based
D. Psychoeducation
E. Supportive

ANSWERS

23.1. C. Having a high frustration tolerance
Good candidates for psychoanalysis must truly wish to understand themselves and not need urgent symptom relief. Being able to withstand frustration and anxiety without acting out are important characteristics to possess in order for psychoanalysis to be successful. Some level of suffering is needed for the therapy to be effective. Antisocial personality disorder, low intelligence, and being in the middle of a major life crisis (i.e., divorce or loss of a job or being diagnosed with a major medical condition) are all potential contraindications to psychoanalysis. (745)

23.2. E. Psychoanalysis
Health, intelligence, good financial means, and being able to commit to long-term treatment are some factors which can lead to success in psychoanalysis. An absence of need for urgent symptom relief and a lack of safety concerns would also make this patient a good candidate. Psychanalysis is suitable for those with depression, anxiety, sexual dysfunction, and some personality disorders, along with those with chronic suffering, as described in the case. (745, 747)

23.3. A. Free association
Free association is a predominant technique in psychoanalysis. The fundamental rule of free association is for the patient to tell the analysis everything that comes to their mind, the unimportant and nonsensical, and it does not mirror normal conversation. A conversation leading from, "cabbages to kings" is a good example of free association. (748)

23.4. C. Face-to-face sessions
Psychoanalytic psychotherapy is derived from psychoanalysis. It uses insight-oriented methods such as expressive techniques along with supportive ones. It is shorter compared to psychoanalysis and the brief treatment is focused on a select problem. Instead of utilization of the couch, sessions are done with the therapist and patient looking at one another face-to-face to help prevent regression and to aid with receiving cues. Free association is rarely used. (749)

23.5. A. A focused understanding of problems is achieved by modifying ego function
While both expressive psychotherapy and psychoanalysis increase awareness, expressive psychotherapy does so by improving object relationship and exploring current interpersonal events. Structural changes in ego function and defenses are achieved in expressive psychotherapy. Unlike psychanalysis which uncovers hidden and past motives dating back to origins in infancy, expressive psychotherapy focuses on how the preconscious or conscious conflicts manifest in the present day. (750)

23.6. E. Supportive psychotherapy
Supportive psychotherapy focuses on external rather than intrapsychic events and on how stressful environmental and interpersonal influences can damage the self. It is useful for those patients with poor ego strength, who are in an acute crisis. Those who are medically ill and/or cognitively limited, or unmotivated and are looking for immediate symptom relief are good candidates for supportive psychotherapy. (751)

23.7. A. A new diagnosis of paranoid schizophrenia with active delusions
There are relatively few contraindications to participating in group therapy. A patient with active delusions, who incorporate the group into the delusions, and a patient who is threatening with frequent outbursts are some examples of patients who should be excluded from the group setting. Bipolar disorder, or mania, is not contraindication to group therapy if manic symptoms are controlled on medication. Those patients with depression and suicidal thoughts can benefit from group therapy. However, if any acute safety concerns are present, individual treatment should be conducted as well. Those with antisocial personality disorder might struggle in a group setting unless other patients with the same diagnosis are in the group, since these patients are thought to respond better to their peers than authority figures. (755, 756)

23.8. D. Narrative
Narrative family therapy involves resolution of a presenting problem through focusing on outcomes and externalizing the problem and helping the family members to create new meaning via "restorying." Therapeutic letters are often written to one another as part of the therapeutic process. Cognitive behavioral family therapy focuses on communication and problem solving and change, along with acceptance and helping members to learn reattribution techniques. Experiential-humanistic therapy focuses on increasing differentiation and on detriangulation by using genograms and the therapist acts as a coach. Integrative family therapy combines cognitive behavioral and psychodynamic methods

to improve communication and problem solving. Psychodynamic family therapy aims to improve insight and enhance empathy by analyzing transference, countertransference, and resistance and relies on interpretation and emphasizes the therapeutic alliance. (761)

23.9. C. Reframing
This is an example of a therapist using a technique called reframing. It is also known as positive connotation and involves relabeling of all negatively expressed feelings or behaviors as positive. It helps the family member to have a new frame of reference and can lead to change. (762)

23.10. C. Dialectical behavioral therapy (DBT)
The patient described above most likely has borderline personality disorder (BPD). DBT is the gold standard to help those with BPD live a life worth living and can help with self-injurious and parasuicidal behavior. DBT includes individual, group, telephone, and team consultation, and helps increase skillful behavior, improve motivation for changing maladaptive behaviors, and improve emotional dysregulation. (764)

23.11. B. Autogenic training
Autogenic training can help with relaxation by having the patient direct attention to specific body areas and think phrases to help them relax (i.e., My forehead is cool.). The patient progresses through six themes including heaviness, warmth, cardiac regulation, breathing adjustment, solar plexus, and forehead. Applied tension involves tensing the muscles and releasing them, but not to the point of relaxation. It can help with situations such as fainting. Progressive muscular relaxation involves tensing and then relaxing the muscles working the way up the body. Relaxation therapy involves immobilizing the body, drawing focus and attention, and cultivating a nonjudgmental, contemplative state of mind. Biofeedback involves the recognition and display of small changes in physical levels (i.e., electromyography [EMG], electroencephalography [EEG] monitoring) to help bring the autonomic nervous system under voluntary control through operant conditioning. (766)

23.12. D. Overgeneralization
Cognitive distortions, also known as automatic thoughts, are the thoughts that occur between external events and a person's emotional reaction to the event. The vignette above is an example of overgeneralization in which an overwhelmingly negative conclusion is drawn from a relatively minor event. All-or-nothing thinking is also known as black-and-white thinking and involves putting a situation into only two categories instead of on a continuum or seeing the gray area in the middle. Labeling is putting a fixed label on yourself or others without examining the evidence fully which could lead to a less disastrous conclusion. Mind reading involves believing you know what others are thinking and not considering more likely possibilities. Tunnel vision involves seeing only the negative aspect of a situation. (769)

23.13. B. Cognitive behavioral therapy
Behavioral techniques can help challenge maladaptive cognition. One of the first behavioral techniques in cognitive therapy for the treatment of depression is to have the patient schedule activities on an hourly basis and keep records of them and rate mastery and pleasure. Often, this leads the patient to realize they had more pleasure than they thought while doing the activity and it helps them to experience a sense of mastery. (770, 771)

23.14. E. Systematic desensitization
Systematic desensitization is the behavioral principle of counterconditioning, which helps the patient to overcome anxiety by gradually exposing them to the feared situation while they learn to be in a state that inhibits anxiety, called reciprocal inhibition. Relaxation training, hierarchy construction, and desensitization of the stimulus are the steps in systematic desensitization. It is commonly used to treat phobias, obsession or compulsions, and some sexual disorders as well. (771, 772)

23.15. D. Participant modeling
Just as a person can develop fears by learning, the principle of participant modeling is that these fears can be unlearned by observing a fearless model confront the feared object. In participant modeling, the patient can learn a new behavior by imitation by observation, without having to perform the behavior until they feel ready. Children respond well to this technique of watching other peers enjoy a feared situation and it is particularly useful therapy for agoraphobia when the therapist accompanies the patient to various places. (772, 773)

23.16. C. Paranoia
Some risks of hypnosis can include developing a strong transference or attachment. On the other

hand, negative emotions can also surface in patients with poor reality testing. As a result, caution should be used in performing hypnosis in those with paranoia, or a high need for control. Patients who lack capacity for basic trust are not good hypnosis candidates. Self-hypnosis can be used to treat post-traumatic stress disorder (PTSD) and can help with memory retrieval. (778)

23.17. C. Interpersonal psychotherapy (ITP)
ITP is a time-limited treatment for major depressive disorder that helps to eliminate symptoms and improve the quality of the patient's interpersonal relations and social functioning. The initial phase focuses on assigning the patient to be in the sick role and describing the diagnosis and treatment expectations. The patient is given permission and responsibility to recover. An interpersonal inventory is conducted, and a formulation is made linking the patient's symptoms to one of four problem areas—grief, interpersonal deficits, interpersonal role disputes, or role transitions. (778)

23.18. B. Intermediate phase of interpersonal psychotherapy (ITP)
Group therapy for ITP has many benefits versus individual treatment. It helps the patient feel that they are not the only one with a psychiatric disorder and gives them a social environment to interact with others with like symptoms. The intermediate phase is where the work is done to facilitate connections among the members and helps them to practice their newly acquired social skills by doing activities with others outside of the session and to share their experience in the group setting. The therapist connects the relationships the patients have in the group with their outside relationships and their psychiatric symptoms. (781)

23.19. B. Be a good listener and connect empathically with the patient's story
Narrative medicine focuses on an open-ended invitation to tell a story to help recognize and interpret and be moved by the story of the patient's illness. The major task of the therapist is being a good listener and connecting empathically with the patient's story. The main goal is to truly understand the patient and the story to help bring the clinician and patient together into a shared experience of the patient's world. (781, 782)

23.20. C. Mentalization-based treatment (MBT)
MBT is a psychotherapy developed for the treatment of borderline personality disorder. It focuses on the mentalizing vulnerabilities of the patient in helping them to understand the attachment process. it involves learning the ability to understand the actions of others and oneself in terms of mental states, thoughts, feelings, wishes, and desires. (786)

23.21. D. Psychoeducation
The description above of helping the patient and family to understand the psychiatric illness, treatment options, prognosis, and recovery, is best consistent with psychoeducation. Psychoeducation also involves providing interventions to help the patient and family strategize how to adjust to living with the illness, and also covers common areas including treatment adherence, identifying signs of relapse, and instructions on how to help manage a crisis situation. (787)

24

Psychiatric Rehabilitation and Other Interventions

24.1. Which term best describes interventions aimed at helping those with mental illnesses to improve function and quality of life by helping them live independently, attend school, or work, and maintain social relationships?

A. Behavioral therapy
B. Multidisciplinary treatment
C. Psychiatric rehabilitation
D. Psychoeducation
E. Token economy system

24.2. Supportive employment programs differ from other vocational approaches in which of the following ways?

A. They actively facilitate acquiring a job
B. They effectively screen for people who are ready for work
C. They offer intermediate work experiences
D. They provide transitional employment opportunities
E. They terminate services once the person is employed

24.3. What is the primary modality of social skills training?

A. Group work
B. Job shadowing
C. Narrative telling
D. Processing work
E. Role-playing

24.4. Which skill is considered the first step in effective interpersonal problem solving?

A. Generalization
B. Generating solutions
C. Nonverbal responsiveness
D. Social perception
E. Verbal conversation

24.5. Which is the last step to achieve in an information-processing model of training patients to handle an interpersonal difficulty and to improve communication and social skills?

A. Adopt a problem-solving attitude
B. Brainstorm solutions to a problem
C. Evaluate efficacy and choose an alternative
D. Identify the problem
E. Pick a solution and implement it

24.6. What is the role the therapist should play in working with a patient for psychiatric rehabilitation?

A. To act as a parental figure
B. To be a shared decision maker
C. To make medical appointments for the patient
D. To suggest a variety of potential jobs for the patient
E. To take a stance on the patient not using alcohol or drugs

24.7. The concept of a complex disease considers the interplay of the environment and which factor?

A. Comorbidities
B. Economic factors
C. Social relations
D. The genome
E. Treatment

24.8. Which is the most likely outcome on mental health of those persons undergoing genomic testing?

A. Experience of a major depressive disorder
B. Increased rates of anxiety
C. Higher rates of suicide
D. Lower rates of employment
E. No long-term adverse effects

ANSWERS

24.1. C. Psychiatric rehabilitation
Psychiatric rehabilitation is the larger term that encompasses a wide variety of interventions aimed at helping those with disabilities from mental illnesses to function and live a good quality life. It focuses on helping patients to function as adults and live independently, finish school, get jobs, and to maintain relationships with family and friends. A goal of psychiatric rehabilitation is to focus on independence and community interventions, rather than on a relationship with an individual professional. (792)

24.2. A. They actively facilitate job acquisition
Federal run supportive employment programs differ from other vocational approaches by helping anyone who wants work to actively acquire a job. Supportive employment program approaches include accompanying clients on interviews and providing ongoing support once the person is employed. Intermediate prevocational, transitional employment, or sheltered workshops are not provided by supportive employment programs. (792)

24.3. E. Role-playing
Social skills rehabilitation can help improve social perceptions, or receiving skills, social cognitions, or processing skills, and behavioral responses, or expressive skills, via focusing on role-playing of simulated conversations. A trainer provides instruction on how to perform the skills and models them. The trainer then encourages the patient to engage in role-play and provides feedback and positive reinforcement. (792)

24.4. D. Social perception
Acquiring good social perception is considered the first step in effective interpersonal problem solving. Training someone to perceive and interpret social and cognitive cues can help with more specific communication and coping skills. (793)

24.5. C. Evaluate efficacy and choose an alternative
The information-processing model of training helps the patient take on different cognitive perspectives. It involves a six-step approach to help one overcome an interpersonal dilemma. The steps include (1) adopting a problem-solving attitude, (2) identifying the problem, (3) brainstorming solutions, (4) evaluating solutions and picking one to implement, (5) planning the implementation and carrying it out, and (6) evaluating the efficacy of the effort, and if ineffective, choose another alternative: (794)

24.6. B. To be a shared decision maker
Psychiatric rehabilitation strategies involve maintaining confidentiality and making sure to not infantilize patients. The patients should be viewed as adults who can make their own choices in terms of where to live, whether to work or not, and whether to use substance. The practitioner's role is to be in a partnership with the patient to help improve their quality of life and collaborate with them and to work as a shared decision maker, rather than a parental or authority figure. (794)

24.7. D. The genome
The concept of complex disease replaced the term, "multifactorial" as an etiologic category for common disorders. It considers the interplay of the genome and environment. The concept includes biologic and physiologic mechanisms of evolution and development within societies and cultures. It is thought that various genomic and environmental risk factors can trigger developmental, growth, and maturational differences and increase the risk of psychiatric illnesses. (795)

24.8. E. No long-term adverse effects
While on one hand physicians don't want to make light of the negative psychological impact that can sometimes occur with testing, physicians do think it is an important point to know that the majority of the times the info is well received with no negative consequences. (797)

25

Consult to Other Disciplines

25.1. Why was the term, "psychosomatic medicine" deleted from the DSM and changed to the term, "consultation–liaison psychiatry"?

A. Insurance companies mandated the change
B. It implied the disorders were all in the individual's head
C. It included religious connotations
D. It separated psychological factors from physical ones
E. The focus was more so on the body, rather than the mind

25.2. Rates of suicide are typically highest in which of the following populations?

A. Late adolescent females
B. Young adolescent males
C. Females over 60 years old
D. Males over 45 years old
E. Midadolescent males

25.3. Which treatment is thought to be safest and most beneficial for hospitalized patients with excessive agitation due to substance use?

A. Antipsychotic medications
B. Mechanical restraints
C. Physical restraints
D. Sedation with opioids
E. Sleeping medications

25.4. Benzodiazepines can often cause sundowner syndrome in a patient with delirium, resulting in which of the following symptoms?

A. Ataxia
B. Fever
C. Hypertension
D. Lethargy
E. Tachycardia

25.5. A son takes his elderly father to neuropsychiatry clinic for a follow-up appointment and mentions that his father has had worsening memory problems and falls and that he is struggling with taking care of him due to him constantly wetting himself. He is afebrile with a normal urinalysis, blood urea nitrogen, and creatinine levels. Which of the following diagnoses is highly suspected?

A. Hydronephrosis
B. Hyperthyroidism
C. Normal pressure hydrocephalus (NPH)
D. Subdural hematoma
E. Urinary tract infection

25.6. A landmark study found that women with metastatic breast cancer receiving which treatment survived an average of 18 months longer compared to control patients?

A. Family based
B. Group therapy
C. Individual cognitive behavioral therapy
D. Individual dialectical behavioral therapy
E. Selective serotonin reuptake inhibitor

25.7. Which of the following is the most common comorbid psychiatric disorder among cancer patients?

A. Adjustment disorder
B. Delirium
C. Generalized anxiety disorder
D. Major depressive disorder
E. Substance use disorder

25.8. Which best describes the incidence of suicidal thoughts, or suicide rates, among cancer patients compared to the general population?

A. A comparable rate of completed suicides
B. A comparable risk of suicidal thoughts
C. A decreased risk of completed suicides
D. A decreased risk of suicidal thoughts
E. A slightly higher risk of completed suicides

25.9. Which demographic group is thought to have the highest rate of suicide?

A. Young African American males
B. Elderly Caucasian females
C. Elderly Caucasian males
D. Middle-aged Caucasian males
E. Middle-aged Hispanic females

25.10. Which is the most common cause of disability among adults 65 years and older?

A. Arthritis
B. Alcoholism
C. Chronic obstructive pulmonary disease
D. Diabetes
E. Dementia

25.11. Depression with which of the following features is more common in the elderly population compared to younger patients with depression?

A. Atypical
B. Increased appetite
C. Insomnia
D. Manic
E. Melancholic

25.12. Which is the most common type of delusion?

A. Grandiose
B. Jealous
C. Mixed
D. Persecutory
E. Sexual

25.13. Which is the single most important factor associated with an increased prevalence of sleep disorders?

A. Advanced age
B. Being in college
C. Depression
D. Malnutrition
E. Psychosis

25.14. Which medication can be helpful in the treatment of vertigo in the elderly?

A. Clonazepam
B. Diphenhydramine
C. Lorazepam
D. Meclizine
E. Propranolol

25.15. Dose adjustments in psychiatric medications should be made in the elderly for many reasons, including which of the following?

A. Decreased presence of lean body mass
B. Lower rates of orthostasis
C. Higher hepatic clearance
D. Increased metabolism
E. Increased gastric secretions

25.16. Which factor is correlated with an increased risk of suicide and should be included in emergency room (ER) screens for suicide?

A. Anhedonia
B. A family history of bipolar disorder
C. Increased sleep
D. Psychomotor retardation
E. Pervasive hopelessness

25.17. A patient with a history of schizophrenia and depression, currently on psychotropic medication, is seen in the emergency room for evaluation of a high fever. Vital signs are also significant for tachycardia. The physical exam is significant for pharyngitis and ulcers in the oral and perianal area. Which psychiatric medication is the most likely culprit of these symptoms?

A. Carbamazepine
B. Clozapine
C. Selegiline
D. Thioridazine
E. Venlafaxine

25.18. After discontinuing the medication in the patient above, administration of which of the following treatments is the most appropriate measure?

A. A blood transfusion
B. Chlordiazepoxide
C. Cyproheptadine
D. Granulocyte colony-stimulating factor
E. Lorazepam

25.19. A patient presents to the emergency room (ER) intoxicated with an unknown substance. He presents with ataxia and is highly somnolent on mental status examination, with low blood pressure, heart rate, and respiratory rate. Which of the following substances is the toxicology screen most likely to come back positive for?

A. Amphetamines
B. Benzodiazepines
C. Lithium
D. Lysergic acid diethylamide (LSD)
E. Phencyclidine (PCP)

25.20. Administration of which of the following treatments is the most appropriate measure in the case above?

A. Charcoal
B. Flumazenil
C. N-acetylcysteine
D. Naloxone
E. Naltrexone

25.21. A patient had a recent gastrointestinal illness and has had poor appetite for the past few days. He remained compliant with psychiatric medication and now presents in the emergency room (ER) with acute worsening of diarrhea, gait instability, and a tremor and is noted to be confused on mental status examination and has a seizure. Which psychiatric medication is the most likely culprit?

A. Divalproex sodium
B. Fluoxetine
C. Lithium
D. Methylphenidate
E. Venlafaxine

25.22. Which of the following treatments is most appropriate to reverse the medication toxicity noted in the previous case?

A. Outpatient dialysis
B. Outpatient neuro follow-up and benztropine
C. Intensive care unit (ICU) transfer and benzodiazepines
D. ICU transfer and charcoal administration
E. ICU transfer and osmotic diuresis

25.23. A 25-year-old female presents with hot flashes and reports feeling shaky and tingling in her fingers. She reports a rapid heartbeat, lasting a few minutes at a time, multiple days a week for the past few months. She presents to the emergency room after another episode. Which medical test should be obtained to rule out an organic cause for this disorder?

A. Chest x-ray
B. Complete blood count
C. Electrocardiogram (EKG)
D. Magnetic resonance imaging of the brain
E. Urinalysis

25.24. Which of the following medication strategies is the best long-term treatment for the patient in the previous case, provided her medical tests are all normal?

A. Alprazolam
B. Fluoxetine
C. Gabapentin
D. Lorazepam
E. Propranolol

25.25. An elderly patient with a history of schizophrenia and a medical history significant for strokes has been stable on fluphenazine for many years. Her psychiatrist decides to lower the dose, and at the next session, abnormal movements of her mouth and tongue are noted, along with twitching and writing movements of her arms. Which is the best course of treatment?

A. Add amantadine
B. Continue to decrease and taper off the medication
C. Cross taper with haloperidol
D. Increase the medication dose backup
E. Start Cogentin

25.26. A child repeatedly sets fires and leaves them burning without any attempt to extinguish them. Which of the following psychiatric or medical disorder is most commonly comorbid with this presentation?

A. Borderline personality disorder
B. Conduct disorder
C. Enuresis
D. Migraines
E. Posttraumatic stress disorder

25.27. Which of the following is often the primary site for human immunodeficiency virus (HIV) infection in children?

A. Brain
B. Lymphatic system
C. Lungs
D. Kidneys
E. Skin

25.28. Which is a specification of the weight criteria for anorexia nervosa in the DSM?

A. A minimum of a 15% loss of body weight must occur
B. At least a loss of 25% of one's body weight must be present
C. Failure to meet expected weight gain must occur, though one does not have to lose weight
D. The weight loss must be severe enough to result in a loss of menses for at least 3 months
E. The weight loss must result in a severe nutritional deficiency

ANSWERS

25.1. B. It implied the disorders were all in the individual's head
The term psychosomatic is derived from the Greek words for psyche (soul) and soma (body). It refers to how the mind affects the body. The term psychosomatic ended up having a negative connotation in those with medical complaints where no physical cause could be found, implying that they were crazy, and the symptoms were all in their head. In 2018, the Academy of Psychosomatic Medicine changed its name to the Academy of Consultation–Liaison Psychiatry and the American Board of Psychiatry and Neurology (ABPN) changed the name of psychosomatic medicine as a specialty to consultation–liaison psychiatry. (799)

25.2. D. Males over 45 years old
Suicide rates are highest in males over 45 years of age. Other risk factors include those with medical illnesses, a history of alcohol dependence, decreased social support, severe pain, and previous suicide attempts. (801)

25.3. A. Antipsychotic medications
Antipsychotic medication may be beneficial for excessive agitation in hospitalized patients with various disorders, including cognitive disorders, or those withdrawing from substances. Physical restraints should be used as a last resort. While sedation is typically safer than physical restraints, opioids should be avoided in a patient with a history of substance use. (801)

25.4. A. Ataxia
Benzodiazepines and other sedatives can worsen delirium, leading to sundowner syndrome. Symptoms include ataxia and disorientation, along with agitation, anxiety, and confusion. While benzodiazepines are sedatives and can cause lethargy, often when used in patients with delirium, they can worsen confusion and lead to agitation. (801)

25.5. C. Normal pressure hydrocephalus (NPH)
Central nervous system disorders, such as NPH can cause delirium and is an urgent medical issue that surgery may cure. The classic triad for presentation of NPH is gait disturbance, incontinence, and dementia. Normal renal labs and a uranalysis would rule out a urinary tract infection and hydronephrosis, which might also cause confusion in the elderly. While a subdural hematoma and hyperthyroidism could also cause some confusion and memory impairment, incontinence is not typical for those disorders. (802)

25.6. B. Group therapy
A study by David Spiegel showed that women with breast cancer receiving weekly group psychotherapy lived an average of 18 months longer, compared to control patients. Other studies on those with cancer show increased activity of NK cells in those receiving a group behavioral intervention for breast cancer and also for patients with malignant melanoma. (803)

25.7. A. Adjustment disorder
About half of all cancer patients have a psychiatric disorder, with an adjustment disorder being the most common, at around 68%. Major depressive disorder is the next most common comorbid diagnosis (i.e., around 13%), followed by delirium (8%). (804)

25.8. E. A slightly higher risk of completed suicides
Though suicidal thoughts are frequent in cancer patients, compared to the general population, the risk of suicide is only slightly higher. (804)

25.9. C. Elderly Caucasian males
The prevalence of major depressive disorder is lower in the elderly compared to younger age groups. However, the incidence of suicide is the highest among elderly persons, in particular, for elderly white males. (804)

25.10. A. Arthritis
Only arthritis is a more common cause of disability among those aged 65 years and older than dementia. Dementia increases with age, with about 20% having severe dementia by 80 years old. (805)

25.11. E. Melancholic
Elderly patients with depression present differently from that seen in younger patients. Typically, there is more of an emphasis placed on somatic complaints in the elderly. Depression with melancholic features is common in the elderly. Some common features of depression with melancholia include hypochondriasis, low self-esteem, worthlessness, self-accusatory trends, paranoia, and suicidal ideation. (805)

25.12. D. Persecutory
While delusional disorder is most common between 40 and 55 years old, it can occur at any time, including in the elderly. Delusions can be seen with medical issues such as Alzheimer disease and can occur with psychiatric illnesses, including schizophrenia and depression. Persecutory delusions are the most common type. (806)

25.13. A. Advanced age
Advanced age is the single most important factor associated with an increased prevalence of sleep disorders. Daytime sleeping, napping, and use of hypnotic drugs are commonly found in the elderly. Higher rates of breathing-related sleep disorders are also found in the elderly. (807)

25.14. D. Meclizine
Vertigo, or dizziness, is a common complaint in the elderly. Various medical causes include anemia, cardiac arrhythmias, Meniere disease, etc. Most cases have a psychological component as well. Anxiolytics and other medications that cause dizziness and daytime somnolence should be avoided. Meclizine 25 mg to 100 mg daily can be helpful in treating vertigo in the elderly. (808)

25.15. A. Decreased presence of lean body mass
Dose adjustment should be made in the elderly when utilizing psychiatric meds due to increased renal and hepatic clearance, along with decreased cardiac output and decreased gastric secretions and absorption. Orthostasis is common, especially from psychotropic meds in the elderly, and often necessitates a decrease in the dose. In general, pretreatment medical clearance and an electrocardiogram (EKG) are recommended before starting psychiatric medications in the elderly. (809)

25.16. E. Pervasive hopelessness
A clinician evaluating a patient in a psychiatric ER setting should always ask the patient about suicidal ideation and assess suicide risk. Some examples of factors that increase the risk of suicide include pervasive hopelessness or pessimism, along with family history of suicide, verbalization of suicidal ideation, and previous attempts. (812)

25.17. B. Clozapine
The patient described above with a high fever, pharyngitis, and oral and perianal ulceration likely has clozapine-induced agranulocytosis. When the number of absolute neutrophil count (ANC) is low, it can cause life-threatening infections. (815)

25.18. D. Granulocyte colony-stimulating factor
The first step in the treatment of Clozaril-induced agranulocytosis, as described in the previous case, is discontinuing the medication immediately. After that, administration of granulocyte colony-stimulating factor may be helpful. Though it is similar to a blood infusion, granulocytes, not red blood cells, can be infused in rare cases of agranulocytosis. (815)

25.19. B. Benzodiazepines
Benzodiazepine intoxication can present with sedation, somnolence, and ataxia, as described in the case above. Risks of intoxication include suppression of blood pressure, heart rate, and respiratory rate. LSD and PCP are hallucinogens that can affect perception. LSD intoxication can present with hypertension, mydriasis, and diaphoresis. PCP intoxication presents with nystagmus, hypertension, and dissociative symptoms and agitation. Unlike benzodiazepines, which are sedatives, amphetamines and stimulants, can cause agitation, tachycardia, hypertension, and dilated pupils. Lithium toxicity causes nausea, vomiting, confusion, and tremors. (816)

25.20. B. Flumazenil
Supportive measures and administration of Flumazenil can be helpful in reversing benzodiazepine overdoses, if skilled personnel are delivering it and resuscitation equipment is nearby. (816)

25.21. C. Lithium
The patient described in the case has lithium toxicity, which can often occur with dehydration, such as that caused by the recent sickness in the case above, given Lithium has a small therapeutic window and fluid shifts can lead to toxicity. Sings of toxicity include vomiting, ab pain, diarrhea, tremor, ataxia, and in more severe cases, seizures, focal neurologic signs, and a coma. (817)

25.22. E. ICU transfer and osmotic diuresis
The previous case describes lithium toxicity. Lithium toxicity can be deadly and often requires an ICU admission. Osmotic diuresis and lavage with a wide-bore tube can help reverse the toxicity. (817)

25.23. C. Electrocardiogram (EKG)
Mitral valve prolapse can be associated with panic disorder, as it can cause heart palpitations, dyspnea, fear, and anxiety. An EKG should be obtained to rule out mitral valve prolapse in cases of panic disorder. (818)

25.24. B. Fluoxetine
While short-acting benzodiazepines might be useful for short-term management of panic disorder, the best long-term management medication wise is an antidepressant, such as fluoxetine, which is U.S. Food and Drug Administration (FDA) approved to treat panic disorder. In cases of mitral valve

prolapse-induced panic symptoms, propranolol could be helpful. (818)

25.25. B. Continue to decrease and taper off the medication

The patient above likely has tardive dyskinesia. Abnormal movements of the mouth, tongue, face, neck, and trunk are common. The elderly and those with underlying brain damage are most at risk. Often, the symptoms come about after the antipsychotic dose is lowered after long-term treatment. No effective medication can treat tardive dyskinesia, but the patient should be managed on the lowest dose possible. Ideally, the medication should be discontinued, or if need be, switched to an antipsychotic less likely to cause tardive dyskinesia in the future. The older typical antipsychotics, such as fluphenazine and haloperidol, are most likely to cause tardive dyskinesia. Increasing the dose might mask the tardive dyskinesia short term, but it is not the best long-term solution. (820)

25.26. B. Conduct disorder

While it used to be thought of that fire setting is associated with a triad of symptoms, fire setting, enuresis, and cruelty to animals, it is now known that no evidence exists indicating that these symptoms are linked. However, conduct disorder has been found to be the most frequent psychiatrist disorder co-occurring with pathologic fire setting. (821)

25.27. A. Brain

In children, the brain is often a primary site for HIV infection, leading to decreased brain development and often presenting with encephalitis, memory, concentration, and attentional issues. The virus often presents itself in the cerebrospinal fluid before it shows up in the blood. Mood disorders, personality changes, and psychosis can also occur with HIV infections. (822)

25.28. C. Failure to meet expected weight gain must occur, though one does not have to lose weight

While weight loss is commonly a feature of anorexia nervosa, and a suggested body weight less than 85% was noted in the DSM-IV, in the current DSM-5, there is no required cut-off for a percentage of weight that must be lost to meet criteria. While prior versions of the DSM required amenorrhea as a criterion, we now know that even those of very low weight still get their periods at times. This led to the elimination of the amenorrhea criterion from the DSM-5. (822)

26

Level of Care

26.1. A patient with bipolar disorder has been intermittently complaint with medications and has had previous hospitalizations and a recent residential stay. He can go to work a few days a week, though struggles at times with routines and activities of daily living (ADLs) on other days. He has persistent suicidal thoughts and self-harm off and on but does not have a plan and reports motivation to get help and stay safe. Which of the following is the most appropriate level of care?

A. Inpatient hospitalization
B. Intensive outpatient treatment
C. Outpatient
D. Partial hospital program
E. Residential

26.2. The Mental Retardation Facilities and Community Mental Health Centers Construction Act of 1963 helped pave the way for which of the following changes in the mental health system?

A. Creating intensive outpatient programs as an alternative to inpatient programs
B. Designing of centralized school-based mental health clinics
C. Funding of local mental health centers to minimize long-term institutionalization
D. Instituting more funding to state child protective services
E. Opening more state hospitals to increase bed availability

26.3. An adolescent has been struggling with anorexia for the past 2 years and her parents feel unable to get her to gain weight despite attempts at daily supervised meals, including taking her home from school for lunch, and restriction of physical activity. Parents noted that she recently started to vomit a few times a week. They struggle with pushing her food intake because she self-harms regularly. She has denied any history of suicidal thoughts or attempts. Parents are also concerned that she might be using substances to help with her anxiety, and they are struggling more with getting her to go to school and therapy. She was recently started on fluoxetine with minimal effect. A few days ago, she was seen by her pediatrician and her labs were within normal limits, heart rate was found to be 68, and blood pressure 110/78. Which of the following levels of care is most appropriate?

A. Inpatient psychiatry
B. Intensive outpatient
C. Medical inpatient
D. Partial hospital
E. Residential

ANSWERS

26.1. D. Partial hospital program
Partial hospital programs are indicated for moderate, but not imminent risk and the patient above feels that he can contract to safety and his suicidal thoughts and self-harm seem chronic. His ADLs are moderately impaired, given he is able to work a few days a week and he is voluntarily willing to get help, indicating partial hospital program is best. Returning to inpatient would be indicated if he is at imminent risk of danger to himself and others, had consistently poor ADLs, and needs continuous monitoring or an involuntary stay. Intensive outpatient treatment would offer even less support than a partial hospital program and safety concerns should not be present for an intensive outpatient program (IOP) level of care. Those of moderate risk with severe ADL impairment are good residential candidates. The patient has previously been to residential and often partial hospital programs are good step downs to help patients transition back to life. (826, 827)

26.2. C. Funding of local mental health centers to minimize long-term institutionalization
In the 1960s, most psychiatric care took place in hospitals. The social justice movement and push for government-funded alternatives to institutionalization occurred in the 1960s. The Mental Retardation Facilities and Community Mental Health Centers Construction Act of 1963 led to the establishment of a grant program for states to fund local mental health centers under the overview of the National Institutes of Health. The goal was to build community-based mental health centers to help minimize long-term institutionalization. (825)

26.3. E. Residential
An inpatient medical admission is not necessary since the patient is medically stable. Inpatient psychiatry on an eating disorder unit is not necessary as she is not a significantly low weight and there are no acute safety concerns. Given the patient struggles with self-harm, purging, and substance use, a residential setting is indicated. Another benefit to a residential level of care is that she can be monitored closely while her medication is adjusted. Though she doesn't have a huge amount of weight to gain and there are no imminent safety concerns, given the history of school refusal, compliance with attendance of a partial or intensive outpatient program is unlikely. In a partial or intensive outpatient settings cessation of vomiting, while remaining abstinent from other substances, would also likely be challenging. (827)

C

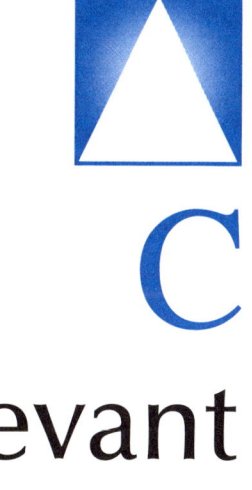

Other Issues Relevant to Psychiatry

27

Ethics and Professionalism

27.1. A 26-year-old man with a diagnosis of schizophrenia has been hospitalized on the inpatient psychiatric unit for the last 5 days. This is his sixth hospitalization in 4 years. He has been on haloperidol, risperidone, quetiapine, and asenapine, each of which was started during a hospitalization. He continued taking the medications until he felt better, then stopped because "I didn't need it anymore." He has been asked numerous times over the last 3 years if he would like to take a long-acting injection (LAI) instead, and each time he refuses because "I don't want any needles. They hurt." His mother asks the physician to "give him a shot, or he can't come back to live at my house." The treatment team relays this to the patient, who still refuses an injection, but consents to oral medication. The psychiatrist prescribes the oral medication. What ethical principle is demonstrated by the psychiatrist's action?

A. Autonomy
B. Beneficence
C. Nonmaleficence
D. Justice

27.2. An 86-year-old woman in the ICU with acute pneumonia awakens, panicked and confused, during the first night of hospitalization and starts to pull at her IV lines. This is noticed by nursing staff, who talk gently to her and get her to stop. She does not seem to understand the need for the treatment and why it is given intravenously. A few minutes later, the patient removes an IV line that contains an antibiotic which must be given intravenously. The patient's son is called to talk with his mother in hopes of convincing her to stop removing the IV lines so that she does not have to be physically restrained. After a few minutes, the son tells the staff that his mother would prefer an oral antibiotic and to remove the IVs. Temperature is 38.9 C (102.1 F), pulse 89, respirations 22, and BP 140/92. Complying with the son's request would constitute a breach of what ethical principle?

A. Autonomy
B. Beneficence
C. Nonmaleficence
D. Justice

27.3. A 45-year-old man presents to an urgent care with a complaint of right leg pain since falling off of a ladder at home the day before. He is able to bear weight on the leg and rates the pain as a 5 out of 10. He states that he took ibuprofen twice yesterday and once today with moderate effect, but that he needs something stronger so that he can return to his job tomorrow at the post office. He has no medical illnesses and is on no other medications. Vital signs are temperature 37.1 C (98.8 F), pulse 90, respirations 19, BP 130/85. Physical examination reveals diffuse tenderness over the anterior aspect of the right quadriceps, with noticeable bruising and abrasions. He has full range of motion. After the examination, he insists that he needs a narcotic for pain. The physician explains that narcotics can be addictive, so they need to be reserved for the most severe pain. What ethical principle was most demonstrated in the physician's response?

A. Autonomy
B. Beneficence
C. Nonmaleficence
D. Justice

27.4. The American Psychiatric Association's (APA's) *Principles of Medical Ethics with Annotations Especially Applicable to Psychiatry* stipulates that sexual relations with a patient are acceptable under what circumstances?

A. If the appointments are for medication management only and involve no therapy
B. Two years after termination of the doctor–patient relationship
C. Five years after termination of the doctor–patient relationship
D. If the relationship ended in marriage
E. Sexual relations with a patient are never acceptable

27.5. A psychiatrist has been treating a 9-year-old boy for attention-deficit/hyperactivity disorder (ADHD), combined type, over the last 10 months. A trial of methylphenidate resulted in the patient's grades improving from Ds to Bs, and he is no longer getting in trouble in class for excessive talking. As a result, appointment frequency was reduced from monthly for the first 6 months to every 2 months. History during the visit today reveals that the child continues to do well and has made a couple of As at school. He has no medical issues and takes no other medications. Vital signs are normal and physical examination reveals no abnormalities. At the end of the visit, the patient's mother, who divorced 2 months ago, asks the physician, who is also single, out on a date. According to The American Psychiatric Association's (APA's) *Principles of Medical Ethics with Annotations Especially Applicable to Psychiatry*, what would be the most appropriate response by the psychiatrist?

A. "Thank you for asking, but it is unethical for me to date a family member of a patient."
B. "I cannot ethically do so right now, but if your son's medication management is turned over to his pediatrician, I can then."
C. "I would like to, but only if your son is comfortable with the idea."
D. "The divorce only occurred 2 months ago. Let's give it more time. If you're still interested in 4 months, I would love to."
E. "I would like to go on a date with you, but I have to run it by the office's risk management team first."

27.6. A boundary crossing becomes a boundary violation once what circumstance occurs?

A. The patient suffers any type of harm
B. Sexual activity occurs in the relationship
C. The physician benefits at the patient's expense
D. The situation could lead to legal ramifications
E. Clinic or hospital bylaws and guidelines are broken

27.7. A 23-year-old male is brought to the emergency department (ED) by emergency medical services (EMS) following a motor vehicle accident in which he was the driver. On arrival, he is stuporous and unable to respond. Glasgow Coma Scale (GCS) is 5. A urine drug screen (UDS) is positive for amphetamines and fentanyl, and blood alcohol content is .28%. The patient's girlfriend, who was also in the vehicle, is brought into the ED and taken immediately to surgery for injuries sustained in the accident. Thirty minutes later, the driver dies. The girlfriend's parents are upset and demand that the driver be alcohol tested, as they suspect he was driving while drunk because "we know he's done that before." How should the hospital respond to the parents' request?

A. Tell the parents that the driver was drug and alcohol tested, but do not release results
B. Release the information about the drug and alcohol tests, as the patient has died
C. Advise the parents to get a court order to see the driver's medical record
D. Withhold any information unless given permission by driver's next of kin
E. Give the parents only the results of the alcohol test, as they only mentioned prior alcohol use

27.8. Administrative staff tell a psychiatrist at an outpatient clinic that they have witnessed the psychiatrist's colleague coming to work smelling of alcohol on three occasions over the past month. They have received no patient complaints. The psychiatrist talks with the colleague, who promises that "it won't happen again." Two weeks later, the colleague comes to work intoxicated. How should the psychiatrist respond?

A. Talk with the colleague to let them know that this will be reported if it happens again
B. Ask the staff if any patients have complained, and if so, report the colleague to the state medical board
C. Report the colleague to the state medical board
D. Report the colleague to the police
E. Offer to take the colleague to an alcohol and drug rehabilitation center

27.9. A 23-year-old man is discharged from his first hospitalization with a diagnosis of schizophrenia. While inpatient, he was given prn Intramuscular (IM) haloperidol for acute agitation. He was discharged on paliperidone palmitate. One month later when his next injection is due, his insurance company denies the prior authorization, stating that he has not tried a generic long-acting injection first. The patient has been stable on the current medication and would like to continue it. How should the outpatient physician respond to the insurance company's decision?

A. Tell the insurance company that the patient has tried an injectable formulation of haloperidol, which did not lead to schizophrenia symptom management
B. Tell the insurance company that the patient will relapse if he does not continue the current medication
C. Ask for a peer-to-peer consultation to make an appeal for the paliperidone palmitate
D. Change the patient's medication to haloperidol decanoate therapy
E. Report the situation to the patient's local and federal elected representatives

ANSWERS

27.1. A. Autonomy
Though the patient could likely benefit from an LAI, he is given the choice between an LAI and an oral medication. He chose oral, and the psychaitrist obliged his wishes. This situation demonstrates the ethical principle of autonomy. Had his wishes been overridden, that could be seen by some as a demonstration of beneficence, whether or not such an action was legally allowed. The principles of nonmaleficence and justice are not relevant in this scenario, as presumably the LAI would not harm the patient and distribution of social benefits is not in question. (829)

27.2. B. Beneficence
Complying with the son's request would be in accordance with the ethical principle of autonomy. However, it would be a breach of beneficence, which involves acting in the patient's best interests. In this case, the IV antibiotics are deemed medically necessary, and to not give them when she is acutely ill would be a breach of fiduciary responsibility to the patient. The ethical course would be to override the patient's autonomy until no longer medically necessary, or until she has a rational understanding of the need for treatment and its risks and benefits. (829)

27.3. C. Nonmaleficence
Nonmaleficence is expressed by the maxim, "First, do no harm." In this scenario, the physician first sought to avoid creating risk for the patient. Had the physician then given the patient a choice between standard-of-care treatment and a narcotic, that would have been showing respect for autonomy. Though beneficence is also a factor, it is not the best answer here because that does not address the physician's response to the patient. (829)

27.4. E. Sexual relations with a patient are never acceptable
The APA code of ethics states, "Sexual activity with a current or former patient is unethical." Under that code, there are no circumstances in which sexual activity with a patient is acceptable. (830)

27.5. A. "Thank you for asking, but it is unethical for me to date a family member of a patient."
According to The APA's *Principles of Medical Ethics with Annotations Especially Applicable to Psychiatry*, sexual activity with a patient's family member is as unethical as sexual activity with a patient. Child and adolescent psychiatrists usually consider treatment of the family as part of the treatment of the patient, so ethical guidelines would apply to sexual relationships with family members as well. The time course of treatment of the patient is irrelevant, as the *Principles* states that "Sexual activity with a current or former patient is unethical." (830)

27.6. C. The physician benefits at the patient's expense
A boundary violation is a boundary crossing that is exploitative, in which the doctor's needs are gratified at the expense of the patient. A boundary violation does not have to include patient harm. If a physician enters into a business relationship with a patient, that is usually considered a boundary violation, even though the patient is ostensibly unharmed and may even benefit. While sexual activity with a patient is always a boundary violation, there are violations in which sex is not involved. Not all violations would lead to legal consequences, such as with the business relationship described above. A boundary violation does not necessarily involve breaking clinic or hospital policy, and vice versa. (830)

27.7. D. Withhold any information unless given permission by driver's next of kin
Patient confidentiality extends even after the patient has died. Release of information decisions then falls to the next of kin. (831)

27.8. C. Report the colleague to the state medical board
An impaired physician should be reported to the proper authority (state medical board, office manager, department chair, etc.) and relieved of duty in order to reduce the risk of harm to patients. Though many physicians say that they will only talk with the colleague first when presented with a similar scenario, the ethical obligation is to report. (832)

27.9. C. Ask for a peer-to-peer consultation to make an appeal for the paliperidone palmitate
The American Medical Association (AMA) Council of Ethical and Judicial Affairs states that physicians have an obligation to advocate for patient care that they deem appropriate. In this case, advocacy should first come in the form of appealing the insurance company's decision by asking for a peer-to-peer

conversation. Though the patient has technically been exposed to IM haloperidol, to report that as having been exposed to the decanoate formulation would be deceptive. Likewise, it is unknown if the patient would relapse if given haloperidol decanoate instead of paliperidone palmitate. Simply changing to haloperidol decanoate, though possibly effective, is not advocating for the patient for whom the current medication regimen has proven effective. Speaking with the patient's elected representative could be helpful but is not likely to be in the time frame needed. (831)

28

Forensic and Legal Issues

28.1. Which one of the following factors must the plaintiff prove to establish that malpractice has occurred?

A. A patient suffered a side effect from a medication that the doctor explained beforehand
B. Care of the patient was not optimal
C. Deviation from the standard of care caused damage to the patient
D. Safety planning failed to be done
E. That split treatment occurred

28.2. How frequently should a patient be seen for medication follow-up to avoid a malpractice claim?

A. As often as the psychiatrist feels is clinically indicated
B. At least once a year
C. At least once every 3 months
D. Every 2 weeks while medication is being titrated
E. Once a month if at least two medications are prescribed

28.3. Which place or relationship is an exception to the law of privileged communications?

A. Doctor and patient
B. Husband and wife
C. Military courts
D. Priest and penitent
E. Social worker and patient

28.4. Courts scrutinize suicide cases and can hold the psychiatrist liable if the event was deemed to be:

A. Foreseeable
B. Impulsive
C. Predictable
D. Preventable
E. Secretive

28.5. The first part of the Tarasoff law requires a psychiatrist to do which of the following when a patient reports intent to kill someone?

A. Document it and release the information to the courts
B. Hospitalize the patient involuntarily
C. Notify the victim and report the intended homicide
D. Report the patient's fantasies and dreams
E. Review a safety plan with the patient

28.6. The second part of the Tarasoff ruling (Tarasoff II) requires the psychiatrist to do which of the following actions?

A. Call the police
B. Maintain confidentiality
C. Notify family members
D. Prevent
E. Protect

28.7. Which is a key difference between a temporary versus an involuntary psychiatric admission?

A. A judge needs to release the patient
B. A writ of habeas corpus is necessary to be released
C. The patient cannot be held for typically more than 15 days
D. The next of kin must be notified in writing
E. Two physicians are required to sign the patient in

28.8. Which of the following ethical principles should be considered when deciding to use seclusion or restraint for a patient?

A. Autonomy
B. Beneficence
C. Justice
D. Least restrictive alternative
E. Nonmaleficence

28.9. Which of the following measures should occur when utilizing seclusion or restraints?

A. A written order should be documented by a medical official
B. Documentation of evidence of an unstable psychiatric condition should be done
C. Proof of suicidal behavior should be noted
D. Release of the patient if consent is not obtained
E. The order needs to be reviewed every half hour

28.10. Proving malpractice for a failure to obtain informed consent differs from other malpractice claims in which of the following ways?

A. Claims cannot be made if no other violation was performed
B. It can only include adverse medication side effects
C. Only minors can be involved
D. There is no requirement for an expert witness
E. There needs to be proof the patient was harmed

28.11. A consent for treatment form should always include which of the following information?

A. A disclaimer that the patient is free to withdraw at any time
B. At least two patient identifiers
C. Conditions under which treatment must be adhered to
D. Information regarding only the gold standard of treatment
E. Signature by a witness

28.12. What is necessary to declare a patient incompetent?

A. A judge's ruling in a court of law
B. Attestation by a forensic psychiatrist
C. Carrying a diagnosis of a severe mental illness
D. Having a prior guardian ad litem appointed
E. Possessing a physical handicap

28.13. A patient with dementia acknowledges that she will lose ability to make decisions for herself soon. She creates a document while still of sound mind, indicating her sister can make decision for her when she is no longer able to act. This describes which of the following principles:

A. Contractual capacity
B. Durable power of attorney
C. Execution of competence
D. Guardian ad lidum
E. Testamentary competence

28.14. According to the M'Naghten rule, to be found not guilty by reason of insanity, which of the following criteria must be met?

A. An expert witness must prove the defendant has a full, rather than a partial delusion
B. Only a diagnosis of bipolar, a delusional disorder, or schizophrenia can be applied
C. The accused does not know the difference between right and wrong in general
D. The act was caused by a delusion that led the accused to feel he was acting in self-defense
E. The accused must be proven by a psychiatrist to have a severe mental illness

28.15. What is true of the verdict if someone is proven to be guilty, but mentally ill?

A. The accused must go to prison after psychiatric rehabilitation
B. The person is still labeled as a criminal but sent to an inpatient psychiatric unit
C. The person cannot be sentenced, as would be if proven not guilty by reason of insanity
D. The sentence is still imposed, and psychiatric treatment is delivered in prison
E. The sentence must be modified to the least restrictive criteria

28.16. Which of the following actions is most important, as advised by risk management, in recovered memory cases?

A. Avoid prescribing benzodiazepines
B. Begin a course of hypnosis to further help recover memories
C. Notify the police
D. Refer for a sodium amobarbital interview
E. Remain neutral and adhere to treatment boundaries

28.17. The Privacy Rule grants the patient which of the following privileges?

A. A release of information to insurance companies if separate forms are signed
B. Access to their records in only emergent situations
C. Ability to obtain copies of psychotherapy notes
D. Right to complain about violations to the police
E. Written notice of their rights

ANSWERS

28.1. D. Deviation from the standard of care caused damage to the patient

To prove malpractice, The 4 Ds, must be proven—duty, deviation, damage, and direct causation (i.e., the deviation from the standard of care directly caused damage to the patient). If the doctor did not inform a patient of the risks of medication, there may be grounds for malpractice. Thus, it should always be documented that potential medication side effects have been reviewed. While one should strive for excellent care, only the standard of care needs to be met, and if not, malpractice can occur. Split treatment can be allowed, but the psychiatrist should be aware that they assume a collaborative or supervisory role with another mental health worker and that the patient's full responsibility lies in their care in split-treatment situations. (836)

28.2. A. As often as the psychiatrist feels is clinically indicated

There are no standard rules or regulations set regarding how frequently patients should be monitored while on psychiatric medications. However, the longer time interval between visits can mean the higher likelihood of adverse drug reactions or new developments of clinical concerns. Though probably patients on medication should not go more than 6 months without being seen, psychiatrists should monitor patients for follow-up visits according to the patient's individual needs. (836)

28.3. C. Military courts

Privilege, the right to maintain secrecy or confidentiality in the face of a subpoena, does not exist in the military courts, regardless of whether the physician is in the military. Privileged communications include husband–wife, priest–penitent, and doctor/therapist–patient relationships. (837)

28.4. A. Foreseeable

The law assumes that suicide is preventable if it is foreseeable. Courts scrutinize suicide cases to determine if the patient's suicide was foreseeable. It does not imply or require clinicians to be able to predict suicide or prevent it. (838)

28.5. C. Notify the victim and report the intended homicide

The 1976 case Tarasoff v. Regents of the University of California involved a patient reporting intent to kill a student. He was kept for 72 hours in an emergency room and the campus police were notified but upon release, he carried out the act and the girls' parents sued the university for negligence. The Tarasoff I ruling requires the therapist to report the intended homicide, and to notify the intended victim or others that they are in danger. This can include notifying the police to warn the intended victim. (839)

28.6. E. Protect

While the Tarasoff I ruling requires the psychiatrist to warn the intended victim, the Tarasoff II law has broadened the previous ruling requiring the duty to protect as well. The ruling prioritizes public safety over individual privacy. The duty to protect typically involves involuntary hospitalizations. Other steps such as calling the police and notifying family members can be involved with the first Tarasoff ruling. Though concerns that the patient won't be able to trust the doctor if confidentiality is maintained, if there is concern of imminent, serious harm, public safety trumps confidentiality. (839)

28.7. C. The patient cannot be held for typically more than 15 days

Temporary admissions are utilized when a patient is confused and so impaired from a psychiatric standpoint that they need to be admitted on an emergency basis for their safety. One physician can recommend admission, whereas two physicians are required for an involuntary admission. After a temporary admission, the hospital staff must confirm the need for admission and that patients cannot be held against their will for a set period, typically 15 days. However, for an involuntary admission, the person can be held for a lengthy period as defined by the state, often around 60 days. The next of kin must be notified in writing of an involuntary hospitalization. The person can file for petition for a writ of habeas corpus to be released and the court must hear the case immediately. (840)

28.8. E. Least restrictive alternative

The principle of least restrictive alternative holds that patients have the right to receive treatment using the least restrictive means (i.e., they should be treated as an outpatient, if possible, in an open ward, instead of seclusion, etc.). This principle should be considered when utilizing involuntary medication, seclusions, or restraints. (841)

28.9. A. A written order should be documented by a medical official

For seclusion and restraints, a medical official must write an order and it should be time specified and the patient's condition must be regularly reviewed and documented. Extension must be reordered. These measures should only be implemented when the patient is at risk of harming themselves or others. Unless continuously monitored with constant direct observation, those patients with overtly suicidal behaviors should not be in seclusion or restraints. A contradiction to restraints include extremely unstable medical and psychiatric conditions. (841)

28.10. D. There is no requirement for an expert witness

Negligence to obtain informed consent is the one area of claim in which there is no requirement for expert testimony. While typically an expert witness is needed to prove departure from accepted medical practice, given the claim involves consent for treatment only, technically the outcome of the treatment does not need to be considered and there is no need to prove that the accepted standard of treatment was met. However, practically unless the treatment has adverse consequences, the complaint of failure to obtain consent typically does not get far. (842)

28.11. A. A disclaimer that the patient is free to withdraw at any time

Essential elements of a consent form include information about the procedure, purpose, identification of any experimental procedures, discomfort, and risks of the treatment as well as reasonable benefits to expect, alternatives to the procedure, and that the patient is free to withdraw consent and discontinue participation at any time. While more than one patient identifier on the form and a signature by a witness can be included, they are not essential features required for all consent forms. (842)

28.12. A. A judge's ruling in a court of law

Competence is determined based on a person's ability to make a sound judgment, which include weighing in on the decision, reasoning, and making a reasonable decision. Competence is task specific. While physicians, typically psychiatrists, can give opinions of a person's competence, only a ruling by a judge can declare someone competent or incompetent. The diagnosis of a mental disorder alone is not sufficient to warrant incompetence, rather impairment must be noted. While a guardian is often appointed if someone is deemed incompetent, it is not mandatory to have one prior to declaring patient incompetent. (842)

28.13. B. Durable power of attorney

A durable power of attorney is when a person appoints someone else to make decisions for them in anticipation of their loss of decision-making capacity. The patient documents a substitute decision maker that can act on their behalf without needing to involve a court proceeding. (843)

28.14. D. The act was caused by a delusion that led the accused to feel he was acting in self-defense

The M'Naghten rule gives guidelines for pleading insanity as a defense against criminal responsibility. To establish a defense of insanity, it must be clearly proven that at the time of committing the act, the patient acted under a defect of reason from an idea of the mind and did not know what he was doing was wrong. This can apply to a person if they have a partial delusion as well. The question is not whether the defendant knows the difference between right and wrong in general, but at the time of the act if the delusion caused them to not know right from wrong and feel they were acting in self-defense. (844)

28.15. D. The sentence is still imposed, and psychiatric treatment is delivered in prison

As an alternative to the verdict of guilty by reason of insanity, some states have established an alternative verdict of guilty, but mentally ill. However, the verdict if proven guilty but mentally ill is the same for other prisoners, in that if convinced, the accused will receive psychiatric treatment in prison, which is available to all prisoners as well. (844)

28.16. E. Remain neutral and adhere to treatment boundaries

There have been cases of therapist being sued for inducing false memories of sexual abuse. A fundamental allegation is that the therapist abandoned a position of neutrality to suggest or implant false childhood sexual memories. The guiding principle of clinical risk management in recovered memory cases is the maintenance of therapist neutrality and establishment of sound treatment boundaries. (844, 845)

28.17. E. Written notice of their rights

The Privacy Rule, as administered by the Office for Civil Rights, mandates that physician must give the patient written notice of their privacy rights. Other mandates of this rule include that a patient can obtain copies of their medical records and that a physician can't limit a patient signing a release for records for nonroutine use. Patients have the right to complain if this rule is violated to the doctor, their health plan, or to the Secretary of HHS (the Federal Department of Health and Human Services). Patients are not permitted to obtain copies of their psychotherapy notes. Patients do not need to sign consent for release of information to health care plans for payment. (845)

29

End-of-Life Issues and Palliative Care

29.1. Which of the following is a feature of the stages of death and dying as described by Dr Kübler-Ross?

A. All the stages are thought to occur in everybody
B. Depression and possibly suicidal ideation can occur
C. Most people do not reach the phase of acceptance
D. Shock and denial are experienced by all
E. The stages are typically followed in order

29.2. Approximately 75% of those who die in late adolescence do so from which of the following causes?

A. Accidents, homicides, and suicides
B. Blood and skin cancers
C. Brain tumors
D. Eating disorders
E. Heart disease and metabolic disorders

29.3. A patient is suffering from an incurable brain tumor. The patient feels significant guilt for dying and views the treatment as a punishment and struggles with feelings of rejection from the family. A person with this attitude surrounding death is most likely to be in which of the following age groups?

A. Preschool
B. Elementary school
C. Early adolescence
D. Late adolescence
E. Elderly

29.4. Which of the following symptoms is the most lasting manifestation of grief after spousal bereavement?

A. Decreased appetite
B. Guilt
C. Loneliness
D. Suicidal thoughts
E. Worthlessness

29.5. Which symptom is more commonly found in a major depressive disorder compared to bereavement?

A. Dysphoria with thoughts of the deceased
B. Onset within the first 2 months of the loss
C. Psychomotor retardation
D. Symptoms lasting for 1 month
E. Transient functional impairment

29.6. Bereavement has been shown to exacerbate which of the following symptoms in both sexes?

A. Accidents
B. Alcohol consumption
C. Death
D. Ischemic heart disease
E. Suicide

29.7. Which is a distinguishing feature of grief compared to depression after a loss of a loved one?

A. Enduring low mood
B. Positive emotions
C. Protracted course
D. Social withdrawal
E. Trouble going to work

29.8. Which medication is commonly prescribed and may be useful in some forms of grief?

   A. An atypical antipsychotic
   B. A mild sedative
   C. A narcotic
   D. A selective serotonin–norepinephrine reuptake inhibitor
   E. A selective serotonin reuptake inhibitor

29.9. Which criterion is part of the Endicott Substitution Criteria for depression in those experiencing advanced disease?

   A. Anhedonia
   B. Changes in appetite
   C. Increased energy
   D. Suicidal ideation
   E. Worthlessness

29.10. Which of the following is a distinguishing factor between a persistent vegetative state versus brain death?

   A. Absence of respiration
   B. Absence of wave formations on electroencephalography
   C. Lack of reflex eye movements
   D. Mild to moderate response to medical intervention
   E. Smiling, frowning, and yawning can be noted

29.11. Use of which of the following pain-relieving drugs in end-of-life care can help minimize the risk of psychotoxicity leading to delirium?

   A. Hydromorphone
   B. Levorphanol
   C. Meperidine
   D. Methadone
   E. Morphine

29.12. Arguments for euthanasia revolve around which of the following ethical principles?

   A. Autonomy
   B. Beneficence
   C. Justice
   D. Loyalty
   E. Nonmaleficence

29.13. In addition to depression and an incurable medical condition, which of the following factors is part of the triad that exists in almost every case in patients asking to be put to death?

   A. A cancer diagnosis
   B. Alzheimer disease
   C. Fear of losing bodily functions
   D. Intolerable pain
   E. Religious reasons

29.14. Which safeguard has been put in place as a part of Oregon's Assisted Suicide Law?

   A. The doctors and pharmacists must abide by the Death with Dignity Act
   B. The patient must make two witnessed written requests at least 1 month apart
   C. The patient must complete at least 3 months of counseling with a licensed provider
   D. The next of kin must be notified of the patient's decision by the doctor and patient together
   E. Two doctors must confirm the patient is terminally ill and acting of their own free will

ANSWERS

29.1. B. Depression and possibly suicidal ideation can occur

The stages of death and dying, as identified by Elizabeth Kübler-Ross include the following: 1. Shock and Denial, 2. Anger, 3. Bargaining, 4. Depression, and 5. Acceptance. In the stage of depression, patients can show clinical signs of a major depressive disorder including withdrawal, psychomotor retardation, and suicidal ideation. It should be noted that a dying patient rarely follows these stages in order and that not all patients experience all five stages. (847, 848)

29.2. A. Accidents, homicides, and suicides

Almost half of the children who die between 1 to 14 years old, and nearly 75% of those who die in late adolescence and early adulthood do so from a combination of accidents, homicides, and suicides. (848)

29.3. A. Preschool

At the preschool age, the preoperational stage of cognitive development predominates. Preschoolers still see death as incomplete and reversible. Separation from the primary caregiver is the main fear. Terminally ill children often feel guilty and responsible for their own death and don't relate treatment to the illness and view it as punishment and feel family separation as rejection. School-aged children in the concrete operational cognitive stage can realize the finality of death but see it as something that happens to older people. Adolescents often struggle with loss of independence and fears of abandonment by friends. Teenagers are capable and should typically be involved in all decision-making processes surrounding their deaths. Adults have various fears including losing control, being a burden to others, pain, fear of afterlife, etc. Late-aged adults often can accept death. (849)

29.4. C. Loneliness

The most lasting manifestation of grief, especially after spousal bereavement, is loneliness. Typically, it can last for up to many years. Grief often becomes circumscribed throughout time and reemerges when specific triggers are present. The other symptoms listed are indicative of a major depressive disorder, which if present, would typically resolve with treatment. (850)

29.5. C. Psychomotor retardation

Symptoms associated with a major depressive disorder, as opposed to bereavement include classic DSM-5 symptoms such as guilt, worthlessness, suicidal ideation, or psychomotor retardation. Dysphoria independent of thoughts of the deceased is typical for a major depressive disorder and the depression causes clinically significant impairment and distress. With bereavement, the functional impairment is transient and mild, with symptoms lasting for less than 2 months, and the onset is within the first 2 months of the loss. (850)

29.6. B. Alcohol consumption

An increased mortality rate is seen after bereavement, especially for men. Higher mortality rates for men are due to an increased risk of death by suicide. Accidents, ischemic heart disease, and some infectious diseases are also more common among men. In both sexes, increased alcohol consumption, smoking, and use of over-the-counter (OTC) medications can be exacerbated. (851)

29.7. B. Positive emotions

Grief involves both positive and negative emotions. Grief is fluid and gradually lessens over time as the negative feelings lessen and positive ones take their place. With grief, the person can eventually find comfort in memories of their loved one and can resume a satisfying life. Major depressive disorder consists of a protracted course, with enduring low mood and impairment in work and social functioning. (852)

29.8. B. A mild sedative

Most people don't end up seeing a psychiatrist for grief, as it is accepted as a normal reaction. However, the most common request for help with grief often involves a request for sleeping medication from a primary care doctor. A mild sedative might be helpful in certain situations. However, antidepressant medication, antianxiety agents, and narcotics are not indicted and can interfere with the normal grief process. (853)

29.9. B. Changes in appetite

The Endicott Substitution Criteria can help diagnose depression in those with advanced disease. The criteria have been found to perform as well as the DSM criteria. The physical/somatic symptoms listed include changes in appetite or weight, sleep disturbances, fatigue, loss of energy, and memory and concentration deficits. Psychological symptoms include tearfulness, despair, withdrawal, self-pity, a lack of mood reactivity, etc. (854)

29.10. E. Smiling, frowning, and yawning can be noted

A persistent vegetative state is a condition in which no awareness exists of the self or environment and is associated with severe neurologic damage. Brainstem or hypothalamic autonomic functions permit survival and various cranial nerves, and spinal reflexes are preserved, and patients can even smile, frown, or yawn and sleep–wake cycles can return. No meaningful response to a stimulant or receptive or expressive language is possible, and medical treatment proves no benefits to patients in persistent vegetative states. Brain death is accepted criterion for death and involves a loss of all higher and lower brain stem functions, respiration, and no brain waves are seen on electroencephalographies (EEGs). (858)

29.11. A. Hydromorphone

Opioids can cause delirium and hallucinations. Psychotoxicity can occur when these drugs or metabolites accumulate because the duration of the analgesics is shorter than their plasma half-lives. Morphine, levorphanol, and methadone are drugs that can accumulate easily whereas hydromorphone has a half-life close to its analgesic duration. Meperidine's active metabolite, normeperidine, can accumulate in the body. (860, 861)

29.12. A. Autonomy

Most medical, religious, and legal groups in the United States are against active euthanasia and it is considered illegal. Those in support of euthanasia argue the ethical principle of autonomy and a right to a dignified death. Passive euthanasia, a patient requesting the withdrawal of life-sustaining treatment, should be abided by if the patient is competent. (864)

29.13. D. Intolerable pain

In almost every case in which a patient asks to be put to death, the triad of depression, an incurable medical condition, and intolerable pain exists. Every effort should be made to provide treatment with antidepressants or stimulants, opioids for pain control, along with therapy and spiritual counseling and family support. (865)

29.14. E. Two doctors must confirm the patient is terminally ill and acting of their own free will

In 1994, Oregon was the first state to pass the legalization of physician-assisted suicide, known as the Death with Dignity Act. Washington, Montana, and Vermont have also since made it legal. Oregon's physician-assisted suicide laws include that two doctors must agree the patient is terminally ill and acting of their own free will and that the patient is capable of making health care decisions and can change their mind at any time. The patient must make one written request and two spoken ones. While the doctor must ask the patient to tell the next of kin, the patient can decide not to. Other parts of the Law include the person must live in Oregon. Pharmacists must be told of the medication's use. It should be noted that all health care providers are not under any obligation to participate in the act. (865)

30 Community Psychiatry

30.1. In addition to promotion of health, what is the main mission of public health programs?

A. Lobbying for government funds
B. Preventing disease
C. Training health care providers to work in the community
D. Increasing opportunities for research
E. Forming partnerships with for-profit health care entities

30.2. The teacher of an 8-year-old girl notices that she is often disengaged in class and stares absently during lessons. She often gets only halfway through her classwork, while her classmates finish the assignments with time to spare. The teacher is concerned that the child may have an attention problem and would like her to get evaluated. In an ideal collaborative care public health model, what would be the next step in the evaluation of this child?

A. The school will set up an appointment with the child's pediatrician
B. The teacher will relay the concern to the school nurse
C. The child will be seen by a psychiatrist at her pediatrician's office
D. The child will be seen by a psychiatrist at the school
E. The parents will come to the school to observe the child

30.3. A pediatrics office begins screening every adolescent for depression using a nine-item questionnaire. They then offer to enroll the patients who score above a certain threshold but are not yet showing depression symptoms into an online therapy program. The referral to the program is an example of what level of intervention?

A. Universal
B. Indicated
C. Selective
D. Multimodal

30.4. A 54-year-old man is serving 30 days in prison for public drunkenness for the third time in nine months. Prior to incarceration, he stayed at a homeless shelter or slept under an overpass. While in prison, he participated in an alcoholics anonymous (AA) group and substance abuse counseling. Once his sentence has been served and he is released from prison, what is the most likely outcome regarding further addiction treatment?

A. He will be court-ordered to receive treatment from the local mental health center
B. He will be court-ordered into an inpatient rehab facility
C. He will be released to a halfway house
D. He will continue AA groups in the community
E. He will receive no addiction treatment

30.5. A 34-year-old man who was diagnosed with schizophrenia enters outpatient treatment with a community psychiatry multidisciplinary team. He states that he has been homeless off and on since getting out of jail 3 weeks ago, where he was held on a trespassing charge. He has not been on medication since he was released. He has not been employed in the last 10 years. He previously worked at a warehouse stocking shelves and was fired because of symptom exacerbations. He says that his main priority is to be a good father to his 6-year-old son, who lives in the same city, but who he has not seen in over a year. What should be the major focus of communication by the team with the patient regarding the patient's treatment?

A. Securing stable housing
B. Decreasing the chance of rehospitalization
C. Restarting his medication
D. Reuniting him with his son
E. Helping him get a job

30.6. In the system of care model for children and adolescents with severe emotional disturbances, what is the unifying factor of the consortium of community agencies that participate in the patient's treatment?

A. All agencies share the same pool of government-provided resources
B. Team members are employed by the consortium, not the individual agencies
C. Agencies have a common plan of care for treatment of the child and their family
D. Representatives from each agency are present at each encounter with the patient

30.7. What is a characteristic of an assertive community treatment (ACT) team model that differentiates it from standard outpatient psychiatry multidisciplinary team treatment?

A. 24/7 team member availability to the patient
B. Assistance with job placement
C. A working relationship with other community agencies
D. Individualized treatment plans
E. A psychiatrist conducts evaluations and provides pharmacotherapy

ANSWERS

30.1. B. Preventing disease
Public health consists of organized community efforts with the goals of prevention of disease and promotion of health. Lobbying for government funds to support not-for-profit community health care delivery systems is necessary, but not a main mission of public health programs themselves. Similarly, training providers to work in the local area and increasing research are important, but not part of the main mission. (867)

30.2. D. The child will be seen by a psychiatrist at the school
In an ideal collaborative care model, a psychiatrist would be present at the school to serve as a consultant for the faculty and staff there. This psychiatrist would likely not work for the school full time, but may have weekly or monthly hours there. Another example of a collaborative care model would be to have a psychiatrist working in the same office as the pediatrician. However, this would add another step in getting the child evaluated, so it is not as ideal as an in-school psychiatrist. (867)

30.3. C. Selective
Screening every patient is an example of universal intervention, while attempting to prevent depression from occurring in those who may be at higher risk as indicated by the screening tool is an example of selective intervention. If some of the patients progress to develop depression, treatment would be an indicated intervention. A multimodal intervention would involve the patients, their families, peers, school, and the larger community in the intervention effort. (868)

30.4. E. He will receive no addiction treatment
For many low-income and/or minority individuals, the jail/prison system provides the most reliable access to mental health and addiction treatment. An overwhelming majority of individuals with addiction disorders will not receive steady addiction treatment once released from incarceration. (868)

30.5. D. Reuniting him with his son
The success of a public community psychiatry multidisciplinary team depends on successful, effective communication with the patient, with a focus on the patient's stated goals. This ensures that the treatment is patient centered and is most likely to lead to maximum engagement and buy-in by the patient to the services provided. As being a part of his son's life is his stated priority, that should be the focus of the team, which can point out that housing, symptom control, employment, and staying out of the hospital can greatly enhance the probability of him realizing his goal. (870)

30.6. C. Agencies have a common plan of care for treatment of the child and their family
The systems of care model consists of an interagency structure which can include child welfare, juvenile justice, the school system, and medical services which form a consortium to respond to the needs of the child and their family. The consortium agencies agree on a common plan of care and pool their resources to provide the most optimal treatment. Team members are employed by their respective agencies and come together, as needed, during patient and family encounters to care for the child and family. (871)

30.7. A. 24/7 team member availability to the patient
Both standard outpatient multidisciplinary treatment teams and ACT teams employ psychiatrists to evaluate and pharmacologically treat the patient. They also both develop individualized treatment plans based on patient goals, assist with job placement as needed, and can have a working relationship with other community agencies. A differentiating feature of an ACT team is the relatively small caseloads and 24/7 on-call availability of a member of the team to the patient. (871)

31

Global and Cultural Issues in Psychiatry

31.1. The World Health Organization estimates that more than what percentage of individuals worldwide develop at least one or more mental disorders over the course of their lifetime?

A. 5
B. 10
C. 25
D. 50
E. 70

31.2. Which are the most common demographics for a person who commits suicide in China?

A. Elderly male in a high socioeconomic class
B. Elderly female in a low socioeconomic class
C. Young female in a rural area
D. Young female in an urban area
E. Young male in an urban area

31.3. Which psychiatric disorder is rated among the most disabling in both developed and developing countries?

A. Attention deficit hyperactivity disorder
B. Bipolar disorder
C. Intermittent explosive disorder
D. Panic disorder
E. Specific phobia

31.4. Which disease is estimated to be the leading cause of disability for the future?

A. Cataracts
B. Cerebrovascular disorder
C. Generalized anxiety disorder
D. Human immunodeficiency virus/acquired immunodeficiency syndrome (HIV/AIDS)
E. Unipolar Depression

31.5. A patient with a mental illness and which of the following demographic factors is statistically speaking most likely to report feeling discriminated against?

A. A male in a rural area
B. A male in the social area
C. A woman in a rural area
D. A woman in the family setting
E. A woman in the job area

31.6. Even after controlling for substance use, patients with which of the following types of psychiatric disorders are at increased risk of diabetes, heart disease, gastrointestinal disorders, and malignant neoplasms?

A. Anxiety
B. Attention deficit
C. Eating
D. Personality
E. Psychotic

31.7. A strong prospective association exists between depression and which of the following medical illnesses?

A. Asthma
B. Irritable bowel disorder
C. Myocardial infarctions
D. Renal failure
E. Seizures

183

ANSWERS

31.1. C. 25
More than 25% of individuals worldwide develop one or more mental disorders in their lifetime. Depression and generalized anxiety disorder are the most prevalent diagnoses. Though disorders differ in prevalence depending on sex, there were no sex differences in the proportion of people having at least one mental disorder. (875)

31.2. B. Young female in a rural area
In China, suicide is the leading cause of death for people between 15 to 34 years old. China is the only country where suicide rates in women are consistently higher than those in men, especially in rural areas. (875)

31.3. B. Bipolar disorder
According to the Disorder-Specific Global Sheehan Disability Scale Ratings for commonly occurring mental and chronic physical disorders in developed and developing countries, bipolar disorder and depression are the top two mental disorders rated the highest for being severely disabling. (876)

31.4. D. HIV/AIDS
According to the DALY (Disability-adjusted life years) scale, for the year 2030, HIV/AIDS is the leading cause of disability at 12.1%. Depression comes in as the 2nd leading cause of disability at 5.7%. (877)

31.5. D. A woman in the family setting
A study carried out in India by the World Psychiatric Association (WPA) found that women and people living in urban areas were the most stigmatized. Men experienced more discrimination in the job area, whereas women experienced more discrimination within the family and social areas. (878)

31.6. E. Psychotic
Those with mental disorders have a higher prevalence of physical disease compared with the general population. Even after controlling for comorbid substance use disorders, those patients with psychotic disorders were found to be more likely than others to develop diabetes, hypertension, heart disease, asthma, gastrointestinal disorders, skin infections, malignant neoplasms, and acute respiratory disorders. (879)

31.7. C. Myocardial infarctions
A strong prospective association exists between depression and coronary heart disease, including fatal myocardial infarctions. It should also be noted though that after having a myocardial infarction, the risk of depression increases. (879)

D

Contributions from the Sciences and Social Sciences to Psychiatry

32

Normal Development and Aging

32.1. The embryo becomes a fetus by the end of which week of pregnancy?

A. 4
B. 8
C. 12
D. 16
E. 20

32.2. Which of the following is an important milestone that occurs around 16 to 20 weeks of pregnancy?

A. Beginning of the sucking reflex
B. Detection of fetal movement
C. Development of layers in the cerebral cortex
D. Smell development
E. Taste development

32.3. How does the developing fetal brain compare to the adult brain?

A. Apoptosis occurs more frequently
B. Cerebral cortex layers are more numerous
C. Increased number of neuronal connections occur
D. More neurons are generated
E. White matter is less sensitive to injury

32.4. An Obstetrics doctor (OB) brought up concerns of fetal growth delay and the mother was referred for a fetal echo and cardiac concerns were noted. At birth, examination of the infant is noted for small eyeballs, underdevelopment of the midface, and a thin upper lip, along with a large distance between the eyes. Which psychiatric disorder is this patient most likely at risk for later in childhood and adolescence?

A. Attention deficit hyperactivity disorder
B. Anxiety
C. Bipolar disorder
D. Feeding and eating disorders
E. Schizophrenia

32.5. Which reflex does not disappear until the 12th month of life?

A. Abdominal
B. Grasp
C. Knee
D. Plantar (Babinski)
E. Startle (Moro)

32.6. Which is the most common cause of malformations in the first year of life?

A. Autosomal genetic diseases
B. Chemical/drug exposures
C. Maternal endocrine diseases
D. Maternal infections
E. Preconception exposures

32.7. A mother expresses frustration that her 2-year-old cannot put on her shoes and struggles with feeding herself. During play, she can only build a tower of a few cubes and says "no" to her mother often and struggles with taking turns. Which of the following is the net most appropriate intervention by the psychiatrist?

A. Arrange more playdates to focus on turn-taking and playing with other children
B. Have the child evaluated by early intervention services
C. Reassurance that these behaviors are normal for her age and in another year, most of those milestones should be met
D. Recommend a private occupational therapy evaluation
E. Refer for parent management training to help the mother set up a behavioral chart to reinforce positive actions

32.8. An adult is making silly faces and tickling an infant. At which age should the infant be able to smile back?

A. Birth
B. 1 month
C. 4 months
D. 6 months
E. 10 months

32.9. At what maximum age should a child be able to understand complex sentences, pronouns, put two words together when speaking, and though not fully understandable, start to use three words together while speaking?

A. 1 year old
B. 1.5 years old
C. 2 years old
D. 3 years old
E. 4 years old

32.10. A child is detail oriented, very focused, and recently learned how to play checkers well. The child can understand that when his ice cube melts, the same amount of liquid is still present. Which developmental period has this child entered?

A. Sensorimotor
B. Preoperational
C. Preproduction
D. Concrete operational
E. Formal operational

32.11. What is the earliest age that infants can imitate facial movements of adult caregivers?

A. Birth
B. 3 weeks
C. 4 months
D. 6 months
E. 10 months

32.12. A 1- to 2-year-old is most likely to display which of the following emotional behaviors?

A. Altruism
B. Approval seeking
C. Competition
D. Self-regulation
E. Sensitivity to criticism

32.13. Which is a distinguishing factor between stranger anxiety versus separation anxiety?

A. Crying and clingy behavior
B. Developmental ability to distinguish caregiver from others
C. Exposures to multiple caregivers
D. Occurrence when the infant is still in the mother's arms
E. It starts later in infancy

32.14. A toddler looks back at his mother before going ahead and touching a dog in a park. This is an example of which of the following developmental concepts?

A. Insecure attachment
B. Object permeance
C. Secure attachment
D. Social referencing
E. Transitional object

32.15. Gender identity is thought to be fixed by which of the following age ranges?

A. 1 to 1.5 years old
B. 2 to 2.5 years old
C. 5 to 6 years old
D. 5 to 12.5 years old
E. 13 to 15 years old

32.16. Which is a common factor to children who experience imaginary companions?

A. Comorbid psychotic disorders
B. High intelligence
C. Nightmares
D. Occurrence most commonly during school age years
E. Onset around 6 to 8 years old

32.17. What is the typical focus of development for a middle aged child?

A. Distinguishing reality from fantasy
B. Idealizing the opposite-sex parent
C. Interest in relations outside of the family
D. Peer rivalry
E. Repression of sexual impulses

32.18. Which is characteristic of normal dreams for a 6-year-old?

A. Accompaniment by enuresis
B. Belief that they are real
C. Occurrence during stage 4 of sleep
D. Thinking they are shared by more than one person
E. Visions of being killed or injured

32.19. Children of divorced families have higher rates of which medical or psychiatric symptom?

A. Cluster A personality traits
B. Eating disorders
C. Psychosis
D. Seizures
E. Suicide

32.20. Aside from perception as having a high value to peers and family, which other factor is the most important correlate of having good self-esteem?

A. Academic achievement
B. Athletic abilities
C. High number of social media followers
D. Perception of attractive physical appearance
E. Musical abilities

32.21. After accidents, which of the following factors is the second leading cause of death among people aged 15 to 25 years?

A. Cancer
B. Eating disorders
C. Homicides
D. Substance use
E. Suicides

32.22. Which is an imminent warning sign of impending school violence?

A. Affiliation with gangs
B. Drug and alcohol use
C. Serious physical fights with peers or family
D. Social withdrawal
E. Threats of violence

32.23. A patient has been struggling with isolation, and is unable to help others, and contribute to society. Which developmental stage is the patient struggling with and at what stage of life is this typically found at?

A. Generativity versus stagnation; early adulthood
B. Generativity versus stagnation; middle adulthood
C. Identity formation versus diffusion; late adolescence
D. Integrity versus despair; late adulthood
E. Integrity versus. despair, middle adulthood

32.24. Which is a neuropsychiatric change associated with aging?

A. Intelligence quotient (IQ) slowly declines
B. Learning takes longer, but still occurs
C. Recognition of right answer on multiple choice tests declines
D. Transfer of information from short- to long-term memory increases
E. Verbal ability gradually declines

ANSWERS

32.1. B. 8
The prenatal period involves the development of the embryo and fetus. After implantation when the egg divides it becomes an embryo. Rapid growth occurs and by the end of 8 weeks, the embryo can be recognized as human and is referred to as a fetus. (883)

32.2. B. Detection of fetal movement
Women usually detect fetal movements between 16 to 20 weeks into the pregnancy. Taste and smell development occur in the fetus around 7 months. The sucking reflex typically does not appear until 28 weeks. The cerebral cortex layers typically don't appear until 6 months of pregnancy. (883, 884)

32.3. D. More neurons are generated
The fetus develops more neurons than it needs for adult life and pruning occurs to get rid of these neurons and apoptosis, or cell death occurs. White matter in the fetal brain, especially before 22 weeks, is more sensitive to damage, such as from hypoxia. At birth, the number of new neurons is negligible, and the branching of dendrites and new connections will occur afterward. The cerebral cortex does not begin to form layers until 6 months of pregnancy. (884, 885)

32.4. A. Attention deficit hyperactivity disorder
The infant above has symptoms characteristic of fetal alcohol syndrome. It affects about one-third of infants born to alcoholic women and symptoms include growth retardation and dysmorphic faces with microcephaly, hypertelorism (large distance between the eyes), microphthalmia (small eyeballs), short palpebral fissures, inner epicanthal folds, short palpebral fissures, short philtrum, thin upper lip, short, upturned notes, etc. Cardiac defects and central nervous system (CNS) manifestations, including seizures, are often present. Other psychiatric symptoms or central nervous system (CNS) manifestations include hyperactivity, attention deficit, and learning and intellectual disabilities. (886)

32.5. D. Plantar (Babinski)
Reflexes present at birth include rooting, grasp reflex, the plantar (Babinski), the knee and abdominal reflexes, and the startle (Moro) reflex along with the tonic neck reflex. In healthy children, by 4 months old, the grasp, startle, and tonic neck reflex disappear. It takes until 12 months for the Babinski reflex to disappear. (887)

32.6. A. Autosomal genetic diseases
Autosomal genetic diseases are thought to account for most of the malformations in the first year of life (15% to 20%). Cytogenetic or chromosomal abnormalities are thought to account for 5%. Maternal endocrine conditions (4%), maternal infections (3%), and chemicals, drugs, radiation, hyperthermia, and preconception exposures (<1%) are less common causes. (887)

32.7. C. Reassurance that these behaviors are normal for her age and in another year, most of those milestones should be met
At 2 years old, a toddler should be able to pull on simple clothing items and say "no" to their mother. Parallel play, in which they play side by side without interacting with other children is normal for this age. Typically, a 2-year-old can build a tower of six or seven cubes. By 3 years old, a child should be able to do the other things mentioned in the vignette such as put on shoes, feed themselves well, understand taking turns, and build a tower of more blocks (9 or 10) cubes. (888)

32.8. C. 4 months
While an endogenous smile can be noted at birth, the spontaneous social smile, or exogenous smile, does not typically occur until around 4 weeks of life. (888)

32.9. C. 2 years old
A 2-year-old should be able to put two words together for a simple utterance and start to use three-word telegraphic utterances, with only around half being intelligible. A 2-year-old should also refer to themselves by name. (889)

32.10. C. Concrete operational
The four Piaget states of cognitive development include the sensorimotor stage (birth to 2 years old), preoperational (2 to 7 years old), concrete operational (7 to 11 years old), and formal operational (11 to 19 years old). Preproduction is a stage of language, not cognitive development. Cognitive achievements in the concrete stage are highlighted above, including principles of reversibility (i.e., can play games backward and forward), conservation (i.e., can understand conservation of matter), and decentration (i.e., worrying about small details). (890)

32.11. B. 3 weeks
By as young as 3 weeks old, infants can imitate facial movements of adult caregivers. They can open their mouths and thrust their tongues when

adults do the same. By the third and fourth months, this behavior is easily elicited, and the exogenous social smile occurs. (890)

32.12. B. Approval seeking
In terms of emotional development, in early childhood (3 to 6 years old) a child can display empathy, and aggression turns into competition at this age. Self-regulation begins to occur, and children become less reactive. By 5 years old, children typically show sensitivity to criticism and care about the feelings of others. By middle childhood (7 to 11 years old), altruism can be displaced and the superego dominates. At 1 to 2 years old, some indications of empathy are starting, though attention seeking and the need for approval predominate. (891)

32.13. D. Occurrence when the infant is still in the mother's arms
Stranger anxiety is a developmentally normal fear that starts around 26 weeks of life, whereas separation anxiety typically begins later around 10 to 18 months. When babies are approached by strangers, they cry and cling to their mothers. Babies with only one caregiver are more likely to have stranger anxiety. Stranger anxiety occurs when the infant is in the mother's arms, whereas with separation anxiety, the anxiety occurs when the person the infant is attached to separates. (892)

32.14. D. Social referencing
Social referencing, typically occurring around 2 years of age, is when the child looks toward the parents and others for emotional cues as to how to respond to novel events. The child must have object permanence to be able to social reference. Transitional objects (as coined by Donald Winnicott), such as a teddy bear, for example, can offer a secure base as a child investigates the world around them. With secure attachment, children are better adjusted with few problems and receive more consistent and developmentally appropriate parenting. Signs of insecure attachment include being clingy and angry towards the parent, along with ambivalence and disorganization. It is often seen with neglectful parents. (893)

32.15. B. 2 to 2.5 years old
It used to be thought that gender identity, the conviction of being male or female, was a function of social learning. It is now known that rearing does not affect gender identity. Gender identity begins to manifest at 18 months and is typically fixed by 24 to 30 months old. (894)

32.16. B. High intelligence
Imaginary companions most commonly occur in the preschool years and are typically found in those with high intelligence. Typically, they disappear by age 12 years and occur in up to 50% of children. Though the significance is not clear, it is thought to reduce anxiety and the companions are typically described as friendly figures. (895)

32.17. C. Interest in relations outside of the family
During the middle years, age 6 to puberty, peer interactions assume significant importance. Interest in relationships outside of the family predominate during the middle years and the children form a special relationship with the same-sex parent and view them as a role model. Peer rivalry and struggles with aggressive impulses and taking turns typically occur in the preschool years. Distinguishing reality from fantasy and focusing on play is also characteristic of the preschool, not the middle years. The middle years typically were thought of as the latency period, including exploration of sexual play. It is now known that a considerable amount of sexual interest does occur throughout these years. (895)

32.18. E. Visions of being killed or injured
By 5 or 6 years old, children often dream of being killed or injured, fear of flying, being in cars, or of ghosts. At 5 years old, children realize their dreams are not real. At 3 years old, children believe their dreams are shared by more than one person. Sleep disorders, such as parasomnias and enuresis or bedwetting, though common are not part of normal dreaming and actually occur during stage 4 sleep when dreaming is minimal. (896)

32.19. E. Suicide
Children of divorced families have much higher suicide rates compared to intact families. Antisocial personality disorder, conduct disorder, and attention-deficit/hyperactivity disorder (ADHD) are more common in children in homes with absent fathers. Children from divorced homes have more struggles with academic achievement and social relations and are more withdrawn, lonely, anxious, and insecure. Aggression, especially onset boys is common. They also have higher rates of medical issues including injury, asthma, and headaches. (897)

32.20. D. Perception of attractive physical appearance

The most important correlates of a good self-esteem, a measure of one's sense of self-worth, has been shown to be one's perception of attractive physical appearance and high value to peers and family. Secondary features include academic achievement, athletic ability, and unique talents. Positive feedback from peers also contributes to self-esteem. In general, girls have more issues maintaining a positive self-esteem than boys do. (902)

32.21. C. Homicides

Violent crimes by young offenders are on the increase in the United States. Homicides are the second leading cause of death among people aged 15 to 25 years, with accidents being the first cause, and suicide the third. (903)

32.22. C. Serious physical fights with peers or family members

According to Center for Disease Control and Prevention (CDC), in 2010, approximately 2% of deaths occurred due to school violence. Imminent warning signs include serious physical fights with peers or family, severe destruction of property, serious rage, detailed threats of violence, poison, or firearms. Early warning signs include feelings of isolation or withdrawal, rejection, being a victim of violence, having a history of discipline problems, drug and alcohol (EtOH) use, gang affiliation, and threats of violence. (904)

32.23. B. Generativity versus stagnation; middle adulthood

Erikson described middle adulthood (40 to 65 years old) as being characterized by generativity or stagnation. The person can help guide future generations and improve society by helping others, being reactive, etc. or they can end up being stagnant and stop developing. They can end up feeling isolated and focusing on themselves and struggle more with old age. Integrity versus despair occurs in old age and involves the process of reviewing one's life and coming to a sense of peace with how one's life was lived and struggling to do so can cause despair. Identify formation versus diffusion is the developmental task Erikson described for adolescence through early adulthood. It involves defining a sense of self, belonging, hobbies, etc., and continued identify refinement. (909)

32.24. B. Learning takes longer, but still occurs

Neuropsychiatric changes with aging include it taking longer to learn new material but learning new information can still occur. IQ remains stable until 80 years old. Verbal ability is maintained with age in terms of memory, though encoding ability diminishes (i.e., transfer of short- to long-term memory and vice versa). Simple recall declines, though recognition of right answers on multiple choice tests remains intact with aging. (915)

33

Contributions from the Neurosciences

33.1. Which of the following phenomenon seen in individuals with schizophrenia is an endophenotype measure?

A. Auditory hallucinations
B. Ventricular enlargement
C. Anhedonia
D. Suicidal ideation
E. Thought blocking

33.2. What type of glial cell is responsible for removing cellular debris following neuronal death?

A. Astrocyte
B. Microglia
C. Oligodendrocyte
D. Schwann Cell

33.3. A 5-year-old boy is fascinated when he sits in a heated electric chair massager. He says in delight, "Mommy, it feels warm and it's shaking!" In what area of the brain do the neurons that carry the information regarding the boy's physical experience synapse?

A. Thalamus
B. Arcuate fasciculus
C. Hypothalamus
D. Pons
E. Spinal cord

33.4. A 30-month-old girl is playing with an electronic toy that asks her to identify the "blue triangle" from among other differently colored shapes. The part of the visual system that allows her to engage in this activity is in what area of the brain?

A. Parietal
B. Frontal
C. Occipital
D. Temporal

33.5. The first step in the processing of sound occurs in what structure of the auditory system?

A. Endolymph
B. Hair cells
C. Ossicles
D. Cochlear nerve
E. Tympanic membrane

33.6. A 79-year-old man is brought to the emergency department by emergency medical services (EMS). His wife reports that they were eating dinner 30 minutes ago when he began to slur his speech "and his arm drew up." She adds that the patient has hypertension but does not take his lisinopril. Vital signs are temperature 37.2 C (99 F), BP 210/120, pulse 110, and respirations 22. Physical examination reveals a clenched right fist. Right arm and wrist are flexed. Tendons are hyperreflexive. Head CT is pending. Which of the spinal tracts was most likely affected?

A. Spinothalamic
B. Corticospinal
C. Fasciculus cuneatus
D. Spinocerebellar
E. Fasciculus gracilis

33.7. A 42-year-old man presents to the neurology clinic for management of his movement disorder. Five years ago, he noticed that his arms were "drawing up and getting stiff," and he was stumbling and becoming clumsy. He also started having memory lapses and feelings of depression. Over time, he developed trouble with balance. Though he has some physical difficulty with speech, he can state that he is distressed by his word-finding difficulties and trouble focusing on tasks. His mother developed the same symptoms when she was in her 50s and died 20 years later. He is on sertraline for depression. Vitals signs are within normal limits. Physical examination is significant for rigidity in both arms with occasional involuntary writhing movements. A brain scan is most likely to show shrinkage of what brain structure?

A. Putamen
B. Caudate
C. Globus pallidus
D. Substantia nigra
E. Subthalamic nucleus

33.8. A 23-year-old man is walking home alone from work at night when he hears someone walk up behind him. He speeds up and notices that the footsteps speed up as well. He turns around and faces a man holding a knife and demanding his wallet. He starts breathing rapidly and notices his heart beating faster before he turns and sprints away. What brain center was responsible for his physiologic response to the situation?

A. Cerebellum
B. Primitive reflex circuit
C. Hypothalamus
D. Basal ganglia
E. Motor cortex

33.9. A 31-year-old professional football player undergoes neurocognitive testing following his second concussion in 3 months. He is given a computerized continuous performance test in which he is instructed to press the space bar on the keyboard every time the letter "X" flashes on the screen over a period of six, 5-minute trials. His results are in normal range during the first trial, but steadily diminish throughout the remainder of the testing. Damage to what lobe of the brain is the most likely cause for his performance?

A. Frontal
B. Occipital
C. Temporal
D. Parietal

33.10. A 54-year-old man is brought to the emergency department (ED) by EMS following a motor vehicle accident in which he sustained blunt-force head trauma. Prior to the accident, he had never been to the hospital and had no history of physical or mental illness. After an inpatient stay of several weeks due to cortical swelling and multiple bilateral leg fractures, he is discharged to a rehab facility to help with ambulation. Staff there describe him as "snappy, foulmouthed, and hateful." His family notes that he had always been known to be a mild-mannered, kind man who "never cursed a day in his life." Since discharge from the rehab facility 3 months ago, the behavior has continued. What is the most likely lobe of the brain that was affected in the car accident?

A. Frontal
B. Temporal
C. Parietal
D. Occipital

33.11. The rate of synaptogenesis is highest during what decade of life?

A. First
B. Second
C. Third
D. Fourth

33.12. A 20-base-pair gene strand of mRNA contains a substitution point mutation at the fifth base pair. A strand of miRNA is introduced to the mRNA and binds to it. What would be the expected effect of the miRNA on the mRNA strand?

A. It will repair the substitution
B. It will excise the substitution
C. It will silence the gene
D. It will upregulate gene expression
E. It will have no effect

33.13. Parents call EMS for their 36-year-old daughter, who they say has not left her room for 3 days, refusing to come out because she thinks the air in the rest of the house is poisoned. They are worried because she has not eaten anything and because she is "screaming half the night at people on TV." She is on haloperidol and quetiapine, "but she hasn't taken them in weeks. She refuses to take a long-acting injection. She's been on just about every medicine there is for hearing voices, but she never stays on anything for long." They report that she has been hospitalized 10 times for similar symptoms over the last 10 years. She has no medical illnesses. They state that her weight goes up and down depending on the medication she is on. The patient is most likely to have decreased volume of what brain structure?

A. Lateral ventricles
B. Third ventricle
C. Hippocampus
D. Amygdala
E. Hypothalamus

33.14. Compared to that of a child without autism spectrum disorder (ASD), the brain growth of a child with ASD shows what characteristic?

A. Negligible growth during the first year followed by normal growth afterward
B. Growth during the first year, followed by a plateau for the next 2 years
C. Accelerated growth from the end of the first year to age 4 years
D. Linear, steady growth throughout childhood until adolescence
E. Growth during the first 5 years followed by slow cortical shrinking

33.15. The cell bodies of serotonergic nuclei reside in what brain structure?

A. Ventral tegmental area
B. Raphe nuclei
C. Locus ceruleus
D. Basal forebrain complex
E. Tuberomammillary nucleus

33.16. A 45-year-old man who has been addicted to methamphetamine for the past 7 months tells other members in a drug abuse support group that decreasing his drug use is difficult. "Using just makes me feel good, you know? The feeling of that high is what keeps me coming back for more." What dopamine brain pathway is most responsible for the feelings he is describing?

A. Mesolimbic
B. Mesocortical
C. Mesoaccumbens
D. Tuberohypophyseal
E. Nigrostriatal

33.17. Dopamine is synthesized from what amino acid?

A. Tryptophan
B. Tyrosine
C. Histidine
D. Glycine
E. Glutamic acid

33.18. A 62-year-old man with a 30-year history of drinking three to five beers a day would be expected to have what profile of N-methyl-D-aspartate (NMDA) and gamma-aminobutyric acid (GABA) receptor regulation?

	GABA	NMDA
A.	Upregulation	Upregulation
B.	Upregulation	Downregulation
C.	Downregulation	Downregulation
D.	Downregulation	Upregulation

33.19. A 23-year-old woman presents to the outpatient clinic with complaints of "not wanting to do anything or eat anything" and feeling "down" for the past 4 weeks. She has been waking up 2 hours before her alarm goes off and cannot return to sleep. She used to go out with friends but has avoided talking with them for the past 3 weeks because "I just don't have the energy." Some days she does not go to work because she is too tired. She reports trouble focusing. She denies suicidal ideation. She has no chronic illnesses and is on no medications. Vital signs are within normal limits. Physical examination is noncontributory. On mental status examination, she gives her mood as "down, blah." What brain pathway structures are most likely to be affected?

A. Hypothalamus, anterior pituitary gland, adrenal gland
B. Hippocampus, amygdala, hypothalamus, and thalamus
C. Hippocampal formation, fornix, mammillary bodies, anterior thalamus, posterior cingulate gyrus
D. Suprachiasmatic nucleus, pineal gland, retinohypothalamic tract, superior cervical ganglia

33.20. A 44-year-old woman and her husband present to the urgent care clinic. She has a chief complaint of, "I can't breathe!" She states that she has had more than 10 episodes of shortness of breath over the last 3 months during which "my heart feels like it's beating out of my chest," and "I'm shaking and pouring with sweat." The first time it occurred, she thought she was having an allergic reaction to a new food she had tried, but a rechallenge of that food did not produce the same results. The symptoms start abruptly and peak in about 15 minutes. The current episode began 2 minutes ago. She wanted her husband to accompany her to "see that this is real and that I'm not just going crazy, which is how I feel when this happens." She worries that she will have an episode one day at work and "I'll get fired," so she has been working from home as much as her boss will allow. After several minutes, her elevated BP and pulse return to normal limits, and she is no longer acutely distressed. What neuropeptide has been associated with her condition?

A. Neurotensin
B. Cholecystokinin
C. Substance P
D. Neuropeptide Y
E. Thyrotropin-releasing hormone

33.21. A 33-year-old woman presents to the outpatient clinic with a complaint of extreme fatigue, poor appetite, and weight loss of 20 pounds over the past 3 months. She notes that picking up her 4-month-old infant has gotten progressively more difficult over the past month. In addition to feeling weak, she reports muscle pain. She has difficulty getting to sleep most nights. On the infrequent occasions when she can sleep longer, fatigue is unchanged. "I don't want to do anything, and I don't have the energy for it." She has also tried making her favorite foods, "but I'm just not hungry." When she eats, she tends to crave salty foods. She has not had these symptoms before. Vital signs are normal. BMI is in the 30th percentile. Physical examination reveals hyperpigmentation of her elbows, face, and neck. What treatment will be most helpful for her symptoms of apathy, decreased appetite, impaired sleep, and fatigue?

A. Mirtazapine
B. Sleep hygiene
C. Cortisone
D. A high-salt diet
E. Cannabidiol

33.22. What psychiatric disorder has the most evidence for the interaction between the immune system and the nervous system?

A. Major depression
B. Bipolar disorder
C. Schizophrenia
D. Autism
E. Alzheimer disease

33.23. Psychotherapy focused on what subject matter has been shown to serve as a protective factor against stress-induced immune responses?

A. Relaxation techniques
B. Medication adherence
C. Internal locus of control
D. Positive thinking
E. Connection between mind and body

33.24. A researcher studies an uncommon disease found in several blood-related members of a family and determines that the relative risk is 1.2. How should this figure be interpreted?

A. A family member exposed to the conditions for the disease has a 20% chance of developing it
B. The disease is 20% more likely to have a genetic etiology
C. Any family member has a 20% chance of developing the disease
D. 20% of the family members exposed to the conditions for the disease will develop it
E. The disease will affect 20% of any given set of family members

33.25. Several residents in a small town have been diagnosed with Disease X. A researcher suspects that the disease may be correlated with certain genetic variations. What type of study would best test the researcher's hypothesis?

A. Pedigree analysis
B. Sib-pair analysis
C. Linkage
D. Association

33.26. What is a major barrier to performing genetic mapping studies for psychiatric illnesses as opposed to other medical illnesses?

A. Psychiatric illnesses are less heritable than other medical illnesses
B. Many antipsychotic medications interfere with DNA sample viability
C. There are fewer individuals with psychiatric than nonpsychiatric illnesses
D. Individuals with psychiatric illness often cannot give informed consent
E. Defining and assessing phenotypes of psychiatric illnesses is inconsistent

33.27. Association studies discovered an association between the e4 allele of the *apolipoprotein E* gene and the development of what psychiatric illness?

A. Alzheimer disease
B. Autism
C. Bipolar disorder
D. Fragile X
E. Schizophrenia

33.28. Linkage studies have shown consistent evidence for contribution to autism by alleles of what chromosome?

A. X
B. 7
C. 15
D. 22

33.29. A 7-year-old girl presents to the outpatient clinic for an EEG as part of an evaluation for seizures. Her teachers report multiple instances a day of "zoning out" for several seconds, even while she is actively talking. Her parents have noticed the same behavior at home for the last 4 weeks. After a few seconds, she resumes talking or whatever behavior in which she had been engaged. She is on fexofenadine for seasonal allergies which were diagnosed a year ago. Birth and postnatal histories reveal no abnormalities. She is on no medications. Vital signs are within normal limits. Forty-five minutes of EEG recordings show no abnormal tracings. What is the next step in the EEG evaluation?

A. Give a bolus of insulin to induce a seizure
B. Have her return for another EEG after being off fexofenadine for a week
C. Have her hyperventilate for 3 minutes
D. Continue the EEG for another 45 minutes
E. End the study with a conclusion that there is no EEG evidence for seizures

33.30. The presence of what waveform during a normal waking EEG is indicative of a possible physiologic abnormality?

A. Alpha
B. Beta
C. Delta
D. Theta

33.31. A 43-year-old man is being evaluated for obstructive sleep apnea. He is diagnosed with schizophrenia, for which he is taking aripiprazole long-acting injection, and panic disorder, for which he takes escitalopram and alprazolam as needed. He presents for an overnight polysomnogram and tells the technician that he had to take alprazolam because he was nervous about the study. He has been taking the escitalopram daily and his last injection of aripiprazole was 2 weeks ago. He is on no other medications and has no other illnesses. What changes can be expected on his EEG based on his medication regimen?

A. No significant changes
B. Increased delta activity
C. Increased beta activity
D. Increased alpha activity
E. Increased theta activity

ANSWERS

33.1. B. Ventricular enlargement
An endophenotype is an internal phenotype based on neuropsychological, neuroanatomical, cognitive, neurophysiologic, biochemical, and brain imaging data. To qualify as an endophenotype, the biologic marker associated with illness in the population must be heritable, seen in people with and without the active illness (which rules out all answer choices but ventricular enlargement), co-segregates with illness within families, and is present at a higher rate in unaffected family members than in the general population. Endophenotypes are not synonymous with symptoms (which also eliminates all answer choices except for ventricular enlargement). The use of endophenotypes in psychiatric studies assumes that a type of biologic marker is simpler to detect and be determined by fewer genes than that of a whole disease, such as schizophrenia. (923)

33.2. B. Microglia
Astrocytes, the most common type of glial cell, serve as nutrition for neurons, deactivate certain neurotransmitters and integrate with the blood–brain barrier. Dendrocytes and Schwann cells create myelin sheaths in the central and peripheral nervous systems, respectively. Microglia are involved in removing cellular debris after neuronal death. (924)

33.3. A. Thalamus
The signals for pain, temperature, coarse touch, and deep pressure travel along the spinothalamic tract while the signals for proprioception, vibration, and light touch travel along the fasciculus gracilis and cuneatus. All neurons for all somatosensory modalities synapse in the thalamus. However, had this been a reflex arc, such as would occur with the child placing his hand on a hot stove and jerking it away, the synapse would be in the spinal cord. (925)

33.4. D. Temporal
The primary visual cortex cells, located in the occipital lobe, respond specifically to line orientation. Those cells project to the secondary visual cortex, also in the occipital lobe, which responds to angles and movement of lines. The temporal lobe detects shape, form, and color while the parietal lobe detects motion, location, and distance. (926)

33.5. E. Tympanic membrane
The processing of sound begins with changes in ambient air pressure, which are picked up by the tympanic membrane, which then vibrates. The vibrations are transmitted to the ossicles, endolymph of the cochlear spiral, and cilia on hair cells which generate neuronal impulses that travel to the cochlear nerve. (927)

33.6. B. Corticospinal
The patient has most likely suffered a stroke which affected the corticospinal tract. The limb spasticity and hyperreflexia indicate an upper motor neuron lesion in a descending tract. The corticospinal tract, which controls fine motor movements, is the only descending one. The others are ascending. Spasticity usually occurs more often in the upper limbs than the lower ones, and more often following a hemorrhagic stroke than an ischemic one. (928, 929)

33.7. B. Caudate
The caudate shrinks in Huntington disease, which is what this patient has. The substantia nigra is affected in Parkinson disease. Lesions in the subthalamic nucleus can lead to intense ballistic movements, which are different than the rigidity and choreiform movements of Huntington. Damage to the globus pallidus can lead to dystonic posturing and limb flapping. (929)

33.8. C. Hypothalamus
The hypothalamus is responsible for mediating the fight or flight response to danger through the autonomic motor system. This involves an increased heart rate, shunting of blood away from the viscera, and increased respirations. The basal ganglia appear to mediate postural tone. The primitive reflex circuit mediates motor movement without immediate conscious awareness, such as quickly pulling a hand away from a hot stove. The motor cortex cells cause contraction of individual muscles. The cerebellum modulates muscle tone. (929, 930)

33.9. A. Frontal
Continuous performance tests measure attention and are used at times to aid in the diagnosis of attention-deficit hyperactivity disorder (ADHD). An intact right frontal lobe is necessary to do well on this test. Of note, there have not been consistent pathologic findings in individuals with ADHD who have no known brain injury. (932)

33.10. A. Frontal
The frontal lobe is responsible for executive functions such as cognition, personality, and social behavior. Damage to this lobe can therefore lead to personality change, such as from a preinjury mild-mannered person to a postinjury difficult and

abusive person. Temporal lobe damage can result in, among other things, difficulty with words, attention, memory, and identification of objects. Parietal lobe damage can result in difficulty drawing objects, distinguishing left from right, difficulty reading, and spatial disorientation. Occipital lobe damage can lead to vision defects and inability to recognize written words. (935)

33.11. A. First
Synaptogenesis peaks within the first 2 years of life and continues at its highest rate during the first 10 years. Though there have been recent discoveries of neurogenesis in specific brain regions in adults, it is well below the amount seen in young children. (936)

33.12. C. It will silence the gene
A purpose of miRNA is to regulate gene expression through RNA silencing by cleaving the target mRNA. miRNA therefore downregulates, not upregulates, gene expression. Repair proteins, not miRNA, excise bases. (946)

33.13. C. Hippocampus
Neuroimaging studies have shown decreased volume of the prefrontal cortex and hippocampus in the brains of people with schizophrenia. In contrast, the ventricles are enlarged. Interestingly, neuroimaging does not show signs of neurodegeneration. (950)

33.14. C. Accelerated growth from the end of the first year to age 4 years
The brain doubles in size in the first year, reaches 80% of its adult size by age 3, and 90% of its adult size by age 5. The brains of children with ASD most likely start with average size at birth, then grow at an accelerated rate between the end of the first year and ages 2 to 4 years. Most of the differences are seen in the frontal and parietal cortex, cerebellar hemispheres, and amygdala. The mechanism for this difference is not currently known. (951)

33.15. B. Raphe nuclei
Serotonergic nuclei cell bodies are found in the midline raphe nuclei of the brainstem. The rostral raphe nuclei send projections up throughout the brain, while the caudal raphe nuclei send projections down to the medulla, cerebellum, and spinal cord. The ventral tegmental area is where, along with the substantia nigra, dopamine neurons reside. Norepinephrine-producing neurons are in the locus ceruleus and lateral tegmental noradrenergic nuclei. The basal forebrain and mesopontine complexes are where acetylcholine projection neurons are found. Histaminergic cell bodies are located in the tuberomammillary nucleus. (954–956)

33.16. C. Mesoaccumbens
The mesoaccumbens dopamine pathway plays a central role in the feelings of reward and pleasure and is activated by drugs of abuse. The mesolimbic pathway is believed to mediate positive symptoms of schizophrenia. The mesocortical pathway is believed to play a role in negative symptoms of schizophrenia. The tuberohypophyseal system mediates prolactin release, and the nigrostriatal pathway modulates motor control. (955)

33.17. B. Tyrosine
Dopamine, like norepinephrine and epinephrine, is a catecholamine, all of which are synthesized from the amino acid tyrosine. Serotonin is synthesized from tryptophan, while histamine is synthesized from histidine. GABA is synthesized from glutamic acid. Glycine is both an amino acid and inhibitory neurotransmitter. (957–958, 962, 963)

33.18. D. GABA Downregulation, NMDA Upregulation
Long-term ethanol use results in the downregulation of GABA receptors and upregulation of NMDA receptors. The latter leaves the patient in a hyperexcitable state in the case of abrupt alcohol discontinuation, which can contribute to delirium tremens. (964)

33.19. A. Hypothalamus, anterior pituitary gland, adrenal gland
A consistent finding in major depressive disorder is hyperactivity of the hypothalamic pituitary adrenal axis (HPA), which consists of the hypothalamus, anterior pituitary gland, and adrenal gland. The hyperactivity leads to hypercortisolemia and resistance to dexamethasone suppression of cortisol secretion. The hippocampus, amygdala, thalamus, and hypothalamus form the limbic system. The addition of the fornix, mammillary bodies, and posterior cingulate gyrus form the Papez circuit, which mediates fear and aggression, feeding, and other homeostatic activities. The suprachiasmatic nucleus, superior cervical ganglia, retinohypothalamic tract, and pineal gland mediate the release and feedback loop of melatonin. (934, 968, 980)

33.20. B. Cholecystokinin
Cholecystokinin is associated with panic disorder, which is this patient's diagnosis. Neurotensin is associated with schizophrenia. Substance P and neuropeptide Y may play a role in posttraumatic

stress disorder (PTSD) and major depression. Thyrotropin-releasing hormone is associated with depression. (968–970)

33.21. C. Cortisone
The patient is displaying signs and symptoms of primary adrenal insufficiency, or Addison disease. The illness has several psychiatric/behavioral manifestations such as apathy, impaired sleep, fatigue, and decreased appetite. Because these symptoms are secondary to the underlying cause, she should be treated with steroids such as cortisone as opposed to antidepressants or therapy. Though getting enough salt in the diet is helpful, it will not solve the underlying problem. (980)

33.22. A. Major depression
Major depression has years of data showing an interaction with the immune system through a decrease in immunocompetence, and most recently, inflammatory activation. There are now several studies showing that bipolar disorder, particularly mania, can lead to increased plasma concentrations of inflammatory cytokines. Schizophrenia has also been associated with immune system activation. The relationship between autism and immune abnormalities has not been substantiated. There is emerging evidence for a link between Alzheimer disease and an immune response. (985, 986)

33.23. C. Internal locus of control
The ability to see stressors as somewhat under one's control (internal vs. external locus of control) has been shown to be protective against stress-induced immune alterations. This can be accomplished through reframing techniques in cognitive behavioral therapy. Group therapy can provide social support, which has also been identified as a protective factor. (986)

33.24. B. The disease is 20% more likely to have a genetic etiology
Relative risk is the rate of occurrence of a disease among family members of an affected individual divided by the rate of occurrence in the general population. If the number is greater than one, the disease occurs more often in the family than it does in the general population. Therefore, the disease is more likely to be genetic. In this case, the disease is 20% more likely to have a genetic contribution. (987, 988)

33.25. D. Association
An association study examines whether or not a certain allele occurs more frequently than expected in affected individuals in a population. The researcher will collect DNA samples from those with Disease X and those without, then look for certain single-nucleotide polymorphisms (SNPs) to see if they occur significantly more frequently in those with the disease phenotype. If they do, the SNPs are associated with the disease. Linkage studies attempt to find the relationship between a genetic variation and a disease, but within a family or families, not compared to a population. Sib-pair analysis compares the frequency of a trait between siblings to that expected in a random segregation. A pedigree analysis determines if two or more genetic loci are cosegregating within a pedigree. (989, 990)

33.26. E. Defining and assessing phenotypes of psychiatric illnesses is inconsistent
Genetic mapping studies depend on consistent phenotyping algorithms. Psychiatric illnesses are diagnosed most often using the DSM-5-TR, which depends on subjective clinical evaluation and leads to less interrater reliability and variable assignment of participants to a certain disease phenotype. In addition, because the DSM-5-TR is menu based, individuals with the same disease phenotype can have different sets of symptoms, which may have different genetic etiologies. Psychiatric illnesses are among the most common conditions affecting individuals of all ages. Antipsychotic medications do not change DNA sample viability. Psychiatric illnesses do not alter most people's ability to give informed consent to participate in studies, range in heritability, and are often multifactorial, just as most other medical illnesses are. Even if they were not, the purpose of mapping studies is to look for genetic contributors to the disease. (991)

33.27. A. Alzheimer disease
The *apoE-e4* allele has been established through genome-wide association studies as being linked to the development of late-onset Alzheimer disease. The GRB-associated binding protein 2 (*GAB2*) allele has also been shown to increase the risk of developing the disease. (994)

33.28. B. 7
Chromosome 7q has shown the most consistent evidence for linkage in autism families. Genes include *RELN* on chromosome 7q and *WNT2* on 7q31. The *FMR1* gene on the X chromosome is linked to Fragile X syndrome. Chromosome 15q11-13 plays a vital role in Angelman and Prader–Willi syndromes, but has not shown strong support for

autism. There has been a small amount of linkage between autism and the *SHANK3* gene on chromosome 22q13. (994, 995)

33.29. C. Have her hyperventilate for 3 minutes
In addition to photic stimulation, hyperventilation is used to increase the probability that abnormal discharges will occur. This is done by having the patient take exaggerated deep breaths for 1 to 4 minutes, and is considered one of the safest methods for EEG activation. Barring a contraindication for someone with cardiopulmonary disease or cerebrovascular pathophysiology, this activation technique would be tried before ending the evaluation. Insulin therapy was used prior to ECT to cause therapeutic seizures and has no place in current psychiatric treatment. Fexofenadine is not known to alter EEG findings. (998)

33.30. C. Delta
Alpha waves are the most common waveform seen during a normal awake EEG with the eyes closed. Fast-frequency *beta waves* can also be seen in awake EEGs. *Theta waves* are seen mostly in the drowsy state, though they can appear sporadically in the wake state. Excessive appearances of theta should raise suspicion for a pathophysiologic process. *Delta waves* should only be seen during deep sleep and should not be present during a normal awake EEG. (998, 999)

33.31. C. Increased beta activity
Some psychotropic medications produce EEG changes, but usually not at nontoxic doses. Benzodiazepines are an exception, and always generate an increase in beta activity. (999)

34

Contributions from the Behavioral and Social Sciences

34.1. A 7-year-old boy is shown two identical glasses of water. When asked which glass has more water, he says they have the same amount. The water in one glass is then poured into a taller, thinner glass in front of him. When asked which glass has more water, he says the taller glass. The water in the tall glass is poured back into the original glass, and he says the amount of water in the two glasses is the same. What cognitive development skill has the child not yet achieved?

A. Inductive reasoning
B. Deductive reasoning
C. Reversibility
D. Conservation
E. Operational thought

34.2. A 6-month-old child is continuously amused when her father places his hands in front of his face, then moves them to reveal his face. This goes on for a full minute, after which the father is exasperated with the child wanting to repeat the game. When he does the same actions a month later, his daughter shows little interest. What is the most likely explanation for the child's change in reaction?

A. The child has become habituated to the game with her father but would engage with her mother
B. The child is no longer able to pay attention to one stimulus for that length of time
C. The child is now able to crawl away and seek novel stimulation
D. The child realizes her father is still there even when his hands are closed
E. The child now experiences the game as frightening instead of amusing

34.3. After several weeks of therapy, a patient and therapist discover the patient's core belief of "I'm a failure." They are most likely engaging in what psychotherapeutic modality?

A. Psychodynamic psychotherapy
B. Supportive therapy
C. Interpersonal therapy
D. Cognitive therapy
E. Dialectical behavior therapy

34.4. Much like monkeys separated from their mothers and isolated at birth, babies who were separated from their mothers and placed in a hospital or other institution for prolonged periods of time eventually demonstrated what behavioral response?

A. Anger
B. Hyperactivity
C. Acting out
D. Withdrawal
E. Anxiety

34.5. A 60-year-old man starts a new oral medication for cancer treatment that he is supposed to take every morning with food. On the first morning, he takes the medication as he reads the newspaper, and 5 minutes later starts to retch and vomit. This occurs every day of the 30 days he is on the medication. As he walks to the store one afternoon, he passes a newspaper stand and vomits. The newspaper represents what element in classical (Pavlovian) conditioning?

A. Conditioned response
B. Conditioned stimulus
C. Unconditioned response
D. Unconditioned stimulus

203

34.6. A 13-year-old girl presents with her mother to the outpatient clinic for a routine physical examination. While alone with the doctor, she talks about how her mother "nags me all the time about doing my homework. I tell her I'm going to do it eventually, but she keeps bothering me until I finally do it just to get her to be quiet." The child's mother is training her daughter by what method of operant conditioning?

A. Positive reinforcement
B. Negative reinforcement
C. Positive punishment
D. Negative punishment

34.7. A 17-year-old girl who was diagnosed with social anxiety disorder a week ago comes to the outpatient clinic for therapy. She is afraid to shake hands with others because she fears she will "catch a disease from their germs." She describes a racing pulse, sweaty palms, feeling like she will vomit, and shortness of breath "when I even think about touching someone else." The therapist teaches her how to engage in deep breathing, then has her imagine shaking hands with someone else. As her anxiety builds, the therapist guides her through the breathing techniques. This progresses to her watching videos of people shaking hands, followed by shaking hands with gloves on, to finally shaking hands without gloves, while pairing the anxiety with deep breathing each time. What technique is being used to decrease her anxiety?

A. Extinction
B. Preparedness
C. State-dependent learning
D. Reinstatement
E. Counterconditioning

34.8. Parents wish to increase the frequency of their 14-year-old son cleaning his room and decide to use a reinforcer of allowing an extra 30 minutes of video game time before bed. Which reinforcement schedule is most likely to result in the highest number of times he cleans his room?

A. Rewarding him every seventh time he cleans the room
B. Rewarding him on average every seventh time, but varying the number of times needed
C. Rewarding him once every 7 days
D. Rewarding him on average every 7 days, but varying the number of days

34.9. A 7-year-old boy tells his parents that he does not want to eat his vegetables, but instead would rather have ice cream. They try to convince him to eat the vegetables, but he refuses. Using the Premack principle, how should the parents respond to get him to engage in the desired behavior?

A. Make him stay at the table until he eats his vegetables
B. Stop saying anything about the situation and carry on with the meal
C. Tell him he can have ice cream once he eats his vegetables
D. Tell him he cannot have ice cream today, but that he possibly can tomorrow
E. Ask him to eat just half the amount of the vegetables

34.10. A 45-year-old man reports to his supervisor for his quarterly performance review. Despite meeting his sales goals, he is yelled at by his boss, who is known to be unusually harsh. He increases his sales for the next quarter and experiences the same result by his boss. The treatment by his boss continues for the next three quarters. He feels demoralized, and his production drops to the point that he no longer meets his goals. The man is then transferred to a new boss. According to learned helplessness, how will the man most likely perform prior to his next review?

A. He will sell just enough to meet the goal
B. He will sell more than he ever has
C. His sales will remain subpar
D. His sales will drop substantially

34.11. A 25-year-old man presents to the emergency department (ED) one evening by emergency medical services (EMS) following an accident in which the all-terrain vehicle he was riding flipped over. He was thrown backward from the vehicle, landed on his head and lost consciousness. He has no prior medical illnesses and is on no medications. He is a graduate student at the local university. A head CT in the ED shows a lesion in the medial portion of the temporal lobe. When asked if he remembers the accident, he says he does not. He is likely to have difficulty answering which of the following memory questions?

A. "What is your birthdate?"
B. "Can you repeat these three words? Flag, ball, tree."
C. "Who was the first president of the United States?"
D. "What did you have for lunch this afternoon?"
E. "What are you studying in school?"

34.12. Two friends recount during a conversation where they were and what they were doing on 9/11/2011 when they learned that the Twin Towers fell in the United States. They were both in their 20s at the time and recall the disbelief upon first hearing the news. One of them states that she was driving to work, talking with her mother on the phone about the next family vacation. The other states that he was in his physiology class, listening to his professor talk about the heart. Besides the hippocampus, what brain structure is activated in the production of the memories of this event as compared to memories of routine events?

A. Amygdala
B. Dentate gyrus
C. Subiculum
D. Parahippocampal cortex
E. Entorhinal cortex

34.13. Amnesia due to Korsakoff syndrome results from alcoholic damage and thiamine deficiency to the frontal lobe and what other region of the brain?

A. Telencephalon
B. Diencephalon
C. Metencephalon
D. Mesencephalon
E. Myelencephalon

34.14. A person with severe amnesia would be expected to be able to remember which of the following?

A. The name of their spouse
B. How to get from their house to their favorite store
C. The melody of their favorite song
D. How to ride a bicycle
E. What they did last New Year's Eve

34.15. A 40-year-old female with amnesia is shown a picture of a woman in a bright red dress holding an umbrella on a rainy day. Also in the scene is a lake with ducks and a boat in the distance. The next day, she is asked to read out loud a set of words as quickly as possible. The set includes the words "duck," "umbrella," and "dress." A patient without amnesia would read words represented in the picture more quickly than neutral words, and remember being shown the picture. How will this patient most likely perform?

	Quicker reading speed	Remember picture
A.	Yes	No
B.	Yes	Yes
C.	No	Yes
D.	No	No

34.16. A 45-year-old man presents to the outpatient clinic with a complaint of difficulty remembering names, facts, and events. He states that this has been a problem "for as long as I can remember." He works as a welder and denies that the memory problems impact his job. "It's just embarrassing to forget things and it bothers me." He has no chronic medical illnesses and is on no prescription medications. He takes over-the-counter ginkgo biloba "because I heard it might help with memory." Vital signs are within normal limits. Body mass index (BMI) is 31. Physical examination is noncontributory. The physician orders a memory assessment, which should also include what test?

A. Visual field studies
B. Audiologic examination
C. Polysomnogram
D. Intellectual function
E. Adaptive functioning

34.17. A researcher wishes to assess a person's ability to learn new information, and designs a test that involves the participant trying to remember a string of words. What would be a necessary part of the testing procedure for it to be sensitive to detecting deficits in new learning?

A. Distracting the test taker between the learning and recall phases of the test
B. Ensuring the test taker knows the meaning of the words used in the test
C. Consistency in the number of syllables in each word used in the test
D. Presenting words with at least a 5-second pause between them
E. Presenting the words both visually and aurally

34.18. In self-reports of memory difficulty, how do patients with depression report their performance with new learning capacity and immediate and remote recall?

	New learning	Immediate	Remote
A.	Impaired	Normal	Normal
B.	Normal	Impaired	Normal
C.	Normal	Normal	Impaired
D.	Impaired	Impaired	Normal
E.	Normal	Impaired	Impaired
F.	Impaired	Normal	Impaired
G.	Impaired	Impaired	Impaired

34.19. A 56-year-old man presents to the emergency department (ED) with his wife who reports that her husband was accused of embezzling at his job a month ago, and that he has a court hearing tomorrow. She states that they were walking to the car when he slipped on a patch of ice, hit his head, and blacked out. "When he came to, he couldn't remember anything, not even who I was, and we've been married for 30 years!" The man tells the physician that he does not know where he is and does not know the lady who brought him to the ED. What question should the examiner ask that would lead to the most likely diagnosis?

A. "What is your name?"
B. "Who is the lady with you today?"
C. "Who was the first president of the United States?"
D. "Where were you born?"
E. "Where do you work?"

34.20. A 50-year-old woman who is president of a major manufacturing company starts a mentorship program for early-career female managers with a goal of "getting more women into the top positions in business." According to Erik Erikson's model, she is working on what developmental task?

A. Avoiding isolation
B. Mastering integrity
C. Avoiding despair
D. Mastering generativity
E. Mastering intimacy

34.21. What part of the brain is most responsible for feelings of attachment and pairing meaning to past experiences?

A. Medial temporal lobe
B. Amygdala
C. Anterior cingulate gyrus
D. Hippocampus
E. Diencephalon

34.22. A 30-year-old man who has constant urges to steal to "see if I can get away with it" applies for a job with a department store chain to devise ways to decrease vulnerability to merchandise theft. This is an example of what defense mechanism?

A. Repression
B. Altruism
C. Sublimation
D. Displacement
E. Suppression

34.23. Which of the following defense mechanisms is considered immature?

A. Humor
B. Sublimation
C. Suppression
D. Anticipation
E. Projection

34.24. In a famous ethology experiment, researcher Konrad Lentz discovered that if he was the first moving object a newly hatched gosling saw, the gosling responded to him as if he were its mother. This is an example of what ethologic concept?

A. Displacement activity
B. Priming
C. Redirection activity
D. Instinct
E. Imprinting

34.25. In ethologic studies, young rhesus monkeys who were fearful and anxious after being socially isolated or separated showed the strongest response to what source of comfort?

A. Food and nourishment
B. Visual stimulation
C. Aural stimulation
D. Physical touch
E. Increased physical space

34.26. The administration of the drug reserpine in both animals and humans can produce symptoms of what psychiatric illness?

A. Anxiety
B. Psychosis
C. Depression
D. Mania
E. Delirium

34.27. A 57-year-old man presents to the outpatient clinic with a complaint of feeling "tired and run down, and I have headaches and stomach aches every night." He has felt this way for the past 3 weeks, and denies having these symptoms together for this amount of time before. He works two jobs, one from the morning to afternoon as a clerk at an office supply store, and one in the late afternoon to late night as a security guard in a mall. He takes lisinopril for hypertension diagnosed 3 years ago. When the physician comments on stress from work being a contributing factor, he states that he is a first-generation immigrant, and that people in his home country are used to his work hours. How should the physician respond?

A. "I really think you're worn out from constant work."
B. "Let's get some lab work to help see what's going on."
C. "What do you think is causing your symptoms?"
D. "Would you like to get a second opinion?"
E. "Is everyone in your home country tired with headaches?"

34.28. Data from the National Comorbidity Study shows that, in comparison to Whites, African Americans have what relative risk for developing substance use, anxiety, and depressive disorders and what degree of persistence once a mental illness is developed?

	Relative risk	Persistence
A.	Lower	Lower
B.	Lower	Higher
C.	Higher	Lower
D.	Higher	Higher

34.29. A 17-year-old girl is preparing her Indian dress for her senior prom. Her great-grandparents emigrated from India to the United States prior to the birth of her parents. She has been raised in a traditional Indian home, in which the family members speak both English and Hindi. She never hesitates to tell someone that she is "Indian first, American second." That declaration refers to what aspect of her identity?

A. Race
B. Ethnicity
C. Culture
D. Nationality

34.30. Sigmund Freud's infant through adolescent stages focused on what aspect of child development?

A. Physical
B. Cognitive
C. Moral
D. Sexual
E. Social

34.31. A 35-year-old woman presents to a therapist for psychoanalysis to "work out some anxiety I think stems from my childhood." During the session, the therapist will encourage her to talk about what aspect of her life?

A. Her relationship with her mother
B. The effect anxiety has on sexual functioning
C. Her identity as someone with anxiety
D. The effect of her upbringing on her adult life
E. Anything she can think of to say about any subject

34.32. Erik Erikson's psychosocial stages focused on what aspect of an individual's development?

A. Identity
B. Personality
C. Attachment
D. Cognition
E. Morality

34.33. According to positive psychology, what is the factor most associated with being extremely happy?

A. Interpersonal relationships
B. Having at least a high school diploma or GED
C. A marriage lasting over 10 years
D. Age between 30 and 60 years
E. Having a career versus a job

34.34. A 56-year-old woman tells her 57-year-old husband that her sister, who lives in the same town, had her first grandchild. "I'm so happy! I get to be a great-aunt!" According to positive psychology, which of the following responses would correlate with a satisfactory marriage?

A. "That's good to hear."
B. "Do you think her daughter is ready to care for a child?"
C. "That's good news. I bet your sister is thrilled!"
D. "It's been a long day. Let's go out for dinner."

34.35. Increased income has been shown to significantly increase life satisfaction in which of the following circumstances?

A. The increase is attained as a result of a promotion at work
B. The individual feels they have earned the increase in income
C. The individual donates the amount of the increase to charity
D. The increase lifts the individual out of extreme poverty
E. The increase allows the individual to save money for emergencies

34.36. A 34-year-old woman presents to the outpatient clinic with a complaint of "being in a funk" for the past week. She has been diagnosed with major depressive disorder twice before, with the last time being 2 years ago. She was on escitalopram both times and stopped it after she felt better. She is on no medications and has no chronic medical illnesses. She has never had therapy "because the medicine worked so well. I just don't want to be dependent on it. I may be open to therapy, though." She denies current or past suicidal ideation, continues to go to work, and denies problems with sleep or appetite. "I just feel negative." After explaining positive psychology to her, she states that she would be willing to try it. What would be a possible focus in therapy?

A. Exploring her feelings about being dependent on medication
B. Congratulating her for wanting to engage in therapy
C. Having her write out what is going well in her life
D. Reflecting on the difference between feeling depressed and feeling happy
E. Helping her learn to live with occasional bouts of depression

34.37. In addition to a willingness of the patient to engage, the effectiveness of positive psychotherapy is dependent on what factor?

A. The relationship between the therapist and patient
B. The patient's ability to be introspective
C. The degree of severity of the patient's symptoms
D. The patient's willingness to help others
E. The type of illness the patient has

ANSWERS

34.1. D. Conservation
The child has not yet understood the concept of conservation, which is the principle that an object maintains its overall size or volume even if the shape or distribution changes. Reversibility is the understanding that some things can be changed into another state, then back again, such as ice to water. A child who has developed operational thought is able to see things from the point of view of someone else. Deductive reasoning involves using logic to go from the general to the specific, while inductive reasoning moves in the opposite direction. (1008, 1009)

34.2. D. The child realizes her father is still there even when his hands are closed
A child learns object permanence between 7 and 8 months old. Prior to that time, a child does not understand that something still exists even though she cannot see it. Once they develop object permanence, her father revealing his face behind his hands is no longer a surprise, so the game then has little meaning. (1007)

34.3. D. Cognitive therapy
One of the aims of cognitive therapy is to get to the patient's core belief, which is thought to be the ultimate driving force of thoughts, behaviors, and emotions. Patients can talk about feelings of being a failure, but only in cognitive therapy is it called the core belief and is a focus of treatment. (1010)

34.4. D. Withdrawal
Harry Harlow's famous monkey experiment showed that when monkeys were separated from their mother at birth, they became withdrawn, unable to mate or relate to peers, and incapable of caring for their offspring. Similarly, human babies become depressed and withdrawn when separated from their mother, as was described by René Spitz when he studied children who were hospitalized or institutionalized. (1013)

34.5. B. Conditioned stimulus
In classical conditioning, two stimuli, in this case the medication and the newspaper, lead to the same response, vomiting. The natural (unconditioned) stimulus is the medication, which causes the natural (unconditioned) response, vomiting. Newspapers do not usually trigger vomiting, and only do so in this man because it has been consistently paired with the natural trigger prior to the unconditioned response. He has become conditioned to the newspaper (the conditioned stimulus), which now produces a response that does not usually occur, making vomiting *specifically to the newspaper* a conditioned response. (1014)

34.6. B. Negative reinforcement
Reinforcement always increases a behavior, and punishment decreases it. Positive is applying something and negative is taking it away. In this case, the behavior of doing the homework is reinforced by taking something negative (the nagging) away, so it is negative reinforcement. Positive reinforcement would be giving her extra money or privileges for doing her homework, which would also increase the likelihood of her daughter getting it done. Conversely, positive punishment would be placing her on restriction (applying something) for *not* doing her homework, in hopes of reducing the behavior of *not* getting the work done. Negative punishment would be taking away her cell phone (removing something) to reduce the behavior of not doing her work. (1014, 1015)

34.7. E. Counterconditioning
In this example of counterconditioning through systematic desensitization, the conditioned stimulus (shaking hands) is paired with a new stimulus (deep breathing), whereas before, the conditioned stimulus was paired with extreme anxiety. Extinction would involve unpairing the conditioned stimulus and the unconditioned stimulus through a technique such as exposure therapy. Preparedness is the concept that organisms have a predisposition to associate certain stimuli with fear or anxiety. Reinstatement occurs when the current context is associated again with the unconditioned stimulus, leading to a return in fear or anxiety. State-dependent learning is the concept that retention of information is best when tested in the same state in which it was learned. (1016, 1017)

34.8. B. Rewarding him on average every seventh time, but varying the number of times needed
Variable ratio reinforcement schedules, in which the desired behavior is reinforced after an average but unpredictable number of times, generate the highest rate of behavior. In a fixed ratio schedule, the reinforcement occurs after a certain number of times the behavior occurs, which leads to increasing rates of behavior up until the reinforcer is delivered, followed by a drop-off. In a fixed interval schedule, the reinforcer is delivered for the first response after a certain length of time. This leads to the lowest rate of desired behavior, as the deliverance of the reinforcer

is completely predictable and only depends on the behavior being done once. In a variable interval schedule, behaviors are reinforced after an average but unpredictable length of time, leading to a higher behavior rate than on a fixed interval schedule, but lower than on a ratio schedule. (1018)

34.9. C. Tell him he can have ice cream once he eats his vegetables

The Premack principle states that a person may engage in a less-preferred behavior if it grants access to a more-preferred one. The child's more-preferred behavior is eating ice cream. To follow the principle, the parents should tell him that engaging in the less-preferred behavior (eating his vegetables) will result in getting ice cream. (1019)

34.10. C. His sales will remain subpar

In the learned helplessness model, an individual repeatedly exposed to an aversive stimulus with no way to avoid it will have difficulty learning behaviors to escape the situation even when escape is possible. In this situation, the new boss presumably would not deliver the aversive stimulus of yelling if the man performs as expected. Because he has learned that his actions are not connected to the deliverance of the negative stimulus, he is much less likely to change his behavior to try to effect change. Therefore, he will continue performing at a subpar level. (1020)

34.11. D. "What did you have for lunch this afternoon?"

Damage to the medial portion of the temporal lobe can lead to anterograde and retrograde amnesia. Retrograde deficits are often most severe for information most recently learned. Immediate memory is usually preserved, which is why he should be able to repeat three words. The most recent non-immediate information he is asked to recall is what he had for lunch earlier in the day. The other questions involve memories that were consolidated years ago. (1024)

34.12. A. Amygdala

The hippocampus, dentate gyrus, subiculum, parahippocampal cortices, and entorhinal cortices are all normally crucial for any memory. However, memories for emotional or arousing events include the activation of the amygdala. (1024)

34.13. B. Diencephalon

The diencephalon, which consists of the thalamus, hypothalamus, epithalamus, and subthalamus is damaged in Korsakoff syndrome. The frontal lobe damage seen in Korsakoff syndrome produces problems with cognition as well as memory retrieval and evaluation. The diencephalon damage adds problems with being able to remember items of one type after switching categories of information to be recalled, as well as the ability to hold verbal and visual information in mind and sustaining mental control. (1025–1026)

34.14. D. How to ride a bicycle

Amnesia affects only declarative (explicit), not procedural (implicit) memory. Declarative memory is divided into episodic (specific events in a person's history) and semantic memory (recall of facts and concepts). Procedural memory involves being able to carry out muscle actions without much conscious thought, such as with riding a bicycle. (1027, 1028)

34.15. A. Quicker reading speed, not remembering the picture

The patient is participating in an experiment to measure the effect of priming, which is the facilitation of the ability to detect or identify a particular stimulus based on a specific recent experience. Studies have shown that the effect of this type of priming remains intact in participants with amnesia, as demonstrated by increased reading speed of words represented in the priming picture. However, as expected, the participant would not remember being shown the picture. (1027)

34.16. D. Intellectual function

General intellectual functioning testing should be a part of any neuropsychological examination, including one focused on memory. This would give information about the patient's test-taking ability and help test certain types of memory impairment. Though disrupted sleep due to obstructive sleep apnea could impact memory, this is less likely the etiology for him as the problem is longstanding. Audiologic and visual examinations should always be performed in children with learning difficulties, as should adaptive functioning. (1030–1032)

34.17. A. Distracting the test taker between the learning and recall phases of the test

Memory tests can properly assess impairment in new learning ability using one of two strategies. The first is to present more information than can be held in immediate memory. This may be asking the test taker to memorize a string of 14 digits or learn pairs of unrelated words. The second strategy is to distract the test taker between the learning and recall phases, such as is done in the mental status examination with the 5-minute recall of three words. (1032)

34.18. G. Impaired Impaired Impaired
Patients with depression who report problems with memory as a symptom tend to endorse difficulty in all three domains of new learning capacity, immediate recall, and remote recall. In contrast, patients with amnesia do not report difficulty with immediate and remote memory, as those domains are not usually deficient. (1032)

34.19. A. "What is your name?"
In contrast to an individual with psychogenic amnesia or who is malingering, patients with neurogenic amnesia do not forget their name. A patient with neurogenic amnesia would also likely remember their city of birth, which could be used as a question to detect psychogenic amnesia or malingering. However, that is not as specific as asking the person's name. (1033)

34.20. D. Mastering generativity
The developmental task of generativity involves guiding the next generation, which could be accomplished by serving as a mentor. Erikson felt that this stage occurred between young adulthood and senior adulthood. The developmental task of isolation versus intimacy begins in adolescence and is centered on being able to become involved with a partner. Integrity versus despair occurs in old age and is centered on feeling whether or not one is at peace with the life they have lived. (1035, 1036)

34.21. C. Anterior cingulate gyrus
The anterior cingulate gyrus is the area of the brain most responsible for making the past meaningful, and creates attachment by linking memory and the capacity to react and reunite with others. Regarding memory, the amygdala is instrumental in memories with a high arousal or emotional content. The medial portion of the temporal lobe, diencephalon, and hippocampus can all lead to amnesia if damaged. (1037)

34.22. C. Sublimation
Sublimation involves channeling an unacceptable urge or impulse into an acceptable outlet. It is generally not acceptable to steal, but it is acceptable to act as a consultant to help businesses mitigate theft. Repression results when a person unconsciously forgets a threatening stimulus, whereas suppression occurs voluntarily. Displacement occurs when an impulse toward someone is redirected to a powerless substitute target. Altruism involves satisfying one's needs by helping others. (1040)

34.23. E. Projection
Defense mechanisms are responses to anxiety. Healthy, or mature, defense mechanisms are conscious, rooted in reality, and are often constructive. They include humor, altruism, sublimation, suppression, and anticipation. Immature defense mechanisms are out of touch with reality, can be socially undesirable, and can lead to problems with effective coping. Examples include projection, passive aggression, regression, and somatization. (1066)

34.24. E. Imprinting
Imprinting occurs during a particular developmental window during which a young animal is highly sensitive to a particular stimulus. In this case, the young gosling is highly sensitive to the movement of an organism, which it then follows as its mother. Priming is the facilitation of the ability to detect or identify a particular stimulus based on a specific recent experience. Redirection activity occurs when an animal is attacked by the dominant animal, and then fights a less-dominant organism instead. Instinct is a developmental process resulting in species-typical behavior. The imprinting of the gosling is instinctual, but does not explain the specific behavior. Displacement activity occurs when an animal cannot choose between two competing drives, such as fight or flight, and engages in an unrelated activity instead. (1042)

34.25. D. Physical touch
In one of Harry Harlow's experiments, young rhesus monkeys separated from their mother preferred a cloth-covered surrogate that provided no food to a wire surrogate that provided food. Seeing or hearing other monkeys, but not being able to touch them, did not relieve fear and anxiety, and they tended to isolate themselves. In one of Stephen Soumi's experiments, isolated monkeys could sometimes be rehabilitated if exposed to "therapist" monkeys who initiated gentle physical contact. (1043, 1044)

34.26. C. Depression
Reserpine is a catecholamine-depleting drug that was originally used to treat hypertension, and later used as an antipsychotic. It is now rarely used because of a possible side effect of severe depression. (1046)

34.27. C. "What do you think is causing your symptoms?"
For any patient, not just someone who emigrated from another country, a patient's idiom of distress

can be culturally bound. The patient should be asked about their cultural identity to avoid misconceptions based on stereotypes or inadequate information. One way to obtain an explanation of a patient's illness is to ask the patient what they believe is the cause of their symptoms. (1048)

34.28. B. Lower relative risk, higher persistence
Though African Americans were found to have lower rates of substance use disorder, anxiety, and depression than Whites, they tend to have more persistent disorders. A notable exception is schizophrenia, in which African Americans are diagnosed at three times the rate of Whites. (1050)

34.29. B. Ethnicity
Ethnicity is the subjective sense of belonging to a group of people who share commonalities including heritage, homeland, history, and values, and is what the girl is expressing in her statement. Race is a grouping of people largely based on physical characteristics. Culture is a set of meanings, norms, beliefs, values, and behavior patterns shared by people. (One of the aspects of ethnicity is a shared culture.) Nationality is the country of one's citizenship, often the same as their place of birth. (1047)

34.30. D. Sexual
Freud's stages of child development were focused on sexuality and libidinal energy, which he postulated shifted to different parts of the body at different ages of an individual. The oral stage involved erotic activity from chewing biting and sucking, the anal stage focused on bowel function, and the phallic stage focused on urination. After the latent stage, in which he theorized that erotic activity was relatively dormant, came the genital stage in which erotic activity is focused on the penis, vagina, and clitoris. (1061)

34.31. E. Anything she can think of to say about any subject
The cornerstone of psychoanalysis is free association, in which the patient says whatever comes to mind. The goal is to analyze the feelings toward the therapist, called transference, and the resultant resistance to free association. "Tell me about your mother" is a pop-culture punchline often associated with psychoanalysis, but by definition, would not be free association as it is directive. The same directiveness would result from asking the patient any pointed question. (1069)

34.32. A. Identity
Erik Erikson's developmental stages centered around identity, identity crisis, and identity confusion. He postulated that identity was "in the inner core of the individual," and that it emerged at the end of adolescence. (1072)

34.33. A. Interpersonal relationships
The strongest correlation to extreme happiness is good relationships with other people, to the extent that relationships may be a necessary condition for extreme happiness. Employment and being married are robustly correlated with happiness. Education and age have a small association with happiness. (1090, 1091)

34.34. C. "That's good news. I bet your sister is thrilled!"
According to positive psychology, positive communication is strongly correlated with a good relationship. In a marriage, positive communication is shown through active-constructive responses which are enthusiastic, such as "That's good news. I bet your sister is thrilled!" A majority of the other types of responses have been correlated with marital dissatisfaction. These include active destructive, which focuses on the potential downside; passive constructive, which are muted responses; and passive destructive, which conveys disinterest. (1091)

34.35. D. The increase lifts the individual out of extreme poverty
Increase in income has a small correlation to life satisfaction with one exception—when the increase allows the person to be able to meet their basic needs. Once the person is no longer in extreme poverty, employment and engagement on the job are much more strongly correlated with happiness. (1091)

34.36. C. Having her write out what is going well in her life
Positive psychology looks at strengths and areas of competence in one's life, as opposed to deficiencies, weaknesses, and problems. Therefore, therapy is not likely to focus on learning to live with depression or what she does not like about medication. Congratulating her on wanting to engage in therapy does not examine her strengths, nor does reflecting on the difference between feeling depressed and happy. Having her think about and write down what is going well in her life could be a technique employed as an intervention. As noted in the stem, the patient should first be assessed to see how open

they are to therapy in general and to positive psychology specifically before beginning an intervention. (1092, 1093)

34.37. A. The relationship between the therapist and patient

A person can engage in positive psychotherapy whether or not they have a mental health issue. Some techniques do not require a high propensity for introspection, such as noticing and recording things that are going well in someone's life. Helping other people can be a therapeutic technique, but is not the only technique. The common thread among positive psychotherapies is the therapeutic alliance, or relationship between the therapist and the patient. (1093)

Index

A
Abnormal EEGs, 108, 110
Abstract reasoning, 4, 8
Accidents, 176, 178
Acetylcholine, 27, 32, 92, 95
Acute akathisia, 115, 130
Acute dystonia, 115, 130
Acute psychosis, treatment for, 120, 132
Acyclovir, 31, 34
Addiction treatment, 180, 182
Adjustment disorders, 65, 67, 154, 158
Adrenal gland, 196, 200
African Americans, rates of substance use disorder, 207, 213
Agnosia, 6
Agoraphobia, 59, 61
 participant modeling therapy, 146, 149
Alcohol, 21, 26, 30, 33
 correlation between sleep apnea and, 88, 90
 dependence, treatment for, 36
 rehabilitation, 36
Alcohol disorders
 DSM terms, 35, 40
 naltrexone for treating alcohol dependence, 36
 psychiatric diagnosis, 36
Alcohol use
 impact on profile of NMDA and GABA receptor, 195, 200
 induced depressions, treatment for, 36, 41
Alcohol withdrawal
 seizures, treatment for, 36
 signs or symptoms in, 35, 40
 tremors, 35, 40
Aldehyde dehydrogenase inhibition, 128, 137–138
Alpha-1 receptor blockade, 119, 132
Alpha waves, 198, 202
Alzheimer disease, 64, 197, 201

American Indians, lifetime rate of substance abuse, 35, 40
American Psychiatric Association's (APA's) *Principles of Medical Ethics with Annotations Especially Applicable to Psychiatry,* 166, 168
Amitriptyline, 123, 134
Ammonia, 5, 11
Amnesia, 127, 137, 205, 211
Amnestic disorder, 29, 32
Amobarbital, 126, 136
Amphetamine salts, 127, 137
Amygdala, 205, 211
Analytically oriented sex therapy, 93, 96
Anankastic personality disorder, 103, 105
Angelman syndrome, 12, 201
Anorexia nervosa
 atypical antipsychotics for, 78, 81
 binge/purge subtype, 77, 80
 body image concerns, 77, 80
 endocrine findings, 77, 80
 phycologic predisposing factor, 79, 82
 prognosis of, 78, 81
 psychotherapeutic approach to, 78, 81
 vs bulimia nervosa, 77, 80
 weight criteria, 157, 160
Anosognosia, 12
Anterior cingulate gyrus, 206, 212
Anterior pituitary gland, 196, 200
Antidepressants, 55, 57
 anticholinergic effects of, 95
 sexual side effects of, 121, 133
 for somatic disorder, 73, 76
Antipsychotic medications
 adequate trial of, 47, 50
 benefits of, 154, 158
 clozapine, 46–47, 50

family history and, 3
 lamotrigine, 52–53
 quetiapine, 47, 52–53
Antisocial behavior, treatments for, 108, 110
Antisocial personality disorder, 36, 41, 102, 105
 contingency management and rewards-based interventions, 103, 106
Aphasias, 5
apoE-e4 allele, 197, 201
Aripiprazole, 63–64, 115, 117–119, 130–132
Arousal-induced sleep cycle fragmentation, 88, 90
Arsenic poisoning, 31, 34
Arthritis, 155, 158
Aspirin, 93, 95
Assertive community treatment (ACT) team model, 181–182
Association studies, 197, 201
Ataxia, 154, 158
Atomoxetine, 20, 26
 mechanism of action, 127, 137
Attention-deficit/hyperactivity disorder (ADHD), 4, 6, 10, 12, 19, 83, 85, 187, 190
 atomoxetine therapy, 20, 26
 first-line therapy for, 16, 23
Atypical neuroleptics, 71
Auditory hallucinations, 44, 49
Auditory system, 193, 199
Authoritarian parents, 109, 111
Autism spectrum disorder (ASD), 14–15, 23, 195, 200
Autogenic training, 146, 149
Automatic behaviors, 127, 137
Autonomy, 165, 168, 177, 179
Autosomal genetic diseases, 187, 190
Avoidant personality disorder, 102, 105
Avoidant/restrictive food intake disorder (ARFID), 16, 23–24

215

Index

B
Barbiturates, 38, 42, 117, 131
Bath salts, 38, 43
Bayley Scale of Infant Development, 11
Bed-wetting, treatment of, 83–85
Behavior modification, 36, 41
Behavior therapy for fear of sexual interaction, 93, 95–96
Beneficence, 165, 168
Benzodiazepines, 30, 33, 36, 41, 59–61, 126, 136, 198, 202
   intoxication, 156, 159
   side effects, 125, 136, 154, 158
Benztropine, 115, 130
Bereavement, 108, 110
   alcohol consumption and, 176, 178
   spousal, 176, 178
Beta waves, 198, 202
Bipolar disorder, 4, 9, 116, 130, 183–184
   bipolar I disorder, advanced age of onset, 52–53
"Black-box" warning, 18, 25
Body dysmorphic disorder, 62, 64
Body image concerns, 77–78, 80–81
Borderline personality disorder, 78, 80–81, 103, 106
   functional improvement in, 103, 106
   gender differences, 104, 106
Boundary violation, 166, 168
Bradycardia, 77, 80
Brain death, 177, 179
Brain tumor, 30, 33
Breathlessness, 7, 13
Brief Psychiatric Rating Scale (BPRS), 9
Broca aphasia, 5, 10
Bromocriptine, 115, 130
Bruxism, 38
Bulimia nervosa, 77, 80
   body image concerns, 77, 80
   PTSD in, 78, 81
Buprenorphine, 128, 137
Bupropion, 121–122, 133–134
   risk for epilepsy, 122, 134

C
CAGE screening tool, 8
Calcifications, 6, 11
Cannabis, 37, 42
   induced psychotic disorder, 37, 42
Carbamazepine, 41, 117, 125, 131, 136
Cataplexy, treatment of, 88, 90
Catecholamines, 38, 43
Cattell Infant Intelligence Scale, 11
Caudate nucleus activity, 96, 194, 199
Child Behavior Checklist (CBCL), 4
Children of divorced families, suicide rate among, 189, 191
Chlorpromazine, 118, 131
Cholecystokinin, 196, 200
Chromosome 7q, 197, 201
Chronic deterioration, 19, 25
Cingulate cortex, 62, 64
Citalopram, 104, 106, 117, 121, 131, 133
Clang associations, 4, 8
Classical conditioning, 84–85
Clinical diagnosis, 4, 9
Clomipramine, 122, 134
Clonidine, 128, 137–138
Clozapine, 46–47, 50, 115, 118, 130–132
   blood counts for monitoring metabolic side effects, 48, 50
   incidence of agranulocytosis, 50
   induced agranulocytosis, 155, 159
   oral and perianal ulceration from, 155, 159
CNS depressants, 90
Cognitive behavioral therapy (CBT), 17, 19, 24–25, 41, 55, 57–58, 78–79, 81, 146, 149
   for insomnia (CBTi), 88, 90
Cognitive distortions, 146, 149
Cognitive functions, 4
Cognitive processing therapy (CPT), 66–67
Cognitive testing, 22
Cognitive therapy, 203, 210
Colchicine, 123, 135
Collaborative care model, 180, 182
Comfort, touch as source of, 207, 212
Competency of patient, 171, 174
Conditioned stimulus, 203, 210
Conduct disorder, 157, 160
Connors Rating Scale, 4
Consciousness, 32
Consent form for treatment, 171, 174
Conservation, 203, 210
Consortium of community agencies, 181–182
Consultation–liaison psychiatry, 154, 158
Contamination fears in OCD, 62, 64
Contingency management, 103, 106
Conversion disorder, 72, 75
   neurologic or nonpsychiatric medical diagnosis, 73, 76
   prevalence rate, 74, 76
   symptoms of, 110
   tests, 72, 75
Cornelia de Lange syndrome, 11–12
Corticospinal tract, 194, 199
Cortico-striatal-thalamic-cortical (CSTC), 63–64
Cortisol levels, in depressed patients, 55, 58
Cortisone, 196, 201
Counseling, for alcohol rehabilitation, 36, 41
Counterconditioning, 204, 210
Cri-du-chat syndrome, 7, 11–12
Criterion validity, 10
Cross-dressing, 97–98
Cultural identity, 207, 212–213
Cyclothymia, 51, 53

D
Death and dying, stages of, 176, 178
Death with Dignity Act, 179
Declarative memory, 211
Deductive reasoning, 210
Default sex of human embryo, 97–98
Defense mechanisms, 207, 212
Delayed reaction time, 37, 42
Delta waves, 198, 202
Delusional disorder, 45, 49
Dementia
   of Alzheimer type, 28, 30, 32–33
   features of, 28, 32
Denial of intent, 9
Denver Developmental Screening Test, 11
Depersonalization disorder, 68, 70
   serotonin reupdate inhibitors for, 68, 70
   symptoms, 68–71
Depression
   reserpine and, 207, 212
   screening for, 180, 182
Depressive disorder
   alcohol use disorder, 54, 57
   decreased appetite, 77, 80
   hippocampus and, 56, 58
   life stressor associated with, 56, 58
   symptoms of depression, 54, 57
   testing of cortisol levels, 55, 58

Derealization disorder, 68, 70
  serotonin reupdate inhibitors for, 68, 70
  symptoms, 68–71
Desmopressin, 84–85
Desvenlafaxine, 93, 95
Detoxification for alcoholism, 36
Diabetes, 3, 8
Dialectical behavioral therapy (DBT), 69, 71, 103, 106, 146, 149
Diencephalon, 205, 211
Discriminant validity, 10
Disinhibited social engagement disorder, 17, 24
Disposition, least restrictive alternative, 170, 173
Disruptive mood dysregulation disorder (DMDD), 18, 24
Dissociative amnesia, 68, 70
  symptoms, 68, 70
Dissociative identity disorder, 68, 70
  dialectical behavioral therapy (DBT), 69, 71
  psychotherapy for, 68, 70
  somatic treatment strategy, 69, 71
Disulfiram, 128, 137–138
Divorce rate among psychiatrists, 109, 111
Dizziness, 127, 137
Dolutegravir/rilpivirine, 31, 34
Dopamine, 195, 200
Down syndrome, 12, 14
Doxycycline, 31, 34
Dronabinol, 37, 42
Drowsiness, 42
Dual-sex therapy, 93, 95–96
Durable power of attorney, 171, 174
Dyscalculia, 5, 10
Dysgraphia, 5, 10

E

Ebstein anomaly, 124, 135
EEG evaluation, 198, 202
Electrocardiogram (EKG), 156, 159
Electroconvulsive therapy (ECT), 29, 33, 52–53, 139, 142
  risk for complications, 140, 142
Embryo development, 187, 190
Empathy, 3–4
Encopresis
  causes of childhood, 83, 85
  constipation in, 83, 85
  diagnosis of, 83, 85
  DSM-5 criteria for, 83, 85
  initial step in treating child with, 83, 85
  minimum age for treatment of, 83, 85
  treatment of, 84–85
  types of, 84, 86
Endicott Substitution Criteria for depression, 177–178
Enlarged ventricles, 48, 50
Enuresis, 83, 85
Erikson, Erik, 208, 213
Estrogen replacement therapy, 93, 95
Ethical principles
  autonomy, 165, 168, 177, 179
  beneficence, 165, 168
  deciding seclusion or restraint for patient, 170, 173
  nonmaleficence, 165, 168
  obligation to report of impaired physician, 167–168
  related to sexual relations with patient, 166, 168
Ethnicity, 207, 213
Euthanasia, 177, 179
  Oregon's Assisted Suicide Law, 177, 179
Excoriation disorder, 63–64
Executive functioning, 34
Expressive psychotherapy, 144, 148
Extinction, 204, 210

F

Face validity, 10
Factitious disorder, 73, 75
  common signs of, 73, 76
  healing of wounds, 73, 76
  history of anemia, 76
  treating child with, 74, 76
Factor validity, 10
Fantasy, 104, 106
Feeding and eating disorders
  anorexia nervosa, 77–82
  anorexia nervosa, binge/purge subtype, 77, 80
  binge eating *vs* overeating, 77, 80
  bulimia nervosa, 77, 80
  decreased appetite, 77, 80
Female sexual interest/arousal disorder, 92, 95
Ferritin level, correlation with sleeping difficulty, 89, 91
Fexofenadine, 202
15q2 deletion, 6, 11
Finger agnosia, 5, 10
"Five Ds" in pellagra, 34
Flibanserin, 93, 95
Fluency, 5, 10
Flumazenil, 125, 136, 156, 159
Fluoxetine, 93, 95, 156, 159–160
Fluphenazine, side effects, 156, 159–160
FMR-1 gene, 201
  inactivation of, 12
  mutation, 15, 22
fMRI (functional magnetic resonance imaging), 5, 10
Folic acid supplementation, 124, 135
Fragile X syndrome, 201
Free association, 144, 148, 213
Freud, Sigmund, 208, 213
Frontal lobe damage, 194, 199–200

G

Galactosemia, 12
Ganser syndrome, 68, 70
Gender-dysphoric male, 97–98
Gender identity, 94, 96, 188, 191
Genderqueer, 97–98
Generalized anxiety disorder, 59, 61, 126, 136
Generativity, mastering, 206, 212
Genetic etiology, 197, 201
Genetic mapping studies, 201
Genomic and environmental risk factors, 152–153
Genomic testing, 152–153
Gerstmann syndrome, 5, 10
Gesell Infant Scale, 11
Ghrelin, 87, 90
Grammar, 15, 23
Granulocyte colony-stimulating factor, 155, 159
Grief, 176, 178
  medication for, 177–178
Group therapy, 93, 95, 108, 110, 145, 148, 201
  for women with breast cancer, 154, 158
Growth hormone, 87, 90
Guilty verdict, 171, 174

H

Hallucinogens, 38, 43
Haloperidol, 160
Hearing test, 15, 22
Hematocrit, 97–98
Hemodialysis, 116, 130
Hemoglobin, 97–98
Heroin withdrawal symptoms, 21, 26
Hippocampus, 195, 200
Histrionic personality disorder, 102, 105
  gender differences, 104, 106
HIV/AIDS infection, 34
  in children, 157, 160
  as leading cause of disability, 183–184

Hoarding, 62, 64
Homicides, 176, 178, 189, 192
Homosexuality, 97–98
H3 receptor agonism/inverse agonism, 89, 91
Hunter syndrome, 12
Hurler syndrome, 12
Hydromorphone, 177, 179
Hypercholesterolemia, 77, 80
Hypersomnolence disorder, 87, 90
Hyperthyroidism, 3, 8
Hyperventilation, 202
Hypoglycemia, 40
Hypomagnesemia, 6, 11, 40
Hyponatremia, 40
Hyponatremic seizure, 84–85
Hypothalamic–pituitary–adrenal (HPA) axis activity, 58
Hypothalamus, 194, 196, 199–200

I
Identity, 208, 213
Iloperidone, 118–119, 131–132
Immigrants, physician approach to, 207, 212–213
Imprinting, 207, 212
Information-processing model of training, 151, 153
Information processing speed, 31, 33
Inhalants, 39, 43
  effects of, 39, 43
Insight-oriented therapy, 41
Intellectual disability, 14–15, 20, 25
  in children with autism spectrum disorder, 20, 26
  seizures and, 20, 25
Intellectual functioning, 206, 211
Intensive outpatient program (IOP), 162
Intermittent explosive disorder (IED), 99, 101
  diagnosis of, 99, 101
  symptoms of, 99, 101
  treatment for, 100–101
Interpersonal psychotherapy (ITP), 146, 150
  intermediate phase of, 147, 150
Intolerable pain, 177, 179
Intoxication, 35, 40
  benzodiazepines, 156, 159
  legal definition, 35, 40
  lysergic acid diethylamide (LSD), 159
  phencyclidine (PCP), 159
Irritability, 17, 24

J
Judgment, 4, 8

K
Ketamine, 38, 43, 123, 135
Kleptomania, 99, 101
Korsakoff syndrome, 29, 33, 205, 211
Kübler-Ross, Elizabeth, 176, 178

L
Lacrimation, 37, 42
Lamotrigine, 52–53, 116–117, 125, 130–131, 136
Language, 6, 11
Lanugo, 77, 80
Lead poisoning, 31, 34
Learned helplessness, 204, 211
  theory of depression, 56, 58
Learning deficits, 206, 211–212
Least restrictive alternative, 170, 173
Leptin, 87, 90
Lesch–Nyhan syndrome, 12
Levorphanol, 177, 179
Lewy inclusion bodies, 28, 32
Linkage studies, 197, 201
Lisdexamfetamine, 81, 127, 137
Lisinopril, 207
Lithium, 53, 139, 142
  dosage, 124, 135
  side effects, 124, 135, 156, 159
  toxicity, 159
Liver function tests (LFTs), 5, 11
Locus ceruleus, 35, 40
Loneliness, 12, 176, 178
Love Addicts Anonymous, 96
Luria-Nebraska Neuropsychological Battery: Children's Revision (LNNB:C), 7, 13
Lysergic acid diethylamide (LSD), 38, 43
  intoxication, 159

M
Major depressive disorder, 54, 57, 176, 196, 201
  age groups, 155, 158
  goal of treatment, 55, 57
  hyperactivity of HPA axis and, 200
  melancholic, 155, 158
  psychomotor retardation in, 108, 110
  treatment for, 119, 132
Male hypoactive sexual desire disorder, 92, 95
Malingering, 108, 110
  causes of feigning symptoms in, 108, 110

Malpractice, 170, 173
  4 Ds, 173
  negligence to obtain informed consent, 171, 174
Manganese poisoning, 31, 34
Mania, 3–4, 8
Manic episode
  emergency admission to psychiatric facility, 52–53
  treatment duration for, 51, 53
Manic–hypomanic episodes, differences between, 51, 53
Marijuana, 19, 25
Masturbation, 92, 95
Meclizine, 155, 159
Medical workup, 45, 49
Medication toxicity, reversal of, 156, 159
Memantine, 129, 138
Memory difficulty, 206, 211–212
Mental disorders
  as factor for discrimination, 183–184
  prevalence estimates, 183–184
Mentalization-based therapy (MBT), 103, 106, 147, 150
Mental Retardation Facilities and Community Mental Health Centers Construction Act of 1963, 161–162
Mental status examination, 3, 12
  for amnestic disorder, 29, 32
  anxiety in, 4
Meperidine, 37, 177, 179
Mercury poisoning, 31, 34
Mesoaccumbens, 195, 200
Methadone, 128, 137, 177, 179
Methamphetamine, 38, 43
Methylphenidate, 127, 137
Metronidazole, 27, 32
Microglia, 193, 199
Migraines, 39, 43
Military courts, 170, 173
Millon Adolescent Personality Inventory (MAPI), 7, 13
Mindfulness, 93, 95–96
Minorities, negative life experiences of, 109–111
miRNA, 195, 200
Mirtazapine, 122, 134
M'Naghten rule, 171, 174
Monoamine oxidase inhibitors (MAOIs), 5, 37, 42, 71, 123, 134–135
Mood, 7, 13
Morphine, 177, 179
Motivational interviewing, 9, 36, 41
Mullen Scales of Early Learning, 7, 13

Multimodal intervention, 180, 182
Multiple sleep latency test (MSLT), 88, 90
Myocardial infarctions, 6, 11, 183–184

N
Naloxone, 37, 42
Naltrexone, 36, 41, 128, 137
Narcissistic personality disorder, 102, 105
Narcolepsy, 88, 90
Narrative family therapy, 145, 148–149
Narrative psychotherapy, 147, 150
Nefazodone, 122, 134
Negative reinforcement, 204, 210
Neuroleptic-induced movement disorder, 115, 130
Neuroleptic-induced parkinsonism, 115, 130
Neuroleptic malignant syndrome (NMS), 115, 129–130, 138
Neurologic abnormality in criminals, 108, 110
Neuropsychological testing, 31, 33
Neurosyphilis, 34
Nicotine replacement therapy, 43
Nitroglycerin, 93, 95
Nonmaleficence, 165, 168
Norepinephrine reuptake inhibition, 20, 26
Normal development and aging. *See also* Toddler development
 characteristic of normal dreams, 189, 191
 concrete operational period, 188, 190
 emotional development, 188, 191
 Erik Erikson's developmental stages, 208, 213
 Freud's stages of child development, 208, 213
 gender identity, 188, 191
 generativity *vs* stagnation, middle adulthood, 189, 192
 imaginary companions, 188, 191
 imitation of facial movements, 188, 190–191
 intelligence, 188, 191
 middle years, 188, 191
 neuropsychiatric changes with aging, 189, 192
 perception of attractive physical appearance, 189, 192
 smiling back, 188, 190
 stranger anxiety *vs* separation anxiety, 188, 191
 utterances and use of words, 188, 190
 verbal ability, 189, 192
Normal pressure hydrocephalus (NPH), 154, 158

O
Objectivity, 3
Object permanence, 203, 210
Observation, 15, 22
Obsessional thoughts, 13
Obsessive–compulsive disorder (OCD), 19, 70, 78, 81
 new-onset symptoms in older individuals, 62, 64
 therapy and medication for, 63–64, 120, 122, 132–134
 types of obsessions with, 62, 64
Obsessive compulsive personality disorder, 102, 105
 gender differences, 104, 106
 medication management, 104, 106
Occipital lobe damage, 200
Olanzapine, 78, 81, 115, 117, 130–131
Olfactory reference syndrome, 62, 64
μ-opioid agonists, 128, 137
Opioids, 35–36, 40–41
 substitution therapy, 37, 42
 withdrawal, signs or symptoms, 37, 42
Oregon's Assisted Suicide Law, 177, 179
Orexin, 87, 90
Orthostatic hypotension, 37, 42, 119, 132, 159
Overgeneralization, 146, 149

P
Paliperidone, 120
Paliperidone palmitate, 167–169
Panic attacks, 59, 61
Parallel play, 190
Paranoia, 146, 149–150
Paranoid personality disorder, 102, 105
 gender differences, 104, 106
 schizophrenia *vs,* 103, 105
Paranoid schizophrenia with active delusions, 145, 148
Paraphilic disorders, 94, 96
Parental psychoeducation, 16, 23
Parietal lobe, 5, 10
 damage, 200
Paroxetine, 65, 67, 117, 131
Partial hospital programs, 161–162
Participant modeling therapy, 146, 149
Patient confidentiality, 166, 168
Patient consent, 3
Pedigree analysis, 197, 201
Pedophilia, diagnosis of, 94, 96
Peer-to-peer consultation, 167–169
Pellagra, 34
Penicillin, 31, 34
Perceptual disturbances, 13
Permissive parenting, 109, 111
Persecutory delusions, 155, 158
Persistent depressive disorder, 54, 57
Persistent vegetative state, 177, 179
Personality
 cannabis-induced psychotic disorder and, 37, 42
 changes, 30–33
Personality disorders
 anankastic personality disorder, 103, 105
 borderline personality disorder, 103, 106
 categorical approach to, 102, 105
 dependent traits, 103, 106
 dissociation and repression, 102, 105
 histrionic personality disorder, 102, 105
 identity diffusion, 103, 106
 narcissistic personality disorder, 102, 105
 paranoid, 102, 105
 paranoid personality disorder, 102–103, 105
 reward dependence, 104, 107
 schizoid personality disorder, 102–103, 105–106
 schizotypal personality disorder, 102, 105
Phencyclidine (PCP) intoxication, 159
Phenothiazine, 12
Phenylalanine, 7, 12
Phenylketonuria (PKU), 12, 22
Pheochromocytomas, 9
Phone consultation, 103, 106
Phonology, 15, 23
Pitolisant, 89, 91
Plantar (Babinski) reflex, 187, 190

Pleasurable feelings, 94, 96
Polacrilex gum, 38, 43
Positive emotions, 176, 178
Positive psychology, 209, 213–214
Posttraumatic stress disorder (PTSD), 17, 24
　in bulimia nervosa, 78, 81
　diagnosis of, 65, 67
　evidence-based therapy for, 66–67
　risk factors, 66–67
　symptoms, 65, 67
Prader–Willi syndrome, 11, 64, 201
Pragmatics, 15, 23
Prazosin, 65, 67, 71
Pregnancy
　embryo development, 187, 190
　fetal brain development, 187, 190
　milestones, 187, 190
　reflexes present at birth, 187, 190
Premack principle, 204, 211
Preparedness, 204, 210
Preschoolers, 176, 178
Priapism, 122, 127, 134, 137
Privacy Rule, 172, 174–175
Privileged communications, 170, 173
Procedural memory, 211
Projection, 207, 212
Projective identification, 102, 105
Propranolol, 46, 49–50, 126, 136
Prosopagnosia, 12
Psychiatric abnormality, 30–33
Psychiatric admission, temporary vs involuntary, 170, 173
Psychiatric disorders, risks of, 183–184
Psychiatric illnesses, 197, 201
Psychiatric interview
　person-centered approach, 3
　steps, 3
Psychiatric medications
　dose adjustments in, 155, 159
　rules or regulations, 170, 173
Psychiatric rehabilitation strategies, 151, 153
Psychiatric symptoms, 3
Psychoanalysis
　free association, 144, 148
　good candidate for, 144, 148
Psychoanalytic psychotherapy, 144, 148
Psychoeducation, 147, 150
Psychogenic amnesia, 206, 212
Psychomotor retardation, 176, 178

Psychotherapy, 9, 41, 197, 201
　note, 4
Psychotoxicity, 179
Public community psychiatry multidisciplinary team, 181–182
Public health programs, 180, 182

Q
Quetiapine, 47, 52–53, 115, 118, 130–131

R
Radioactive iodine, 31, 34
Ranolazine, 93, 95
Raphe nuclei, 195, 200
Rapid Alcohol Problem Screen 4 (RAPS4) screening tool, 3
Rating scales, 4
Reboxetine, 84–86
Reframing, 145, 149
Reinstatement, 204, 210–211
Relaxation techniques, 60–61
RELN gene, 201
Reserpine, 207, 212
Residential care, 161–162
Retrograde deficits, 211
Reversibility, 210
Rhabdomyolysis, 39, 43
Right–left disorientation, 5, 10
Risperidone, 14, 22, 65, 67, 115, 120, 130
Role-playing, 151, 153
Rotter Incomplete Sentences Blank Test, 7, 13
Rubella, 20, 25
Rubinstein–Taybi syndrome, 11

S
Schizoaffective disorder, 44, 46, 49
Schizoid personality disorder, 102–103, 105–106
　common defense mechanisms, 104, 106
Schizophrenia, 120, 201
　diagnosis of, 45, 49
　hospital admission, 46, 49
　suicide as cause of premature death, 44, 49
　treatment duration, 47, 50
Schizotypal personality disorder, 102, 105
　saccadic eye movements in, 104, 106
School resource officer (SRO), 18
School violence, 189, 192
Scurvy, 34
Seclusion or restraint for patient
　ethical principles, 170, 173
　measures, 171, 174

Sedatives, 177–178
Seizures, 139, 142
　alcohol abuse and, 35, 40
　intellectual disability and, 20, 25
　simple partial, 30, 33
Selective intervention, 180, 182
Selective serotonin reuptake inhibitors (SSRIs), 17, 24, 59, 61, 64, 67–68, 70–71, 81, 121, 133–134
　with benzodiazepine, 60–61
　discontinuation syndrome, 121, 133
　for impulsivity and aggression, 101
　sexual dysfunction as side effect of, 120, 133
　treatment of cataplexy, 90
Semantic memory, 30, 33, 211
Semantics, 15, 23
Senile plaques, 14, 22
Separation anxiety, 18, 24–25, 188, 191
Serotonin, 104, 107, 195, 200
Serotonin–dopamine antagonists, 115–116, 130, 132
Serotonin syndrome, 121, 133
Sex Addicts Anonymous, 96
Sexaholics Anonymous, 96
Sexual fantasies or impulses, 93, 96
SHANK3 gene, 202
Sib-pair analysis, 197, 201
Sildenafil, 93, 95, 129, 138
Simple partial seizure, 30, 33
Single-nucleotide polymorphisms, 201
Sleep disorders, advanced age and, 155, 159
Sleepwalking, 88, 90
Social functioning, 22
Social perception, 151, 153
Social phobia, 78, 81
Social referencing, 188, 191
Social skills rehabilitation, 151, 153
Sodium, 116, 130
Sodium oxybate, 90
Somatic disorder
　antidepressants for, 73, 76
　comorbidities in, 73, 76
　distinction from factitious disorder, 73, 76
　ICD-10 criteria *vs* DSM-5-TR criteria, 72, 75
　similarities between anxiety disorder and, 72, 75
　symptoms, 72, 75
Specific phobia, 59, 61

Speech therapy, 20, 26
Spinal cord, as epicenter of orgasms, 94, 96
Spontaneous remission in enuresis, 83, 85
Spousal bereavement, 176, 178
State-dependent learning, 204, 210
Stevens–Johnson syndrome, 136
Stimulants, 15–16, 23, 38, 43
Stranger anxiety, 188, 191
Sublimation, 207, 212
Substance abuse
 ethnicity and lifetime rate of, 35, 40
 screening tool, 3
Substance use disorder, 94, 96
Suicidality, 18, 25
Suicidal statement, 4
Suicide, 12, 117, 131, 176, 178
 attempt, risk of, 18, 24, 38, 42
 as cause of premature death in schizophrenia, 44, 49
 in China, 183–184
 emergency room (ER) screens for, 155, 159
 foreseeable, 170, 173
 pervasive hopelessness as risk factor, 155, 159
 prevalence rates in children of divorced families, 189, 191
 prevalence rates in males over 45 years of age, 154, 158
 risk in cancer patients, 155, 158
 substance abuse and, 35, 40
Supportive employment program, 151, 153
Supportive psychotherapy, 145, 148
Suprachiasmatic nucleus, 87, 90
Synaptogenesis, 194, 200
Synthetic THC, FDA approval, 37, 42
Systematic desensitization, 146, 149

T
Tarasoff law, 170, 173
Tardive dyskinesia (TD), 115, 130, 160
Temporal lobe, 193, 199
 damage, 200, 205, 211
 tumor, 30, 33
Testosterone supplementation, 98
Tetrabenazine, 115, 130
Thalamus, 193, 199
Thematic Apperception Test (TAT), 7, 13
Therapeutic communities, 108, 110
Therapist–patient relationship, 209, 214
Theta waves, 198, 202
Thiamine deficiency, 34, 36, 41
Thiamine replacement, 29, 32–33
Thought content, 7, 13
Thyroid function, 123, 135
Thyroid-stimulating hormone, 87, 90
Tobacco dependence, 35, 40
Toddler development, 187–188, 190
 social referencing, 188, 191
Toluene, 5, 10–11, 31, 34
Topiramate, 65, 67, 82, 125, 136
Tourette syndrome, 19, 25
Transexual, 97–98
Transference, 213
Transference-focused psychotherapy (TFP), 103, 106
Transgender, 97–98
Transient global amnesia, 68, 70
Trazodone, 122, 134
Treatment boundaries, 172, 174
Treponema infection, 34
Trichotillomania, 62–64
Tricyclic antidepressants (TCAs), 71, 73, 76
 concerns of, 131
 serotonin and norepinephrine reuptake inhibition, 122, 134
 side effects, 123, 134–135
 therapeutic effect of, 122, 134

Tuberoinfundibular pathway, 120, 132
Tympanic membrane, 193, 199
Tyrosine, 195, 200

U
Universal intervention, 180, 182

V
Valbenazine, 115, 130
Valproic acid, 5, 11, 116–117, 130–131
 laboratory test, 124, 135–136
Vascular dementia, 28, 32
Venlafaxine, 65, 67, 121, 133
Ventricular enlargement, 193, 199
Vineland adaptive behavior scale, 6, 11
Vitamin B3 (niacin), 31, 34
Vitamin B12, 5, 11
Vitamin deficiencies, 36
 thiamine, 36, 41
 vitamin A, 34
 vitamin B12, 34
 vitamin C, 34

W
Weight gain, 127, 137
Wernicke encephalopathy, 36, 40
Wernicke–Korsakoff syndrome, 34
Williams syndrome, 12
Withdrawal behavioral response, 203, 210

X
X chromosome, 201

Y
Yale-Brown Obsessive-Compulsive Scale (Y-BOCS), 120
Yohimbine, 93, 95

Z
Ziprasidone, 6, 11, 115, 118, 120, 130–131
Zolpidem, 126, 136